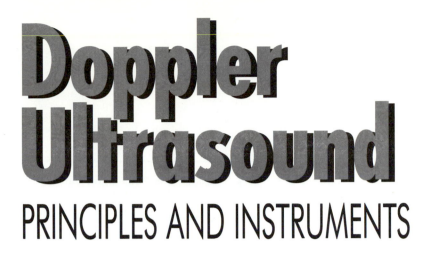

Doppler Ultrasound

PRINCIPLES AND INSTRUMENTS

FREDERICK W. KREMKAU, Ph.D.

Professor and Director
Center for Medical Ultrasound
Bowman Gray School of Medicine
Wake Forest University
Winston-Salem, North Carolina

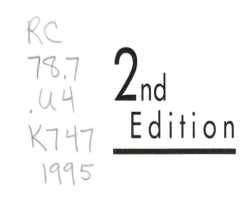

2nd Edition

W.B. SAUNDERS COMPANY
A Division of Harcourt Brace & Company
Philadelphia   London   Toronto   Montreal   Sydney   Tokyo

JR

W.B. SAUNDERS COMPANY
A Division of Harcourt Brace & Company

The Curtis Center
Independence Square West
Philadelphia, Pennsylvania

Library of Congress Cataloging-in-Publication Data

Kremkau, Frederick W.
  Doppler ultrasound:principles and instruments / Frederick W.
Kremkau.—2nd ed.
    p.   cm.
  Includes bibliographical references and index.
  ISBN 0–7216–4869–X
  1. Doppler ultrasonography.   I. Title.
  [DNLM: 1. Ultrasonics. 2. Ultrasonography—instrumentation.   WB
289 K92da 1995]
RC78.7.U4K747   1995
616.07'543—dc20
DNLM/DLC   94-10940

DOPPLER ULTRASOUND: PRINCIPLES AND INSTRUMENTS, SECOND EDITION
ISBN 0–7216–4869–X

Printed in the United States of America

Last digit is the print number: 9   8   7   6   5   4   3   2   1

Some of the same illustrations are also used in Kremkau FW: *Diagnostic Ultrasound: Principles, Instruments and Exercises, 4th edition.* Philadelphia, WB Saunders, 1993. Cover modified from Siemens Medical Systems, Inc.

To the Ultrasound Center
Sonographers and Staff

Pam Burgess
Sharon Hughes
Marie King
Joy Kronenfeld
Kim Malachi
Sherry McNeill
Larry Myers
Louise Nixon
Jo Patterson

Preface

Doppler ultrasound is the field of detection, quantitation, and medical evaluation of tissue motion and blood flow using ultrasound. This book provides vascular technologists, sonographers, and physicians, who need a basic knowledge of the physical principles and instrumentation of Doppler ultrasound, with a simple explanation of how Doppler ultrasound works. It does not describe how to perform diagnostic examinations or how to interpret the results, except in a limited way in the consideration of spectral and color-flow displays in Chapters 5 and 6 and artifacts in Chapter 7. Little background in mathematics and physics is assumed. Many statements in this book are simplifications of the actual situation for the sake of brevity and comprehension.

Exercises are provided at the end of each chapter to check progress, strengthen concepts, and provide practice for registry and specialty-board examinations. Answers to all exercises are given beginning on page 315. A comprehensive multiple-choice examination with explanatory referenced answers is given in Appendix B.

Superscript numbers refer to citations in the reference list starting on page 364.

This book and reference 1 by Kremkau are complementary. That is, this book contains an expansion of Chapter 5 in reference 1, and reference 1 contains an expansion of Chapter 2 in this book (Fig. P.1). They are, therefore, companion texts that together cover in detail the principles of both Doppler ultrasound and sonography.

This second edition expands the treatment of signal processing details of spectral instruments and enlarges the coverage of color-flow instruments from one section in the previous edition to an entire chapter here. Several equations in the previous edition have been eliminated from the text to make the book less mathematic. Qualitative messages from equations are introduced in this edition as up and down arrows.

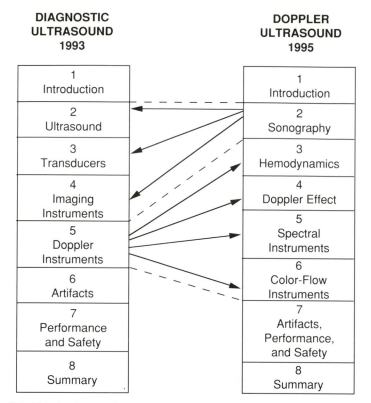

Figure P.1. This book contains an expansion of Chapter 5 in reference 1; reference 1 contains an expansion of Chapter 2 in this book.

A complete set of equations is contained in Appendix A for readers who are interested in the mathematic details.

Chapter 6 is a revision of an earlier one on the subject (reference 39). It, along with reference 32, was used as the basis for the new chapter with the permission of Mosby-Year Book and the Society of Vascular Technology. Section 7.4 is a revision of an earlier chapter on the subject (reference 50), which was used as a basis for this section with the permission of Mosby-Year Book.

The author gratefully acknowledges comments and suggestions from instructors and students who have used the previous edition of this book. For assistance with figure acquisition, he thanks Pam Burgess, Cindy Burnham, Peter Burns, Marge Cappuccio, George Cook, Diane Davis, Tom Dew, Jean Ellison, Rob Gill, Tracey Heriot, Marie King, Jill Leighton, Anne Mansfield, Kristin Martin, Steve Meads, Chris Merritt, Terry Needham, Mohsen Nomeir, Valerie Perry, Delores

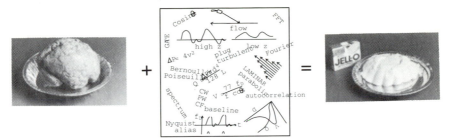

Figure P.2. Is this your opinion of Doppler physics?

Pretorius, Paul Ramsey, Scott Reavis, Joe Roselli, Pam Rowland, Dennis Shields, Jackie Sledge, Gene Strandness, David Taylor, Ken Taylor, Chuck Tegeler, Paul Tesh, The American Institute of Ultrasound in Medicine, and the following companies: Acuson, Advanced Technology Laboratories, Diasonics, General Electric, Hewlett Packard, JJ&A Instruments, Philips, Radiation Measurements, Inc., and Siemens/Quantum. He thanks Louise Nixon for typing the manuscript and Marie King and Jo Patterson for proofreading.

Your view of physics might be as described in Figure P.2. This book is offered in the hope that as you read it, you will not only understand the physics of Doppler ultrasound but will actually enjoy it (maybe just a little bit)! Best wishes for your professional ultrasound future!

Contents

1 Introduction 1

2 Sonography 7

   2.1 Ultrasound 13
   2.2 Transducers 22
   2.3 Instruments 35
   2.4 Artifacts 44
   2.5 Review 51

3 Hemodynamics 63

   3.1 Fluids 64
   3.2 Steady Flow 65
   3.3 Stenoses 72
   3.4 Pulsatile Flow 76
   3.5 Review 77

4 Doppler Effect 89

   4.1 Doppler Effect 89
   4.2 Speed 99
   4.3 Angle 102
   4.4 Frequency 109
   4.5 Review 111

5 Spectral Instruments 121

  5.1 Continuous Wave 122
  5.2 Pulsed Wave 134
  5.3 Spectral Analysis 141
  5.4 Spectral Displays 144
  5.5 Review 159

6 Color-Flow Instruments 177

  6.1 Color-Flow Principle 178
  6.2 Principles of Color Vision 180
  6.3 Instruments 181
  6.4 Displays 198
  6.5 Review 210

7 Artifacts, Performance, and Safety 219

  7.1 Spectral Artifacts 221
  7.2 Color-Flow Artifacts 238
  7.3 Performance 245
  7.4 Safety 248
  7.5 Review 266

8 Summary 279

Glossary 305
Answers to Exercises in the Text 315
Appendix **A**
Symbols, Abbreviations, and Equations 331
Appendix **B**
Comprehensive Examination 337
Comprehensive Examination Answers 359
References 364
Index 367

1 Introduction

The Doppler effect was used by bats, dolphins, and other animals long before humans applied it to their needs. These animals use ultrasonic pulse-echo Doppler information to determine the motion of prey.[2] Human applications of the effect include those involving light, radar, and sound. Doppler shifts in light received from stars and galaxies allow us to conclude that the universe is expanding and to determine the detailed motions of closer bodies, such as the sun. Doppler radar in weather reporting and forecasting, aviation safety, and police highway surveillance has made the term a household word. In addition to experiencing the acoustic Doppler effect in normal everyday life (for example, approaching and receding sirens or vehicle horns), we have applied it to automatic door openers in public buildings and to portable home burglar alarms (Fig. 1.1).

The early investigation into the nature of the effect during the mid-1800s by Christian Andreas Doppler is an interesting story.[3] Because of his work, the effect is named after him. His name is often given incorrectly as Johann in the scientific and medical literature. His father's name was Johann Evangelist Doppler.

Doppler ultrasound has been in use in diagnostic medicine for many years. Long-standing applications include monitoring of the fetal heart rate during labor and delivery and evaluating blood flow in the carotid arteries. Applications that developed largely in the 1980s extended its use to virtually all medical specialties, including cardiology, neurology, radiology, obstetrics, pediatrics, and surgery. Flow can be detected even in vessels that are too small to image with ultrasound. Doppler ultrasound can determine the presence or absence of flow, the direction and speed of flow, and the character of flow (Table 1.1). Doppler instruments provide audible and visual outputs of blood flow informa-

1

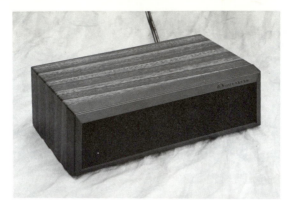

Figure 1.1. An ultrasonic motion-detection burglar alarm that uses the Doppler effect.

tion (Table 1.2). For an intelligent and successful application of the technique to medical diagnosis, an understanding of Doppler principles and instruments is necessary.

The Doppler effect is a change in frequency or wavelength of a wave caused by motion. The motion can be that of the source, the receiver, or a reflector of the wave. The wave can be of any type, including light and sound. In medical applications, it is commonly the motion or flow of blood that is the source of the Doppler effect and

Table 1–1
Types of Flow Information Provided by Doppler Ultrasound

1. Presence of flow
   - □ Yes
   - □ No
2. Direction of flow
   - □ ←
   - □ →
3. Speed of flow
   - □ Slow
   - □ Fast
4. Character of flow
   - □ Normal
   - □ Turbulent

Table 1–2
Presentation of Doppler Information

Audible sounds
Strip-chart recording
Spectral display
Color-flow display

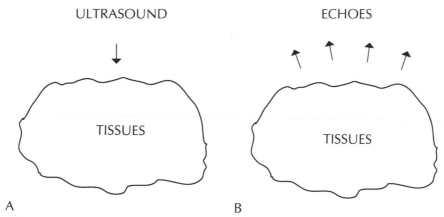

ULTRASOUND

ECHOES

TISSUES

TISSUES

A

B

Figure 1.2. (A) In diagnostic ultrasound, ultrasound is sent into the tissues to interact with them and obtain information about them. (B) Echoes return from the tissues, providing information that is useful for imaging, flow measurement, and diagnosis.

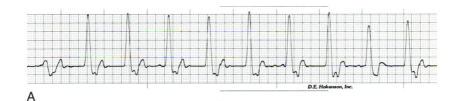

D.E. Hokanson, Inc.

A

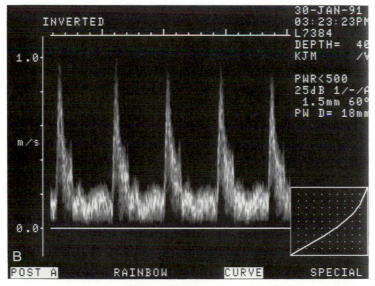

Figure 1.3. (A) Strip-chart recording of Doppler information. (B) Spectral display of common carotid artery blood flow (see Color Plate I).

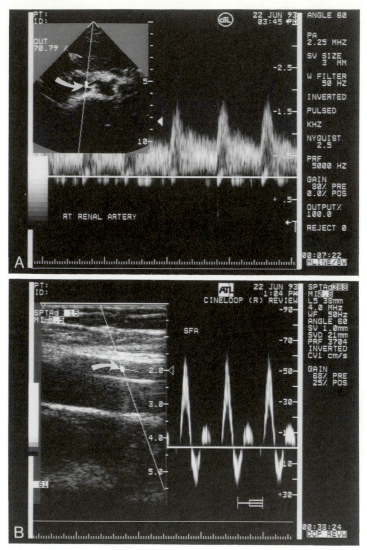

Figure 1.4. Spectral displays of (A) right renal artery and (B) superficial femoral artery blood flow with anatomic images showing the locations (curved arrows) from which the Doppler information was acquired.

about which information is desired. This diagnostic technique is accomplished as follows. Continuous-wave or pulsed-wave ultrasound is transmitted into the patient's body (Fig. 1.2A). Echoes are generated as the sound interacts with the tissues (Fig. 1.2B). When echo-generating structures (heart and blood vessel walls) or blood are moving, Doppler-shifted echoes are generated. These echoes are received and converted into electric voltages that pass into the electronics of the instrument. Here, the voltages that represent the echoes are amplified, and the Doppler shifts are determined. Doppler-shift frequencies that represent the tissue motion or blood flow are applied to loudspeakers for audible analysis and, usually, to a display for visual analysis (Fig. 1.3, Color Plate I). Pulsed-Doppler instruments are commonly combined with pulse-echo imaging[1] to select and evaluate flow data intelligently (Fig. 1.4). Rapid scanning and processing of Doppler data allow two-dimensional, cross-sectional, color-coded, real-time presentations of Doppler flow data to be superimposed on real-time, gray-scale, anatomic images (Fig. 1.5, Color Plate II).

In this book, we consider the following questions. How does blood flow? How does ultrasound detect and measure blood flow? In what ways is flow information presented? How is flow detection localized to a specific site in tissue? How is two-dimensional flow information acquired and presented in real time? Other textbooks dealing with the physics of Doppler ultrasound include references 4 through 8.

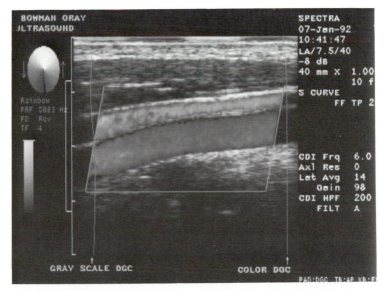

Figure 1.5. Color-flow display of blood flow in the common carotid artery (red) and jugular vein (blue) (see Color Plate II). (From Kremkau FW: Principles and instrumentation. In Merritt CRB [ed]: Doppler Color Imaging. New York, Churchill Livingstone, 1992. Reprinted with permission.)

Exercises

1.1 The Doppler effect is a change in (more than one correct answer)

    a. amplitude
    b. intensity
    c. impedance
    d. frequency
    e. wavelength

1.2 The change in Exercise 1.1 is a result of _____.

1.3 The motion that produces the Doppler effect can be that of the (more than one correct answer)

    a. source
    b. receiver
    c. memory
    d. display
    e. reflector

1.4 In medical applications, it is commonly the flow of _____ that is the source of the Doppler effect. Doppler shift frequencies are applied to _____ for audible analysis and to a _____ for visual analysis.

1.5 The visual display of Doppler information can be in the form of a _____ - _____ recording, a _____ display, or a _____ - _____ display.

The answers to the exercises are given beginning on page 315.

2 Sonography

The information in this chapter is important to understanding Doppler ultrasound for two reasons. First, ultrasound (Section 2.1) and transducers (Section 2.2) are used in Doppler ultrasound. Second, Doppler ultrasound is combined with sonography in most applications. Thus, an understanding of imaging instruments (Section 2.3) and artifacts (Section 2.4) is important. All these subjects are covered in more detail in reference 1.

Ultrasound imaging (sonography) is accomplished with a pulse-echo technique. An image is a representation of the real object. In sonography, the echoes represent the anatomy that generated them. Pulses of ultrasound (generated by a transducer) are sent into the patient (see Fig. 1.2A) where they produce echoes at organ boundaries and within tissues. These echoes return (see Fig. 1.2B) to the transducer and are detected and displayed. Thus, the transducer both generates the ultrasound pulses and detects the returning echoes. The ultrasound instrument processes this information and generates appropriate dots, which form the ultrasound image on the display. The brightness of each dot corresponds to the echo's strength. The location of each dot corresponds to the anatomic location of the echo-generating structure. The positional information is determined by knowing the direction of the pulse when it enters the patient and measuring the time for its echo to return to the transducer. From an assumed starting point on the display (usually at the top), the proper location for presenting the echo can then be determined, knowing the direction in which to travel from that starting point to the appropriate distance. The ultrasound pulse and its echo are assumed to travel at the average speed in tissues, i.e., 1.54 millimeters per microsecond (mm/μs). This means that 13 μs are required for the ultrasound pulse to travel round trip to a structure

7

located 1 centimeter (cm) away from the transducer (26 μs for 2 cm, 130 μs for 10 cm, and so forth).

If one pulse of ultrasound is transmitted into tissue or tissue-equivalent phantom material, a series of echoes returns as the pulse travels through the material. These are converted into a series of voltages by the transducer that are then processed by the electronics in the instrument and displayed as a string of dots on the display, i.e., one scan line (Fig. 2.1). If the process is repeated, but with different starting points for each subsequent pulse, a cross-sectional image builds up (Fig. 2.2). In this case, each pulse travels in the same direction but starts from a different point. The parallel scan lines produce a rectangular display, as shown in Figure 2.3. This image of vessels was produced with vertical parallel scan lines that are so numerous and close together that they cannot be identified individually. The rectangular display resulting from this procedure is often called a linear scan because the pulses originate from a line across the top of the scan, with linear being the adjectival form of the word line. A second approach to sending ultrasound pulses through the object to be imaged is shown in Figure 2.4. Here, each pulse originates from the same starting point,

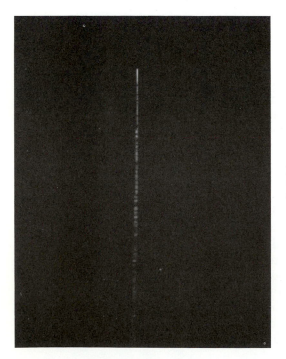

Figure 2.1. A single scan line (series of echoes) results from sending one pulse into tissue.

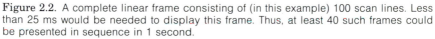

Figure 2.2. A complete linear frame consisting of (in this example) 100 scan lines. Less than 25 ms would be needed to display this frame. Thus, at least 40 such frames could be presented in sequence in 1 second.

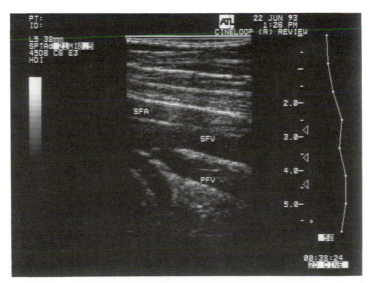

Figure 2.3. Example (lower extremity) of a linear scan with its rectangular shape.

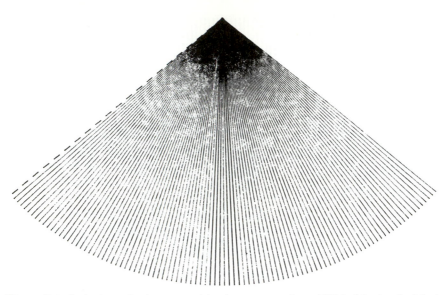

Figure 2.4. A single-sector frame consists of many scan lines (100 in this drawing) that fan out from a common origin.

but subsequent pulses go out in slightly different directions from previous ones. This results in a pie slice—shaped sector scan (Figs. 2.5 and 2.6).

Linear and sector scans are the formats utilized most commonly in the automated scanning techniques described in Section 2.2. Others could be used, but in each case, what is required is that ultrasound pulses be sent, in some manner, through all portions of the cross section that is to be imaged. Each pulse generates a series of echoes, which results in a series of dots (a scan line) on the display. The resulting cross-sectional image is made up of many (typically, 100 to 200) of these scan lines. The scan format determines the starting points and paths for the individual scan lines, according to the starting point and path for each pulse used in generating each scan line. Figures 2.3 and 2.5 are examples of cross-sectional ultrasound images of the linear and sector types, respectively. These are often called "B" scans. This terminology refers to the fact that the images are produced by scanning the ultrasound through the tissue cross section (i.e., sending pulses through all regions of the cross section) and converting the echo's strength into the brightness of each represented echo on the display (thus B or brightness scan). The term "gray-scale imaging" is also used to describe this process. Note that a B scan is a presentation of *echoes,* but it can be viewed as an image of anatomy because the echoes are produced by the anatomy.

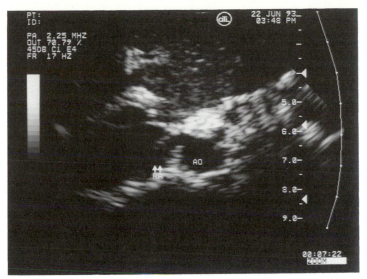

Figure 2.5. Example (transverse aorta and right renal artery) of a sector scan with its pie-slice shape.

Continuous-wave or pulsed-wave Doppler instruments may be combined with imaging instruments to yield what are commonly called duplex instruments. Figure 2.6 shows the flow in a vessel as a function of time (over several cardiac cycles). A cross-sectional image of the vessel and its surrounding anatomy is combined with indicators of the

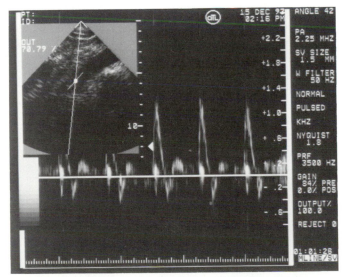

Figure 2.6. Example (aorta) of a sector scan with Doppler blood flow information.

Doppler beam's location and the region (sample volume) within the vessel from which the Doppler information is being obtained. This is discussed in detail in Chapter 5. Color-flow instruments combine two-dimensional Doppler information with anatomic B scans (Chapter 6). Subsequent sections in this chapter deal with the primary aspects of sonography: ultrasound, transducers, instruments, and artifacts.

In this chapter, we consider the following questions. What is ultrasound and how does it behave? How is ultrasound weakened as it travels through tissue? How are echoes generated? How does a transducer generate ultrasound and receive echoes? How are sound beams focused and scanned through tissue? How do sonographic instruments work? How do displays work? What are detail, contrast, and temporal resolutions and on what do they depend? The following terms are discussed in this chapter:

absorption	gain
amplification	gray scale
amplitude	hertz
annular array	impedance
array	intensity
attenuation	kilohertz
bandwidth	linear array
beam	matching layer
beam former	megahertz
cathode ray tube	mirror image
composite	operating frequency
continuous wave	penetration
contrast resolution	phased array
convex array	piezoelectricity
crystal	pixel
cycle	postprocessing
damping	preprocessing
demodulation	pressure
depth gain compensation	propagation speed
detail resolution	pulse
duty factor	pulse repetition frequency
echo	radio frequency
element	refraction
enhancement	reverberation
focus	scattering
frame rate	section thickness
freeze frame	shadowing
frequency	temporal resolution

time gain compensation   video
transducer   wave
ultrasound   wavelength

2.1
Ultrasound

Ultrasound is like ordinary sound, except that it has a pitch higher than humans can hear. Sound is a wave (i.e., a propagating or traveling variation in quantities called acoustic variables). These acoustic variables include pressure, density, and particle motion. They go through repeating cycles of increase and decrease as the sound wave travels. Sound is a mechanical compressional wave in which the back-and-forth particle motion is parallel to the direction of the wave's travel.

Frequency describes how many complete variations (cycles) an acoustic variable goes through in 1 second of time (i.e., how many cycles occur in 1 second). For example, pressure may start at its normal (undisturbed) value, increase to a maximum value, return to normal, decrease to a minimum value, and return to normal (Fig. 2.7). This describes a complete cycle of the variation of pressure as an acoustic variable. As a sound wave travels past some point, this cycle is repeated over and over. The number of times that it occurs in 1 second is called the frequency. Frequency units include hertz (Hz) and megahertz (MHz). One hertz is one cycle per second, and 1 MHz is 1 million Hz. Sound with a frequency of 20,000 Hz or more is called ultrasound because it is beyond the frequency range of human hearing (the prefix ultra means "beyond").

Wavelength is the length of space over which one cycle occurs (Fig. 2.8). If we could stop the sound wave, visualize it, and measure the distance from the beginning to the end of one cycle, that distance would be the wavelength.

Propagation speed is the speed with which a wave moves through a medium. It is the speed at which a particular value of an acoustic variable moves or with which a cycle moves. The average propagation

Figure 2.7. One complete variation (cycle) of an acoustic variable (pressure). This variation may repeat as time passes, as indicated by the dashed lines.

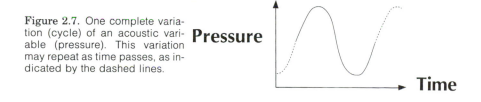

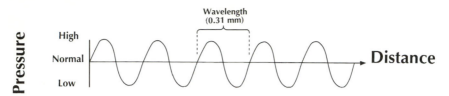

Figure 2.8. The wavelength is the length of space over which one cycle occurs. In this example, each cycle covers 0.31 mm. Thus, the wavelength is 0.31 mm. For a propagation speed of 1.54 mm/μs and a frequency of 5 MHz, the wavelength is 0.31 mm.

speed in soft tissues (excluding the lung and bone) is 1540 m/s or 1.54 mm/μs (about 3500 miles/hr). Wavelength is equal to propagation speed divided by frequency. Thus, if frequency increases, wavelength decreases.

> frequency ↑   wavelength ↓ *

For sonography, short pulses of sound are used. This pulsed ultrasound is produced by applying electric pulses to the transducer. The number of pulses produced per second is called the pulse repetition frequency and is usually given in kilohertz (kHz). One kilohertz is 1000 Hz. The fraction of time the sound is on is called the duty factor.

Spatial pulse length is the length of space over which a pulse occurs. It is equal to the wavelength times the number of cycles in the pulse (typically one to three for imaging, more for Doppler). It decreases with increasing frequency (Fig. 2.9).

> frequency ↑   spatial pulse length ↓

The strength of the ultrasound is described by two terms: amplitude and intensity. These are measures of how loud the sound would be if it could be heard. Of course, it cannot be heard because it is ultrasound.

Amplitude is the maximum variation that occurs in an acoustic variable. It is the maximum value minus the normal (undisturbed) value (Fig. 2.10). The amplitude is given in units appropriate for the acoustic variable considered. Intensity is the power in a wave divided by the area over which the power is spread. It is an important term to describe the sound that is produced and received by diagnostic instru-

---

*This statement is a qualitative presentation of the relationship between variables. The up arrow represents an increase and the down arrow, a decrease. Thus, this statement means that as the frequency increases, the wavelength decreases.

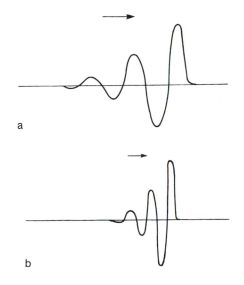

Figure 2.9. (a) A three-cycle pulse traveling from left to right. (b) A higher frequency
pulse is shorter. (From Kremkau FW: Ultrasound instrumentation: physical principles. In Callen PW [ed]: Ultrasonography
in Obstetrics and Gynecology. Philadelphia, WB Saunders, 1982. Reprinted with
permission.)

a

b

ments and to discuss bioeffects and safety. It may be illustrated by an
analogy with the sunlight incident on dry leaves (Fig. 2.11). Sunlight
will not normally ignite the leaves, but if the same power is concen-
trated into a small area (increased intensity) by focusing with a magni-
fying glass, the leaves can be ignited. An effect is therefore produced
by increasing the intensity, even though the power remains the same.
For our purposes, the area is the cross-sectional area of the sound beam
discussed in Section 2.2.

Amplitude and intensity decrease as the sound travels through a
medium (Fig. 2.12). This reduction is called attenuation. It encom-
passes absorption (conversion of sound to heat), reflection, and scattering. Absorption is normally the dominant contribution to attenuation
in soft tissue. The units of attenuation are decibels (dB). The longer
the path over which the sound travels, the greater the attenuation is.
The attenuation coefficient is the attenuation per unit length of sound
travel. Its units are decibels per centimeter (dB/cm). The attenuation

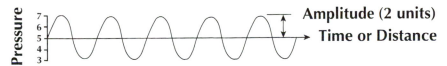

Figure 2.10. The amplitude is the maximum amount of variation that occurs in an acoustic
variable (pressure, in this case). It is equal to the maximum value of the variable minus
the normal (undisturbed) value. In this example, the amplitude is 7 (maximum value) minus
5 (normal value) or 2 units.

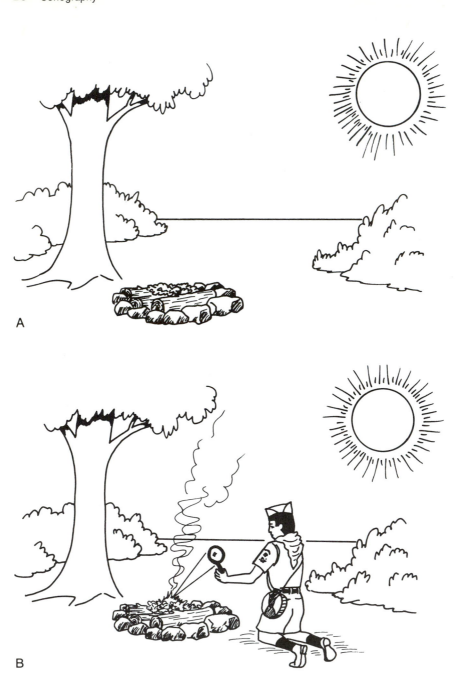

A

B

Figure 2.11. (A) Sunlight does not normally ignite a fire. (B) With focusing of the sunlight (increased intensity), ignition can occur.

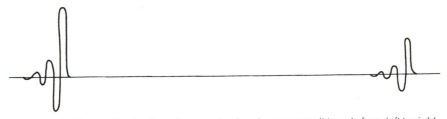

Figure 2.12. The amplitude of an ultrasound pulse decreases as it travels from left to right. (From Kremkau FW: Ultrasound instrumentation: physical principles. In Callen PW [ed]: Ultrasonography in Obstetrics and Gynecology. Philadelphia, WB Saunders, 1982. Reprinted with permission.)

coefficient increases with increasing frequency. Persons who live in apartments or dormitories experience this effect when they hear mostly the bass notes through the wall from a neighbor's sound system. For soft tissues, attenuation coefficients are given by a simple proportional approximation of 0.5 dB of attenuation per centimeter for each megahertz of frequency. Therefore, the average attenuation coefficient in decibels per centimeter for soft tissues is approximately one half the

Table 2–1

Attenuation for Various Intensity Ratios*

Attenuation (dB)	Intensity Ratio
0	1.00
1	0.79
2	0.63
3	0.50
4	0.40
5	0.32
6	0.25
7	0.20
8	0.16
9	0.13
10	0.10
15	0.032
20	0.010
25	0.003
30	0.001
35	0.0003
40	0.0001
45	0.00003
50	0.00001
60	0.000001
70	0.0000001
80	0.00000001
90	0.000000001
100	0.0000000001

* The intensity ratio is the fraction of the initial intensity remaining after the attenuation.

frequency in megahertz. To calculate the attenuation in decibels, simply multiply one half the frequency in megahertz (which is approximately equal to the attenuation coefficient in decibels per centimeter) by the path length in centimeters, and the result is the attenuation in decibels. Various decibel values (along with their corresponding intensity reductions) are listed in Table 2.1.

A practical consequence of attenuation is that it limits the depth to which images and flow data can be obtained. As frequency is increased, attenuation increases, and imaging depth (penetration) decreases (Fig. 2.13).

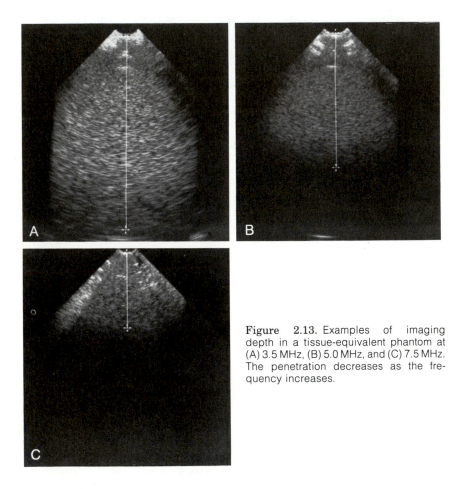

Figure 2.13. Examples of imaging depth in a tissue-equivalent phantom at (A) 3.5 MHz, (B) 5.0 MHz, and (C) 7.5 MHz. The penetration decreases as the frequency increases.

frequency ↑   attenuation ↑   penetration ↓

The usefulness of ultrasound as an imaging tool is the result of reflection and scattering (echo generation) at organ boundaries and scattering within heterogeneous tissues. When an ultrasound pulse is incident on a boundary between two tissues, the incident sound may be reflected, transmitted, or both. The intensities of the reflected and transmitted sound depend on the incident intensity and the impedances of the tissue. Impedance is the density multiplied by the propagation speed. If the two impedances are equal, there is no echo, and the transmitted intensity equals the incident intensity. The more different the impedances are, the stronger the echo is, and the weaker the transmitted sound will be.

Oblique incidence occurs when the direction of travel of the incident ultrasound is not perpendicular to the boundary between two media. This is the common situation in diagnostic ultrasound. Refraction is a change in direction of sound when crossing a boundary. It is caused by a difference in propagation speeds on either side of the boundary. There is no refraction if the propagation speeds are equal.

In the previous discussion, we assumed that the wavelength was small compared with the boundary's dimensions and roughness. The resulting reflections are called specular (mirrorlike) reflections. On the other hand, if the boundary dimensions are comparable to or small compared with the wavelength or the boundary is not smooth (i.e., has surface irregularities comparable in size to the wavelength), the incident sound is scattered. Scattering is the redirection of sound in many directions by rough surfaces or by heterogeneous media (Fig. 2.14), such as tissues or particle suspensions like blood. Both types of scattering are seen in Figures 2.3 and 2.5. These cases are analogous to light, in which specular reflections occur at mirrors. For a rougher surface, such as a white wall, although virtually all the light is reflected (that is why the wall is white), a reflected image is not observed (as in a mirror) because the light is scattered at the surface and mixed up as it travels back to the viewer's eyes. When light passes through a suspension of water droplets in air (fog), it is also scattered. Backscatter (sound scattered back in the direction from which it originally came) intensities vary with the frequency of the sound and the size of the scatterer. Normally, scatter intensities are much less than boundary specular reflection intensities. The intensity received by the transducer from specular reflections is highly angle dependent. This is seen, for example, with echoes from the blood vessel intima. Scattering from

Figure 2.14. A sound pulse may be scattered by (A) a rough boundary between tissues or (B) from within tissues as a result of their heterogeneous character. (C) The four straight arrows show echoes from tissue boundaries (interfaces). The three curved arrows point out regions of scatter (echo generation) from within tissue.

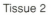

Tissue 1

Tissue 2

A

B

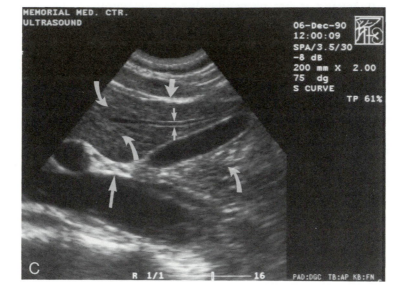

C

boundaries helps to make echo reception less dependent on incidence angle (for example, echoes from plaque). Scattering, thus, permits ultrasound imaging of tissue boundaries that are not necessarily perpendicular to the direction of the incident sound. It also allows imaging of tissue parenchyma in addition to organ boundaries. Scattering is relatively independent of the direction of the incident sound, and therefore is more characteristic of the scatterers (i.e., the tissue).

The average speed of sound in tissues (1.54 mm/μs) leads to the important round-trip travel time rule of 13 μs/cm. That is, it takes

13 μs of round-trip travel time for each centimeter of distance from the transducer to the reflector or scatterer of sound (Fig. 2.15). Thus, in clinical imaging, the deepest echoes (approximately 20 cm for abdominal imaging) will return approximately 250 μs after the pulse leaves the transducer. This allows time for 4000 pulses (and, thus, 4000 scan lines) to be generated in 1 second.

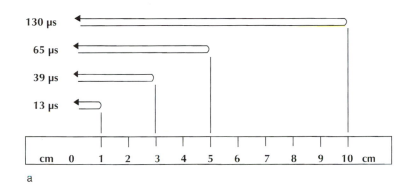

a

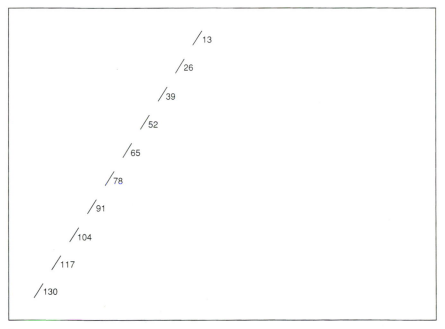

b

Figure 2.15. (a) Echo arrival times for 1-, 3-, 5-, and 10-cm reflector distances. (b) Echoes from 1-, 2-, 3-, 4-, 5-, 6-, 7-, 8-, 9-, and 10-cm depths arrive at the times (in microseconds) indicated.

2.2

Transducers

Transducers (Fig. 2.16) convert energy from one form to another. Ultrasound transducers have no special name, such as microphone or loudspeaker, which are the names applied to devices that accomplish similar functions with audible sound. Rather, they are simply referred to by the generic term, transducer. Ultrasound transducers convert electric energy into ultrasound energy and vice versa. The electric voltages applied to them are converted to ultrasound. The ultrasound (echoes) incident on them produces electric voltages. Ultrasound transducers operate on the piezoelectric principle, which states that some materials (ceramics, quartz, and others) produce a voltage when deformed by an applied pressure. Piezoelectricity also results in the production of pressure when these materials are deformed by an applied voltage. Various formulations of lead zirconate titanate are commonly used as materials for the production of modern transducer elements. Ceramics such as these are not naturally piezoelectric (as quartz is). They are made piezoelectric during production by placing them in a strong electric field while they are at a high temperature. They are often combined with a nonpiezoelectric polymer to create materials that are called composites. These composites have improved sensitivity and resolution.

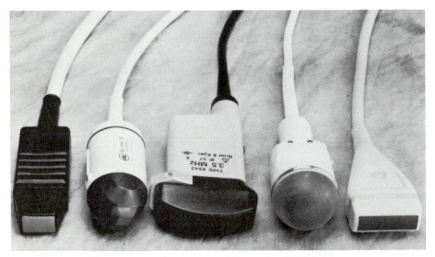

Figure 2.16. Several transducers of various types.

Single-element transducers are in the form of disks (Fig. 2.17). When an electric voltage is applied to the faces of an element, its thickness increases or decreases, depending on the polarity of the voltage. The term transducer element (also called piezoelectric element, active element, or crystal) refers to the piece of piezoelectric material that converts electricity to ultrasound and vice versa. The element, with its associated case and damping and matching materials, is called a transducer assembly, scanhead, or probe (Figs. 2.16 and 2.17). Both the transducer element and the transducer assembly are commonly referred to as the transducer. Source transducers operated in the continuous mode are driven by a continuous alternating voltage and produce an alternating pressure that propagates as a sound wave (Fig. 2.18a).

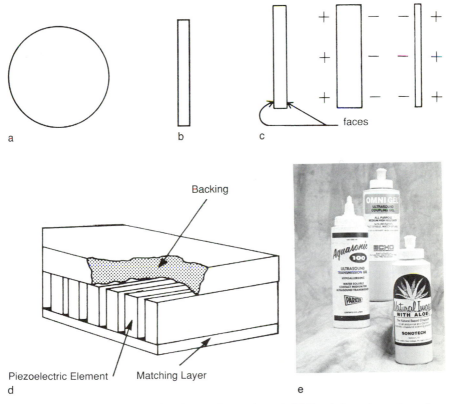

Figure 2.17. (a) Front view of a disk transducer element. (b) Front view of a rectangular element. (c) Side view of either element with no voltage applied to faces (normal thickness), voltage applied (increased thickness), and opposite voltage applied (decreased thickness). (d) A transducer assembly (scanning head or probe). The damping material reduces pulse duration, thus improving axial resolution. The matching layer increases sound transmission into the tissues. (e) Coupling gel improves sound transmission into the patient.

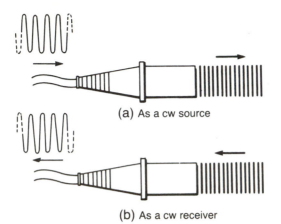

(a) As a cw source

(b) As a cw receiver

Figure 2.18. A transducer assembly operating in the continuous-wave mode. The device converts (a) a continuous-wave voltage into continuous-wave ultrasound or converts (b) received continuous-wave ultrasound into a continuous-wave voltage.

The frequency of the sound produced is equal to the frequency of the driving voltage. The operating frequency (sometimes called resonance frequency) of the transducer is its preferred (most efficient) frequency of operation. The operating frequency is determined by the thickness of the transducer element. The thinner the element is, the higher the operating frequency is. This is analogous to the familiar fact that small bells produce a higher frequency sound than do large ones. Continuous-wave sound entering a receiving transducer is converted to a continuous alternating voltage (Fig. 2.18b). For instruments that use the continuous-wave mode, separate source and receiver transducer elements are required because they each must continuously perform their function. These elements are built into a single transducer assembly (Section 5.1).

Source transducers operated in the pulsed mode (pulsed ultrasound) are driven by voltage bursts (Fig. 2.19) or pulses (Fig. 2.20) and produce ultrasound pulses. These transducers convert received echoes into voltage pulses (Figs. 2.19 and 2.20). The pulse repetition frequency is equal to the voltage pulse repetition frequency, which is determined by the instrument driving the transducer. Damping material (usually a mixture of metal powder and a plastic or epoxy) is attached to the rear face of the transducer element to reduce the number of cycles in each pulse and, thus, the pulse length (Fig. 2.21). Reducing the pulse length improves the resolution. This method of damping is analogous to packing foam rubber around a bell that is rung by a tap with a hammer. The rubber reduces the time that the bell rings following the tap. Typically, pulses of one to three cycles are generated with the transducers used for sonography. Longer pulses are used with pulsed Doppler instruments (Section 5.2).

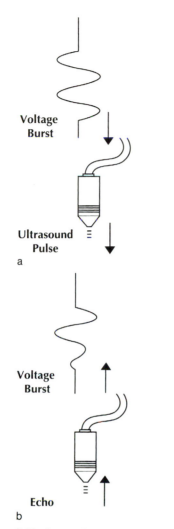

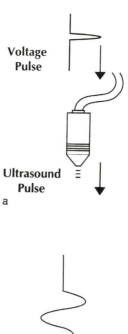

Figure 2.19. A transducer operating in the burst-excited mode. This device converts electric voltage bursts into ultrasound pulses (a) and converts received echoes into electric voltage bursts (b).

Figure 2.20. A transducer assembly operating in the shock-excited mode. This device converts electric voltage pulses into ultrasound pulses (a) and converts received echoes into electric voltage bursts (b).

A matching layer is commonly placed on the transducer's face (Fig. 2.17d). This material has an impedance intermediate between those of the transducer element and the tissue. It reduces the reflection of ultrasound at the transducer element's surface, improving sound transmission across it in both directions (into and out of the tissues).

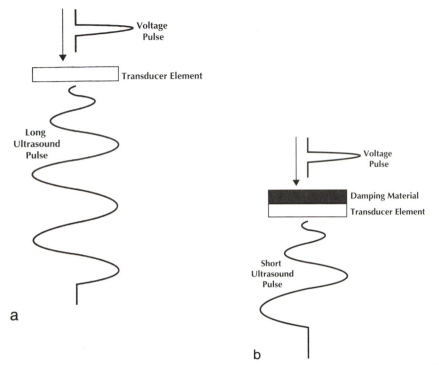

Figure 2.21. (a) Without damping, a voltage pulse applied to the transducer element results in a long ultrasound pulse of many cycles. (b) With damping material on the rear face of the transducer element, application of a voltage pulse results in a short pulse of a few cycles. This figure shows each pulse traveling (down) away from the transducer in space so that the bottom end is the beginning or leading edge of the pulse as it travels down.

Because of its very low impedance, even a very thin layer of air between the transducer's face and the skin's surface would reflect virtually all the sound, preventing penetration into the tissue. For this reason, a coupling medium, usually an aqueous gel, is applied to the skin before transducer contact (Fig. 2.17e). This eliminates the air layer and permits the sound to pass into and out of the tissue.

A single-element flat-disk transducer operating in the continuous-wave mode produces a sound beam with a beam diameter that varies according to the distance from the transducer face, as shown in Figure 2.22. Sometimes, significant intensity travels out in some directions that are not included in the beam as pictured. These additional "beams" are called side lobes. They are really "cone" or "ring" beams for a disk transducer.

The region from the disk out to a distance of one near-zone length is called the near zone. The near zone is longer for larger diameter transducers and for higher frequency transducers. The region beyond a distance of one near-zone length is called the far zone. The beam's diameter at any point depends on the frequency, transducer diameter, and distance from the transducer. It is important to realize that even for flat, unfocused transducer elements (Fig. 2.22), there is some beam narrowing or "focusing."

For improved resolution, the beam's diameter is reduced by focusing the sound in a manner similar to the focusing of light. The sound may be focused by using a curved transducer element, a lens, or a phased array (Fig. 2.23). The focal length is the distance from the transducer to the center of the focal region (Fig. 2.24). It cannot be greater than the near-zone length of the comparable unfocused transducer. Most diagnostic transducers are focused to some degree.

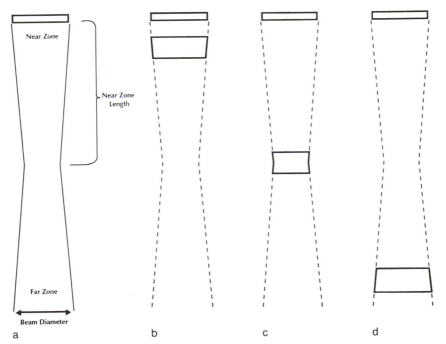

a b c d

Figure 2.22. (a) Diameter of the beam for a single-element, unfocused disk transducer operating in the continuous-wave mode. This diameter approximates the region of that portion of the sound produced that is greater than 4 percent of the spatial peak intensity. The near zone is the region between the disk and the minimum beam diameter. The far zone is the region beyond the minimum beam diameter. The intensity is not constant within the beam; the intensity variations are greatest in the near zone. The beam's diameter in (a) approximates the changing pulse's diameter as an ultrasound pulse travels away from the transducer. (b) A pulse shortly after leaving the transducer. (c) Later the pulse is located at the end of the near-zone length, where its diameter is at a minimum. (d) Still later the pulse is in the far zone, where its diameter is increasing as it travels. This figure assumes a nonscattering, nonrefracting medium, such as water.

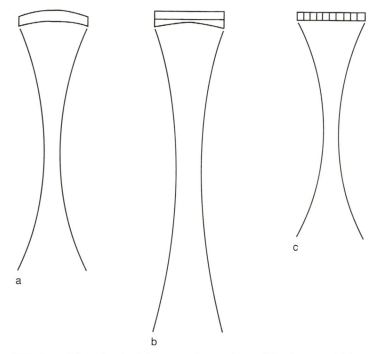

Figure 2.23. Sound focusing by (a) a curved transducer, (b) a lens, and (c) a phased array. Lenses focus because the propagation speed through them is higher than that through tissues. Refraction at the surface of the lens forms the beam such that a focal region occurs. The degree to which the beam's diameter is reduced by focusing is described qualitatively as weak or strong focusing.

There are two ways in which automatic scanning of a sound beam can be performed: mechanical and electronic. Both methods provide a means for sweeping the sound beam through the tissues rapidly and repeatedly. The first method may be accomplished by oscillating a transducer's angle or by rotating a group of transducers (Fig. 2.25). In most mechanical, real-time transducers, the rotating or oscillating component is immersed in a coupling liquid within the transducer assembly. The sound beam is thus swept at a rapid rate without movement of the entire transducer assembly.

Electronic scanning is performed with arrays. Transducer arrays are transducer assemblies with several transducer elements. The elements are rectangular in shape and arranged in a line (linear array) or are ring shaped and arranged concentrically (annular array, Fig. 2.26).

A linear-sequenced array (sometimes called a linear-switched array and commonly called simply a linear array) is operated by

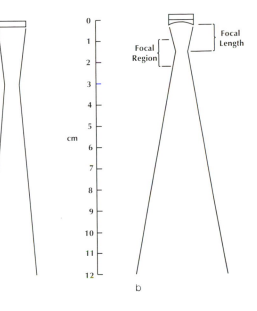

Figure 2.24. Diameter of the beam for a 6-mm 5-MHz disk transducer without (a) and with (b) a focusing lens. Focusing reduces the minimum diameter of the beam compared with that produced without focusing. However, beyond the focal region, the focused beam's diameter is greater than that of the unfocused one. (c) A focused beam from a 5-MHz, 19-mm diameter transducer. This is an ultrasound image of a beam-profile test object that contains a thin vertical scattering layer down the center. Scanning this object generates a picture of the beam profile (the pulse width at all depths). In this case, the focus occurs at about a 4-cm depth (this image has a total depth of 15 cm). The 1-cm depth markers are indicated on the left edge.

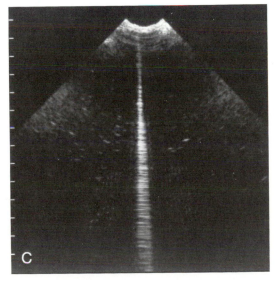

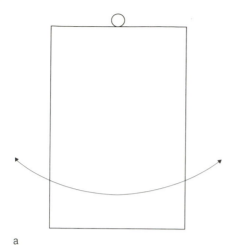

a

Figure 2.25. (a) An oscillating mechanical transducer. (b) A rotating mechanical transducer. (c) An image from a mechanical transducer.

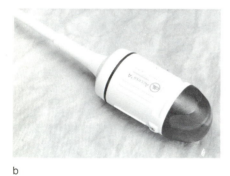

b

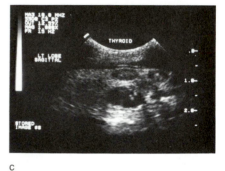

c

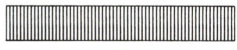

(a)

Figure 2.26. Front views of (a) a linear array with 64 rectangular elements and (b) an annular array with four elements.

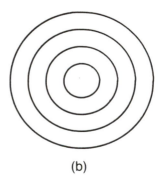

(b)

applying voltage pulses to groups of elements in succession (Fig. 2.27). The origin of the sound beam moves across the face of the transducer assembly and thus produces the same effect as manual linear scanning with a single-element transducer. Such electronic scanning, however, can be done more rapidly and consistently. If this electronic scanning

Figure 2.27. A linear-sequenced array (side view). Voltage pulses are applied simultaneously to all elements in a group: first to elements 1 through 4 (for example) as a group (a), next to elements 2 through 5 (b), and so on across the transducer assembly (c–e). Then the process is repeated (f). (g) An image from a linear-sequenced array. (h) A linear array.

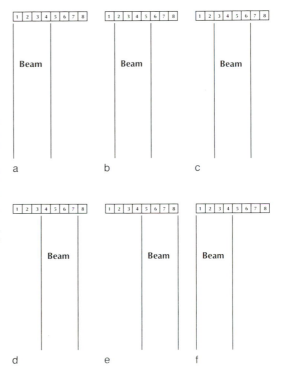

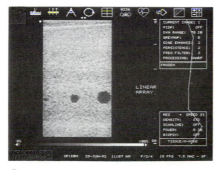

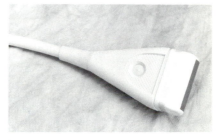

is repeated rapidly enough, a real-time presentation of information can result. That is, several frames or images can be presented per second in rapid sequence. Convex arrays operate similarly to linear arrays but have a curved array surface. They produce sector images.

A linear-phased array (commonly called a phased array) is operated by applying voltage pulses to all elements in the assembly as a complete group but with small time differences (phasing); therefore, the resulting sound pulse may be electronically steered (Fig. 2.28). If the same time differences are used each time the process is repeated,

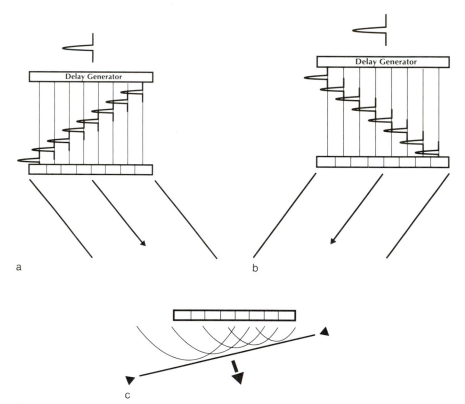

Figure 2.28. A linear-phased array (side view). (a) By applying voltage pulses in rapid progression from left to right, one ultrasound pulse is produced that is directed to the right. (b) Similarly, by applying voltage pulses in rapid progression from right to left, one ultrasound pulse is produced that is directed to the left. The delays in (a) produce a pulse whose combined pressure wavefront (arrowheads) is angled from lower left to upper right as shown in (c). A wave always travels perpendicular to its wavefront, as indicated by the arrow.

the same beam direction will result repeatedly. However, the time differences may be changed with each successive repetition so that the beam's direction (Fig. 2.29) can continually change. This can then result in sweeping of the beam (i.e., the beam's direction changes with each pulse). Phasing also enables variable focusing (the focal length changes with each pulse). Multiple focus can be used to achieve, in effect, a long focus. A separate pulse is required for each focus. Phased arrays can be of the linear-array or annular-array type. Annular arrays provide two-dimensional focusing, shaping the beam like a cone. However, they must be mechanically scanned.

There are three aspects to resolution in imaging: detail (geometric) resolution, contrast (gray-scale) resolution, and temporal (frame-rate) resolution. The latter two are discussed in the next section and the first one, here. If two reflectors are not sufficiently separated, they will not produce separate echoes and, thus, will not be separated on the instrument's display. The characteristics of the instrument's electronics and display may further degrade this detail resolution. It is apparent, however, that if separate echoes are not initially generated, the reflectors will not be separated on the display. In ultrasound imaging, there are two aspects to detail resolution: axial and lateral. They depend on pulse length and pulse width, respectively. The shorter the pulse is,

Diagnostic Ultrasound

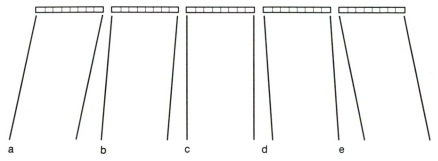

a   b   c   d   e

Figure 2.29. A five-pulse sequence in which each pulse travels out in a different direction. (a) The firing sequence is from right to left across the array. (b) A right-to-left sequence with shorter time delays. (c) No delays (all elements fire simultaneously). (d) A left-to-right sequence. (e) A left-to-right sequence with longer delays.

Figure 2.30. The axial resolution improves as frequency increases. (a) 3.5 MHz; resolution, 2.0 mm. (b) 5.0 MHz; resolution, 1.0 mm. (c) 7.0 MHz; resolution, 0.5 mm. Detail resolution is like a golf score (d); i.e., smaller is better.

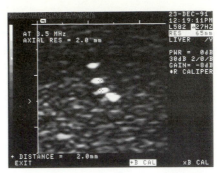

a

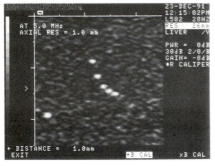

b

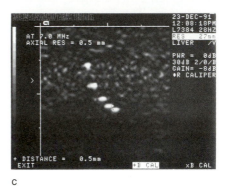

c

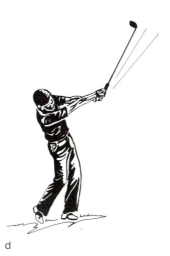

d

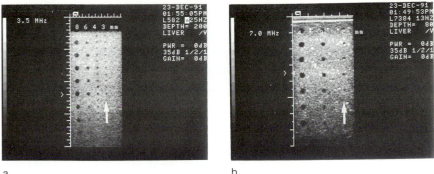

a   b

Figure 2.31. (a) An image of a resolution penetration phantom that contains circular an-echoic regions ("cysts") in tissue-equivalent material. From left to right, the cysts are 8, 6, 4, 3, and 2 mm in diameter and occur every 1 or 2 cm in depth of the image. Close examination shows that 3-mm cysts are the smallest that can be resolved. This image was produced using a 3.5-MHz transducer. (b) The same phantom imaged with a 7.0-MHz transducer. In this instance, 2-mm cysts can be seen. Note the loss of penetration compared with (a) (8 versus 20 cm). Detail resolution can be improved by increasing the frequency of the ultrasound beam but at the expense of decreasing the imaging depth.

the better the axial resolution is; the narrower the pulse is, the better the lateral resolution is. Damping and the use of higher frequencies shorten the pulse, improving the axial resolution. Focusing narrows the pulse, improving the lateral resolution (at least in the focal region). The axial resolution is equal to one half the pulse length. The lateral resolution is equal to the pulse width. Both are like a golf score, i.e., the lower they are, the better. Improved resolution with higher frequency (Figs. 2.30 and 2.31) is accompanied by decreased imaging depth as a result of increased attenuation (Section 2.1).

2.3
Instruments

Imaging systems (Fig. 2.32A) produce visual displays from the electric voltages (representing echoes) received from a transducer. A diagram of the components of a pulse-echo imaging system is given in Figure 2.32B.

The pulser is where the action originates. It produces electric voltage pulses that drive the transducer through the beam former. In response, the transducer produces ultrasound pulses. The pulse repetition frequency of the pulser is the number of electric pulses produced per second. It is typically a few thousand hertz. The beam former is

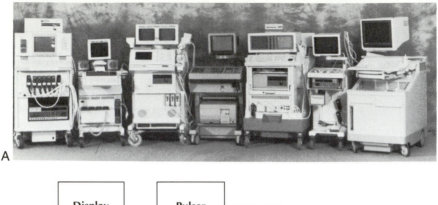

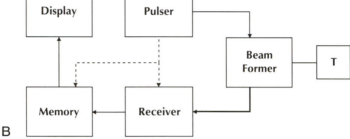

Figure 2.32. (A) Several sonographic instruments. (B) The components of a pulse-echo imaging system. The pulser produces electric pulses that drive the transducer (T) through the beam former. It also produces pulses that tell (dashed line) the receiver and memory when the transducer has been driven. The transducer (acting as a source) produces an ultrasound pulse for each electric pulse applied. For each echo received from the tissues, an electric voltage is produced by the transducer (acting as a receiving transducer). These voltages go through the beam former to the receiver where they are processed to a form suitable for driving the memory. Electric information from the memory drives the display, which produces a visual image of the cross-sectional anatomy interrogated by the system. Some authors consider the clock or timing circuit separately in a diagram such as this. The clock determines the pulse's repetition frequency and causes the various components of the instrument to work together. In this diagram and in Section 2.3, the clock is considered to be part of the pulser.

responsible for the production of the sequencing, delays, and variations in pulse amplitudes necessary for the electronic control of beam scanning, steering, and focusing, as described in the previous section.

Voltages produced by the transducer in response to echoes are sent to the receiver for processing. The receiver performs amplification, compensation, and other functions on these voltages, which represent the echoes. Amplification increases the small voltages received from the transducer to larger ones suitable for processing and storage (Fig. 2.33). Receiver amplifiers usually have 60 to 100 dB of gain (Table 2.2). Compensation (also called gain compensation, swept gain, time

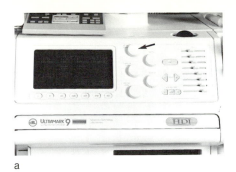

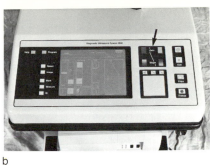

a

b

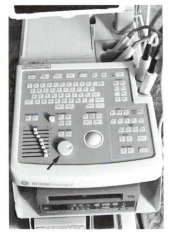

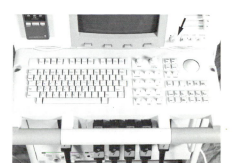

c

d

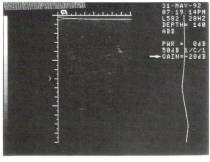

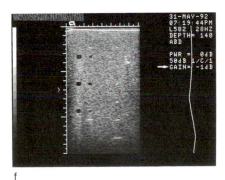

f

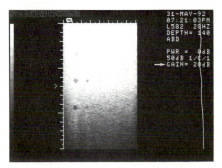

e

g

Figure 2.33. (a–d) Gain controls (arrows) on several control panels. (e) Gain too low. (f) Proper gain. (g) Gain too high; saturation is occurring.

Table 2–2

Gain for Various Power Ratios*

Gain (dB)	Power Ratio
0	1.0
1	1.3
2	1.6
3	2.0
4	2.5
5	3.2
6	4.0
7	5.0
8	6.3
9	7.9
10	10.0
15	32.0
20	100.0
25	320.0
30	1000.0
35	3200.0
40	10,000.0
45	32,000.0
50	100,000.0
60	1,000,000.0
70	10,000,000.0
80	100,000,000.0
90	1,000,000,000.0
100	10,000,000,000.0

* The power ratio is the output power divided by the input power.

gain compensation, or depth gain compensation) equalizes differences in received echo amplitudes because of the reflector's depth. Comparable reflectors do not result in equal-amplitude echoes arriving at the transducer if their travel distances are different (the distances from the transducer to the reflectors are different). This is because attenuation depends on length of the path. It is desirable to display echoes from comparable reflectors in a similar way (comparable brightness). Because these echoes may not arrive with the same amplitude, as a result of different path lengths, their amplitudes must be adjusted to compensate for path-length differences. Larger path lengths result in later arrival times. Therefore, if voltages from echoes arriving later are amplified more than earlier ones are, attenuation compensation is accomplished. This is what compensation does (Fig. 2.34). The rate of increase of gain as echoes return from a pulse is called the time gain compensation slope.

Storing each cross-sectional image in memory as the sound beam is scanned through the tissue permits the display of a single image (scan) out of the rapid sequence of several images (frames) normally

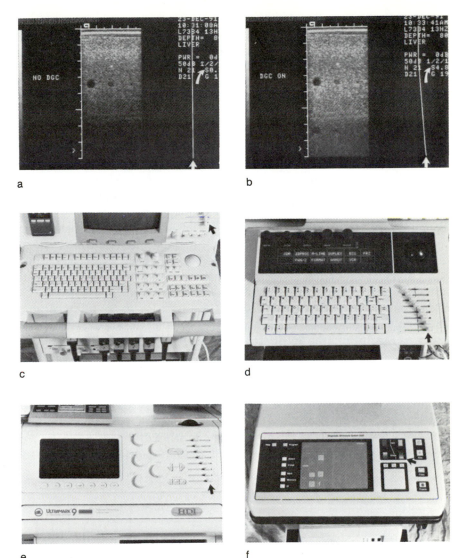

Figure 2.34. Two scans of a tissue-equivalent phantom imaged at 7 MHz with and without depth gain compensation (DGC). These scans show (a) no compensation and (b) correct compensation. Without DGC, the echo's brightness (amplitude, intensity, and strength) falls off with depth (top to bottom). On the display, DGC settings are shown graphically (arrow). The slopes (curved arrow) are (a) 0 dB/cm and (b) 4.8 dB/cm. The average tissue attenuation is 0.5 dB/cm/MHz (see Section 2.1). This is per centimeter of sound propagation. The average attenuation is then 1 dB/cm/MHz, with the distance in centimeters from the transducer to the reflector. The sound must travel twice this distance (round trip) so that the attenuation number doubles. Typical DGC slopes are then about 1 dB/cm/MHz. (c–f) DGC controls on several instruments (arrow).

acquired each second in dynamic (real-time) ultrasound instruments. Displaying one scan out of the sequence is called freeze frame. Some instruments have enough memory to store the last several frames acquired; this is sometimes called cine review, cine loop, or image review. Ultrasound instrument memories are computer memories that store the echoes in the form of numbers. They are called digital scan converters because they provide a computerized means for displaying a scan using a television scan format from information acquired by a linear or sector ultrasound scanning technique. The image is divided (like a checkerboard) into squares called pixels (picture elements), commonly 512 × 512 squares on each side. In each of these spaces, a number is stored that corresponds to the echo intensity received from the point within the body corresponding to that storage position (Fig. 2.35). To image in gray scale (several shades of gray or brightness), it is necessary to have more than one layer of memory. In a four-bit (binary digit) memory, there are four "checkerboards" back to back so that each pixel has four bits associated with it (Fig. 2.36). Any pixel can store a number from 0 to 15 (16-shade system with a four-bit memory). Other examples are given in Table 2.3. Eight-bit memories are now common in sonography. Increasing the number of shades improves contrast resolution (the ability to distinguish echoes of slightly different intensity).

The procedure for storing the information required for the display of the two-dimensional, cross-sectional image for a digital scan converter is as follows: The beam is scanned through the patient in such a way that the ultrasound beam "cuts" through the tissue in a cross section. Echoes received from all points on this cross section are converted into numbers, which are stored at corresponding places in the

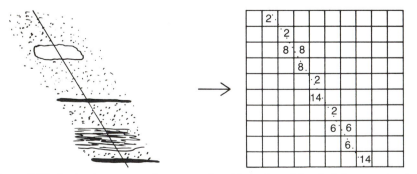

Figure 2.35. Anatomic cross section scanned and front view of the digital scan converter. Numbers are stored in the memory's elements, according to the intensity of the echoes received from corresponding anatomic locations.

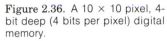

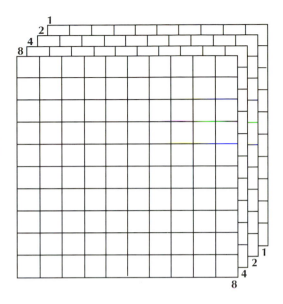

Figure 2.36. A 10 × 10 pixel, 4-bit deep (4 bits per pixel) digital memory.

digital memory. All the information necessary for displaying this cross-sectional image is then stored in memory. The information can then be taken out of memory and applied to a two-dimensional display in such a way that the numbers coming out of memory are displayed with corresponding brightnesses on the face of the tube (Fig. 2.37). Examples of such displays are shown in Figure 2.38.

The display device is a cathode ray tube. This tube generates a sharply focused beam of electrons that produces a bright spot on the phosphor-coated front face (screen) of the tube (Fig. 2.39). This spot can be moved across or up and down the face by applying voltages to deflection plates or electric currents to magnetic deflection coils. If the voltage or current is properly varied, the spot can be made to move across the face at constant speed. At the completion of this motion (i.e., when an image line is completed), the spot can be made to jump rapidly

Table 2–3

Characteristics of Digital Memories

Bits per Pixel	Lowest Number Stored	Highest Number Stored	Number of Shades
4	0	15	16
5	0	31	32
6	0	63	64
7	0	127	128
8	0	255	256

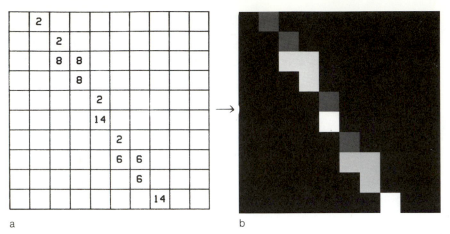

Figure 2.37. For the display of scanned anatomic structures, numbers are read out of pixel locations in digital memory (a) and applied to the display in such a way that brightness corresponds to the stored number (b).

back and down slightly to begin the next line. B-mode operation causes a brightening of the spot for each echo. The greater the echo intensity (the larger the number in memory) is, the brighter the spot.

Television monitors are often used as the display devices for ultrasound imaging instruments. A television monitor is a cathode ray tube in which the horizontal electron beam scanning format (described earlier) is used. The electron beam current is continually changed as the beam is scanned to provide varying brightness of the spot, thus providing gray-scale imaging capability. The television scanning format consists of a left-to-right and top-to-bottom scanning pattern, similar to the way in which this page of text is read. The resulting display consists of 525 horizontal display scan lines that produce one frame of a dynamic image (Fig. 2.40). This picture is updated (dynamic imaging) 30 times each second (real-time or dynamic imaging instruments must produce several cross-sectional images per second). This requires the use of mechanical or array real-time transducers (Section 2.2). External monitors connected to the ultrasound instrument use the television scan format described here. By comparison, some internal displays in instruments use more horizontal scan lines to improve resolution and higher frame rates for improved imaging of rapidly moving structures. In all cases, however, the images consist of horizontal scan lines on the display.

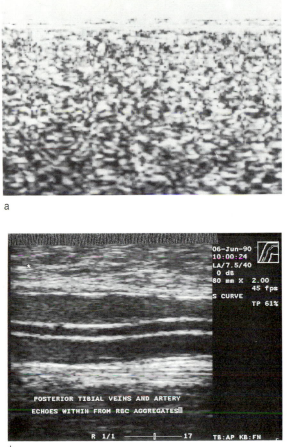

a

b

Figure 2.38. Display of pixels of various brightnesses representing various numbers in the corresponding memory locations. The display is magnified (zoom) here to make the square pixels easily seen. Normally, they are too small and numerous to be noticed individually. (a) Magnified image of tissue-equivalent phantom. (b) Magnified image of leg vessels.

Figure 2.39. A cathode ray tube (side view). The electron beam produces a bright spot where it strikes the phosphor-coated face of the tube. The set of horizontal deflection plates is not shown.

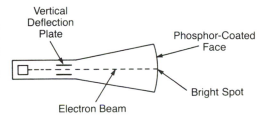

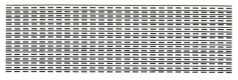

Figure 2.40. The television display format has 525 horizontal display scan lines, which are written out in one thirtieth of a second. One half of these (alternate solid lines) are written first, followed by the remaining (dashed) ones. Each of these sets of lines (solid and dashed on this illustration) makes up a "field." Two fields make a frame. Writing the frame in the format of two fields reduces flicker.

Each complete scan of the sound beam produces an image on the display that is called a frame. Each frame is made of scan lines (one for each time the transducer is pulsed). For each focus on each scan line in each frame, a pulse is required. More focuses or more scan lines per frame thus slow down the imaging process (lower frame rate). Deeper imaging requires more time per scan line, also lowering the frame rate. Temporal resolution (the ability to distinguish closely spaced events in time) improves with an increased frame rate.

> number of focuses ↑   frame rate ↓
> penetration ↑   frame rate ↓

2.4
Artifacts

In sonography, an artifact is anything not properly indicative of the structures imaged. It is caused by some characteristic of the imaging technique. Because some artifacts are useful, imaging can at times be better than direct viewing of the anatomy (if that were possible). This is because some ultrasound imaging artifacts, although errors from an anatomic imaging standpoint, give valuable information on the nature of objects or lesions that might not be apparent with other imaging methods or even direct viewing. In addition to helpful artifacts, there are several that hinder proper interpretation and diagnosis. These must be avoided or properly handled when encountered. Artifacts in ultrasound imaging occur as structures that are one of the following: not real; missing; improperly located; or of improper brightness, shape, or size.[1] Only a few of the recognized sonographic artifacts are discussed here.

With two or more reflectors in a sound path (one may be the transducer face), multiple reflections (reverberations) occur. These may be sufficiently strong to be detected by the instrument and to cause confusion on the display. The process by which they are produced is shown in Figure 2.41. This results in the placement on the image of reflectors that are not real. They are placed beyond the second real reflector at separation intervals equal to the separation between the first and second real reflectors (Fig. 2.42).

Refraction can cause a reflector to be positioned improperly on the display (Fig. 2.43). A common site for this occurrence is in abdominal scanning with the transducer over the rectus abdominis (Fig. 2.44).

In a mirror-image artifact, objects that are present on one side of a strong reflector are presented on the other side also (Fig. 2.45). This

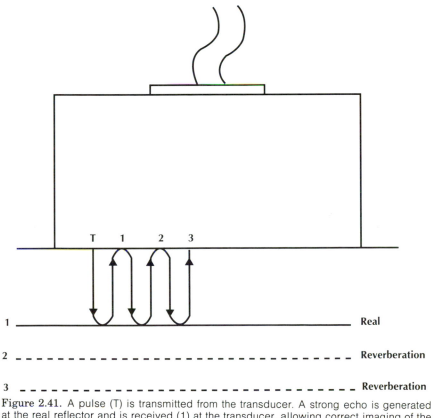

Figure 2.41. A pulse (T) is transmitted from the transducer. A strong echo is generated at the real reflector and is received (1) at the transducer, allowing correct imaging of the reflector. However, the echo is partially reflected by the transducer so that a second echo (2) is received and also a third (3). These later echoes appear deeper on the display where there are no reflectors.

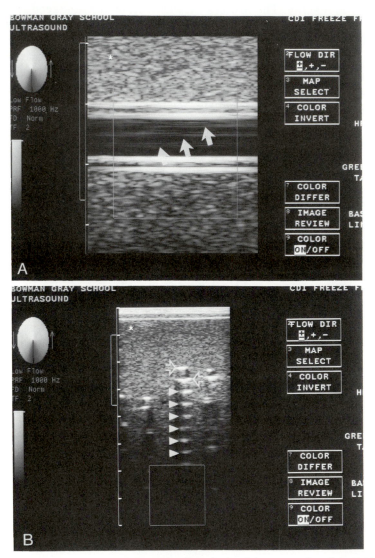

Figure 2.42. Reverberation. (A) Reverberations (arrows) from vessel wall appear within the lumen. (B) Transverse view of vessel. Vessel wall (open arrows) produces reverberations (arrowheads).

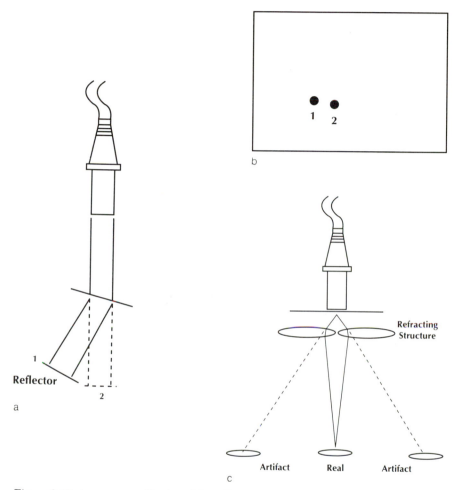

Figure 2.43. Improper positioning of the reflector on the display (b) because of refraction (a). The system places the reflector at position 2 because that is the direction from which the echo was received. The reflector is actually at position 1. (c) One real structure is imaged as two artifactual objects because of the refracting structure closer to the transducer. If unrefracted pulses can propagate to the real structure, a triple presentation (one correct and two artifactual) can result.

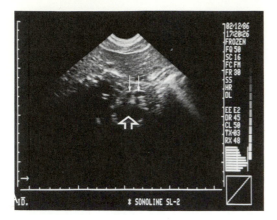

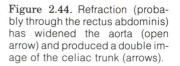

Figure 2.44. Refraction (probably through the rectus abdominis) has widened the aorta (open arrow) and produced a double image of the celiac trunk (arrows).

commonly occurs around the diaphragm, pleura, and vessel walls (Fig. 2.46). Examples in color-flow imaging are given in Section 7.2.

Shadowing is the reduction in an echo's amplitude from reflectors that lie behind a strongly reflecting or attenuating structure (Fig. 2.47). Enhancement is the increase in an echo's amplitude from reflectors

Figure 2.45. The mirror-image artifact occurs around strong reflectors (SR). The reflector that is located at position (1) is imaged at position (2) because that is the direction in which the transducer is pointing.

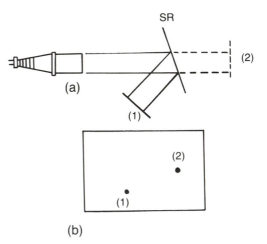

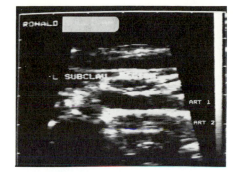

Figure 2.46. Subclavian artery (ART 1) and mirror image (ART 2).

that lie behind a weakly attenuating structure (Fig. 2.48). Shadowing and enhancement result in reflectors being placed on the image with amplitudes that are too low and too high, respectively. Shadowing and enhancement are useful artifacts for determining the nature of masses.

Interference from electronic equipment can add unwanted noise to the image (Fig. 2.49).

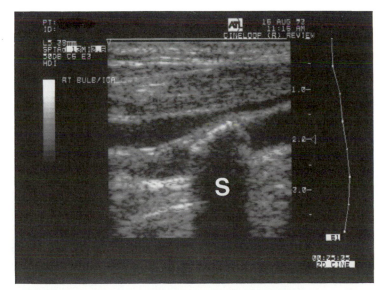

Figure 2.47. Shadowing (S) from a high-attenuation calcified plaque in the common carotid artery.

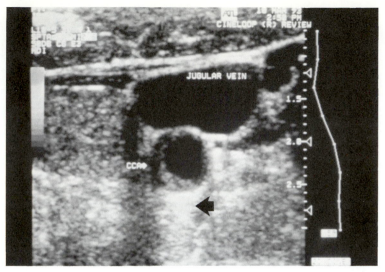

Figure 2.48. Enhancement (arrow) from the low attenuation of blood in the common carotid artery (CCA) and jugular vein in transverse view.

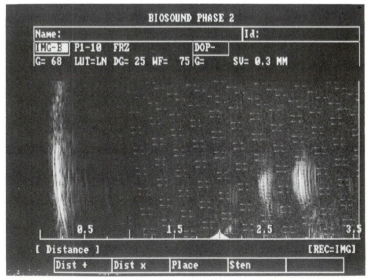

Figure 2.49. Interference (repeating white specks) from nearby electronic equipment.

2.5
Review

By sending short pulses of ultrasound into the body and using echoes received from tissue interfaces and within tissues to produce images of internal structures, ultrasound is used as a medical diagnostic tool. Ultrasound is a wave of traveling acoustic variables described by frequency, wavelength, propagation speed, amplitude, intensity, and attenuation. Diagnostic ultrasound commonly uses the frequency range of 2 to 10 MHz.

Pulsed ultrasound is used in sonography. It is described, in addition, by pulse repetition frequency and spatial pulse length.

For perpendicular incidence at boundaries, echoes are produced if media impedances are different. For oblique incidence, refraction occurs if media propagation speeds are different. Scattering occurs at rough boundaries and within heterogeneous media. The distance to reflectors is found from the round-trip travel time.

Transducers convert electric energy to ultrasound energy, and vice versa, by piezoelectricity. Axial resolution is equal to one half the pulse length, which can be reduced (improving resolution) by damping and increasing frequency. Lateral resolution is equal to the beam's diameter, which can be reduced (improving resolution) by focusing. Disk transducers produce sound beams with near and far zones. Focusing can be accomplished only in the near zone of the comparable unfocused transducer. Arrays can scan, steer, and shape (focus) beams electronically, permitting dynamic imaging. Dynamic imaging can also be accomplished with mechanically driven, single-element transducers or mirrors.

Pulse-echo systems use the amplitude, direction, and arrival time of echoes to produce images. Imaging systems consist of pulser, beam former, transducer, receiver, memory, and display. The pulser delivers the energizing voltages to the transducer, which responds by producing ultrasound pulses. Receivers amplify voltages that represent returning echoes and compensate for attenuation. Digital memories store gray-scale image information and permit their display on a television monitor. The number of bits per pixel in the digital memory determines the number of gray shades that can be displayed by the system. Dynamic imaging instruments display a rapid sequence of images (frames).

Display artifacts include reverberation, refraction, mirror image, shadowing, and enhancement.

The definitions of terms used in this chapter are listed below:

Absorption. Conversion of sound to heat.

Amplification. Increasing small voltages to larger ones.

Amplitude. Maximum variation of an acoustic variable or voltage.

Annular array. Array made up of ring-shaped elements arranged concentrically.

Array. Transducer array.

Attenuation. Decrease in amplitude and intensity as a wave travels through a medium.

Beam area. Cross-sectional area of a sound beam.

Beam former. The part of an instrument that accomplishes electronic beam scanning, steering, and focusing with arrays.

Cathode ray tube. A display device that produces an image by scanning an electron beam over a phosphor-coated screen.

Compensation. Equalizing received echo amplitude differences caused by attenuation.

Composite. Combination of piezoelectric ceramic with nonpiezoelectric polymer.

Continuous wave. A wave in which cycles repeat indefinitely. Not pulsed.

Contrast resolution. Ability of a gray-scale display to distinguish between echoes of slightly different amplitudes or intensities.

Convex array. Linear array with a curved (bowed out) shape.

Crystal. Element.

Cycle. Complete variation of an acoustic variable.

Damping. Material placed behind the rear face of a transducer element to reduce pulse duration. Also, the process of pulse duration reduction.

Depth gain compensation. Compensation.

Detail resolution. Ability to image fine detail and to distinguish closely spaced reflectors.

Duty factor. Fraction of time that pulsed ultrasound is on. Sometimes called duty cycle.

Echo. Reflection.

Element. A small piece of piezoelectric material in a transducer assembly.

Enhancement. Increase in echo amplitude from reflectors that lie behind a weakly attenuating structure.

Focus. To concentrate the sound beam into a smaller beam area than would exist otherwise.

Frame rate. Number of frames displayed per second.

Freeze frame. Constant image of the last frame entered into memory.

Frequency. Number of cycles per second.

Gain. Ratio of output to input electric power.

Gray scale. Continuous range of brightnesses between white and black.

Hertz. Unit of frequency, one cycle per second. Unit of pulse repetition frequency, one pulse per second.

Impedance (acoustic). Density multiplied by sound propagation speed.

Intensity. Power divided by area.

Kilohertz. One thousand hertz.

Linear array. Array made up of rectangular elements in a line.

Matching layer. Material placed in front of the front face of a transducer element to reduce the reflection at the transducer surface.

Megahertz. One million hertz.

Mirror image. In sonography, duplication of an object on the opposite side of a strong reflector.

Operating frequency. Preferred frequency of operation of a transducer.

Penetration. Imaging depth.

Phased array. An array that steers and focuses the beam electronically (with short time delays).

Piezoelectricity. Conversion of pressure to electric voltage.

Pixel. Picture element. The unit into which imaging and Doppler information is divided for storage and display in a digital instrument.

Postprocessing. Signal processing done after memory.

Preprocessing. Signal processing (gain, time gain compensation, etc.) done before memory.

Pressure. Force divided by area.

Propagation speed. Speed with which a wave moves through a medium.

Pulse. A brief excursion of a quantity from its normal value. A few cycles.

Pulse repetition frequency. Number of pulses per unit time. Sometimes called pulse repetition rate.

Refraction. Change of sound direction on passing from one medium to another.

Reverberation. Multiple reflections.

Scattering. Diffusion or redirection of sound in several directions on encountering a particle suspension or a rough surface.

Shadowing. Reduction in echo amplitude from reflectors that lie behind a strongly reflecting or attenuating structure.

Sound. Traveling wave of pressure and other acoustic variables.
Temporal resolution. Ability to distinguish closely spaced events in time. Improves with increased frame rate.
Time gain compensation. Compensation.
Transducer. Device that converts energy from one form to another.
Ultrasound. Sound of frequency greater than 20 kHz.
Wave. Traveling variation of wave variables.
Wavelength. Length of space over which a cycle occurs.

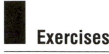

Exercises

2.1 The diagnostic ultrasound imaging method has two parts:

    a. Sending _____ of _____ into the body.

    b. Using _____ received from the tissues to produce an _____ of internal structures.

2.2 Ultrasound B scans are _____-_____ images of tissue cross sections.

2.3 The brightness of an echo, as presented on the display, represents its _____ .

2.4 A linear scan is made up of many _____ scan lines.

2.5 A sector scan is made up of many scan lines with a common _____ .

2.6 A linear scan has a _____ shape.

2.7 A sector scan is _____ _____ shaped.

2.8 Sonography is accomplished by using a _____-_____ technique. The information of importance in doing this is the _____ from which the echo origi-

nated and the _____ _____ of the echo.
From these, the echo _____ and _____
on the display are determined.

2.9 Which of the following is a characteristic of a medium through
which sound is propagating?

a. impedance
b. intensity
c. amplitude
d. frequency
e. period

2.10 Match the following:

_____ a. frequency
_____ b. period
_____ c. wavelength
_____ d. propagation speed
_____ e. amplitude

1. time per cycle
2. maximum variation per
   cycle
3. length per cycle
4. cycles per second
5. speed of a wave through a
   medium

2.11 If no refraction occurs as an oblique sound beam passes through
the boundary between two materials, the _____
_____ of the materials are known to be
_____ .

2.12 What must be known to calculate distance to a reflector?

a. attenuation, speed, density
b. attenuation, impedance
c. attenuation, absorption
d. travel time, speed
e. density, speed

2.13 With perpendicular incidence, if the impedances of two media are
the same, there will be no

a. inflation
b. reflection
c. refraction
d. calibration
e. both b and c

2.14 No reflection occurs with perpendicular incidence if the media _____ are equal.

2.15 Scattering occurs at smooth boundaries and within homogeneous media. True or false?

2.16 Match the following transducer assembly parts with their functions:

_____ **a.** cable	**1.** reduces reflection at
_____ **b.** damping material	transducer surface
_____ **c.** piezoelectric	**2.** converts voltage pulses to
element	sound pulses
_____ **d.** matching layer	**3.** reduces pulse duration
	4. conducts voltage pulses

2.17 Which of the following improve sound transmission from the transducer element into the tissue? (More than one correct answer.)

a. matching layer
b. Doppler effect
c. damping material
d. coupling medium
e. refraction

2.18 Lateral resolution is improved by

a. damping
b. pulsing
c. focusing
d. reflecting
e. absorbing

2.19 For a focused transducer, the best lateral resolution (minimum beam diameter) is found in the _____ region.

2.20 Beam diameter may be reduced in the near zone by focusing. True or false?

2.21 Beam diameter may be reduced in the far zone by focusing. True or false?

2.22 The axial resolution of a transducer can be improved most by

    a. increasing the damping
    b. increasing the diameter
    c. decreasing the damping
    d. decreasing the frequency
    e. decreasing the diameter
    f. attaching a dopple

2.23 The principle on which ultrasound transducers operate is the

    a. Doppler effect
    b. acousto-optic effect
    c. acoustoelectric effect
    d. cause and effect
    e. piezoelectric effect

2.24 The lower and upper limits of the frequency range that are useful in diagnostic ultrasound are determined by _____ and _____ requirements, respectively.

2.25 The range of frequencies useful for most diagnostic ultrasound applications is _____ to _____ MHz.

2.26 The compensation (time or depth gain compensation) control

    a. compensates for machine instability in the warm-up time
    b. compensates for attenuation
    c. compensates for transducer aging and the ambient light in the examining area
    d. decreases the patient's examination time

2.27 A gray-scale display shows

    a. gray color on a white background
    b. reflections with one brightness level
    c. a white color on a gray background
    d. a range of echo amplitudes

2.28 A digital scan converter is a _____ .

    a. compressor
    b. receiver
    c. display
    d. computer memory
    e. none of the above

2.29 Television monitors produce _____ frames per second with _____ lines in each.

    a. 30, 60
    b. 30, 525
    c. 60, 512
    d. 512, 512
    e. 60, 120

2.30 In a digital instrument, echo intensity is represented by

    a. positive charge distribution
    b. a number stored in memory
    c. electron density of the scan converter writing beam
    d. a and c
    e. all of the above

2.31 If there were no attenuation in tissue, _____ would not be needed.

    a. rejection
    b. compression
    c. demodulation
    d. compensation

2.32 Reflection imaging includes ultrasound generation, propagation, and reflection in tissues and the reception of returning _____ .

2.33 Sonographic instruments determine three things: the _____ , _____ , and arrival _____ _____ of echoes that occur in tissues.

2.34 Imaging systems produce a visual _____ from the electric _____ received from the transducer.

2.35 The transducer is connected to the memory through the _____ .

2.36 The transducer receives voltages from the _____ in pulse-echo systems.

2.37 The _____ receives voltages from the transducer.

2.38 Increasing gain generally produces the same effect as

  a. decreasing attenuation
  b. increasing attenuation
  c. increasing compression
  d. increasing rectification
  e. both b and c

2.39 Voltage pulses occur at the output of the

  a. pulser
  b. transducer
  c. receiver
  d. display
  e. both a and b
  f. both c and e

2.40 Ultrasound pulses from the pulser are applied to the transducer through the

  a. pulser
  b. beam former
  c. transducer
  d. receiver
  e. display

2.41 Gain and attenuation are usually given in

  a. dB
  b. dB/cm
  c. cm
  d. cm/3 dB
  e. none of the above

2.42 Compensation (swept gain) makes up for the fact that echoes from deeper reflectors arrive at the tranducer with greater amplitude. True or false?

2.43 A real-time B-mode display may be produced by rapid _____ transducer scanning or by _____ scanning of a transducer array.

2.44 Each complete scan of the sound beam produces an image on the display that is called a _____ .

2.45 The number of lines in each frame is equal to the number of times the transducer is _____ while the frame (single focus) is produced (while the sound beam is scanned).

2.46 Real-time imaging permits imaging of the motion of moving structures but cannot present static (freeze-frame) images. True or false?

2.47 To correct for attenuation, the time gain compensation must (increase or decrease) _____ the amplification (gain) for increasing depth.

2.48 If a higher frequency is used, resolution is (improved or worsened), imaging depth (increases or decreases), and the time gain compensation slope must be (increased or decreased)?

2.49 Memory is necessary to have _____ _____ capability.

2.50 If an instrument produces 1000 pulses per second and 20 frames per second, how many scan lines make up each frame?

2.51 Which of the following can cause improper location of objects on a display? (More than one correct answer.)

  a. shadowing
  b. enhancement
  c. reverberation
  d. mirror image
  e. refraction

2.52 Match these artifact causes with their results:

  a. reverberation   **1.** unreal structure displayed
  b. shadowing   **2.** structure displayed with
  c. enhancement   improper brightness

2.53 Reverberation results in added reflectors being imaged with equal _____ .

2.54 In reverberation, subsequent reflections are _____ than previous ones.

2.55 Enhancement is caused by a

    a. strongly reflecting structure
    b. weakly attenuating structure
    c. strongly attenuating structure
    d. refracting boundary
    e. propagation speed error

2.56 Shadowing results in decreased echo amplitudes. True or false?

2.57 Which artifact should be suspected if observing twin blood vessels in transverse section when scanning through the rectus abdominis? _____

3 Hemodynamics

The word hemodynamics is derived from two Greek words meaning blood and power. The word, thus, refers to the forces and motion of blood flow and the science concerned with the study of blood circulation. An associated word is rheology, the science dealing with the deformation and flow of matter. It comes from the Greek word rhein, meaning to flow.

Doppler ultrasound is used primarily for detecting and evaluating blood flow in the body. It is, therefore, important to understand the principles of this flow to use this diagnostic tool effectively.

The circulatory system consists of the heart, arteries, arterioles, capillaries, venules, and veins, containing about 5 L of blood. Flow in the heart, arteries, and veins can be detected with Doppler ultrasound. The capillaries are the smallest (a few micrometers in diameter) vessels. There are approximately 1 billion of them in the human body. It is across their walls that the exchange of gases and nutrients takes place with the body's cells. We consider here the characteristics of fluids, such as blood, and their behavior when they flow through tubes, such as blood vessels, in steady and pulsatile flow forms.[9–11]

In this chapter, we address the following questions. What is a fluid? What are pressure and resistance, and how do they affect flow? What are plug, laminar, parabolic, disturbed, turbulent, and pulsatile flows? How does a stenosis affect flow? The following terms are discussed in this chapter:

acceleration	critical Reynolds number
Bernoulli effect	density
bruit	disturbed flow
compliance	eddies

energy   pressure
energy, kinetic   resistance (flow)
energy, potential   Reynolds number
flow   speed
flow rate   stenosis
flow speed   stoke
force   streamline
heat   turbulence
inertia   turbulent flow
laminar flow   velocity
mass   viscosity
parabolic flow   viscosity, kinematic
plug flow   volume flow rate
poise   vortices
Poiseuille's law

3.1
Fluids

Matter is generally classified into three categories: gas, liquid, and solid. Gases and liquids are fluids, i.e., substances that flow and conform to the shape of their containers. To flow is to move in a stream, continually changing position and, possibly, direction. Rivers flow downstream. Water flows through a garden hose. Air flows through a fan. Blood flows through the heart, arteries, capillaries, and veins.

Blood is a liquid (therefore a fluid), the function of which is to supply nutrients and oxygen to the cells of the body and remove their waste products. Blood is a body tissue, i.e., a group of similar cells specialized to perform certain functions. It is comprised of plasma, erythrocytes, leukocytes, and platelets. Plasma is primarily water (approximately 90 percent) and proteins. About 40 percent of the blood's volume is cells. This percentage is called the hematocrit. Erythrocytes (red cells) are the dominant (about 99 percent) cells in the circulation. They contain hemoglobin, which is responsible for the transport of oxygen. Leukocytes (white cells) are larger than erythrocytes but less numerous in the blood. Their chief function is to protect the body against disease organisms. Platelets are smaller than erythrocytes and are important in the process of blood clotting.

Two important characteristics of fluids are density and viscosity. The density of a fluid is its mass per unit volume, commonly given in grams per milliliter (g/mL). Mass is a measure of an object's resistance to acceleration. This resistance is called inertia. The greater the mass

Table 3–1	
Blood Properties	
Density	1.05 g/mL
Viscosity	0.035 poise
Kinematic viscosity	0.033 stoke
Sound speed	1.57 mm/μs
Impedance	1.62 Mrayl
Attenuation	0.21 dB/cm·MHz

is, the greater the inertia is. If two different masses are to be accelerated at the same rate, more force must be applied to the greater mass. The density of blood (1.05 g/mL) is slightly greater than that for water (1 g/mL) because of the presence of proteins and cells. Viscosity is the resistance to flow offered by a fluid in motion. It is given in units of poise (honoring Poiseuille) or kg/m·s. One poise is 1 g/cm·s or 0.1 kg/m·s. Water has a relatively low viscosity (0.0069 poise at 37°C); that of molasses is high. The viscosity of blood plasma is about 50 percent greater than that of water. The viscosity of normal blood is 0.035 poise at 37°C, approximately five times that of water. Blood viscosity can vary from about 0.02 (with anemia) to about 0.10 poise (with polycythemia). It also varies with flow speed. The viscosity divided by the density is a sometimes useful quantity that is given the name kinematic viscosity. For blood, its value is about 0.033 stoke. One stoke is 1 cm^2/s or 0.0001 m^2/s. Several properties of blood are listed in Table 3.1.

3.2
Steady Flow

Pressure is the driving force behind fluid flow. Pressure is the force per unit area. It is equally distributed throughout a static fluid and exerts its force in all directions (Fig. 3.1). A pressure *difference* is required for flow to occur. Equal pressures applied at both ends of a liquid-filled tube result in no flow. If the pressure is greater at one end than it is at the other, the liquid flows from the higher pressure end to the lower pressure end. This pressure difference can be generated by a pump (for example, the heart in the circulatory system). Flow can also be produced by the force of gravity, that is, by raising one end of a tube above the other. (Because this is the situation in lower extremity veins when standing, these vessels have valves in them to prevent reverse flow.) The greater the pressure difference is, the greater the flow rate is. This pressure difference is sometimes called a pressure gradient, although strictly, a pressure gradient is the pressure differ-

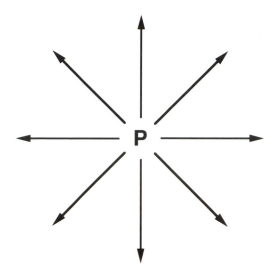

Figure 3.1. Pressure (P) is uniformly distributed throughout a static fluid and exerts its force in all directions.

ence divided by the distance between the two pressure locations. Gradient comes from grade and refers to the upward or downward sloping of something. As the pressure drops from one end of the tube to the other, this decrease can be thought of as a slope (i.e., the pressure difference divided by the distance over which the pressure drop occurs, Fig. 3.2). In this section, we consider a constant driving pressure that produces steady flow (unchanging with time). The driving pressure produced by the heart varies with time. This is considered in Section 3.4.

Figure 3.2. The pressure gradient or slope is the pressure difference $(P_1 - P_2)$ divided by the separation (L) between the two pressure locations.

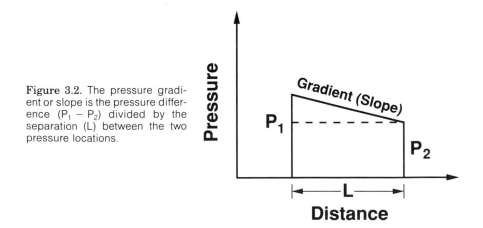

The flow rate in a long, straight tube is determined not only by the pressure difference but also by the resistance to flow.

$$\text{volume flow rate (mL/s)} = \frac{\text{pressure difference (dyne/cm}^2)}{\text{flow resistance (g/cm}^4\cdot\text{s)}}$$

$$Q = \frac{\Delta P}{R}$$

pressure difference ↑ volume flow rate ↑
flow resistance ↑ volume flow rate ↓

Volume flow rate is the volume of blood passing a point in a unit of time, usually given in milliliters (mL)* per minute or per second. The total adult blood flow (cardiac output) is about 5000 mL/min (i.e., the total blood volume [5 L] circulates in about 1 minute). The flow resistance in a long, straight tube depends on the fluid's viscosity and the tube's length and radius, as follows:

$$\text{flow resistance} = \frac{8 \times \text{length} \times \text{viscosity}}{\pi \times \text{radius}^4} \qquad R = \frac{8L\nu}{\pi r^4}$$

length ↑ resistance ↑
radius ↑ resistance ↓
viscosity ↑ resistance ↑

As expected, an increase in viscosity or tube length increases the resistance and an increase in the size (radius or diameter) of the tube decreases the resistance. The latter effect is particularly strong, with the resistance depending on the radius to the fourth power. Thus, doubling the radius of a tube decreases its resistance to one sixteenth of the original value. By experience, we know that a longer or smaller-diameter garden hose reduces water flow, and we could guess that, if we tried to force molasses through the hose, we would not get nearly the flow rate we get with water.

---

*In the International System of Units, L and l are recognized as alternative symbols for the volume unit, liter. In the United States, to avoid confusion with the numeral 1, only L is recommended.

Substituting the equation for flow resistance into the first equation and using tube diameter rather than the radius yields Poiseuille's law:

$$\text{volume flow rate} = \frac{\text{pressure difference} \times \pi \times \text{diameter}^4}{128 \times \text{length} \times \text{viscosity}}$$

$$Q = \frac{\Delta P \pi d^4}{128 L \nu}$$

pressure difference ↑ flow rate ↑
diameter ↑ flow rate ↑
length ↑ flow rate ↓
viscosity ↑ flow rate ↓

The units for this equation are dynes per centimeter squared for pressure, centimeters for diameter and length, poise for viscosity, and milliliters per second for volume flow rate. Note the appearance of the pressure gradient (pressure difference divided by length) in this equation. The resistance of the arterioles accounts for about one half of the total resistance in the systemic circulation.[9] Their muscular walls can constrict or relax, producing dramatic changes in their flow resistance. They can thus control blood flow to specific tissues and organs in response to their needs.

Steady flow can be divided into five spatial categories: plug, laminar, parabolic, disturbed, and turbulent. At the entrance to a tube, the speed of the fluid is essentially constant across the tube (Fig. 3.3). This is called plug flow. After some distance, which depends on the tube's diameter, the average flow speed, and the viscosity, laminar flow is achieved (Fig. 3.3). Laminar flow is a flow condition in which stream-

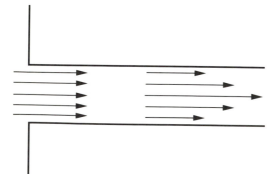

Figure 3.3. At the entrance to a tube or vessel, plug flow exists. After some distance, laminar flow is achieved.

lines (describing fluid particle motion) are smooth and parallel to each other. There is maximum flow speed at the center of the tube and minimum or zero flow at the tube walls. A decreasing profile of flow speeds from the center to the wall exists. Successive cylindric layers (laminae) of fluid slide on each other with relative motion. The pressure difference at the ends of the tube overcomes the viscous resistance to this relative motion, maintaining the laminar flow through the tube. For steady flow in a long straight tube, a parabolic flow profile results (Fig. 3.4). This means that the pattern of varying flow speeds across the tube is in the shape of a parabola (dashed line in Fig. 3.4). For parabolic flow, the average flow speed across the vessel is equal to one half the maximum flow speed (at the center).

Nearly plug flow is found in larger vessels (e.g., the aorta) (Fig. 3.5a). Laminar flow is found in smaller vessels (e.g., the ovarian artery) (Fig. 3.5b). An intermediate-flow character is found in intermediate-sized vessels, such as the common carotid artery. Even helical flow is likely to be present in vessels.[12–14]

Disturbed flow occurs when the parallel streamlines that describe the flow (Fig. 3.3) are disturbed (Fig. 3.6). This occurs, for example, in

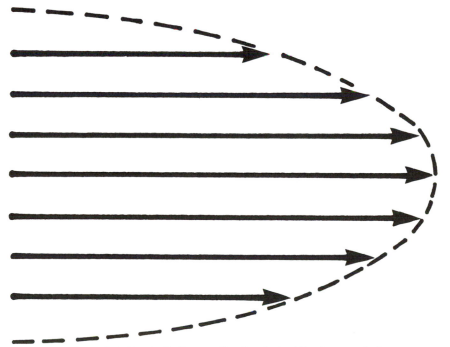

Figure 3.4. Parabolic flow profile. The dashed line is a parabola.

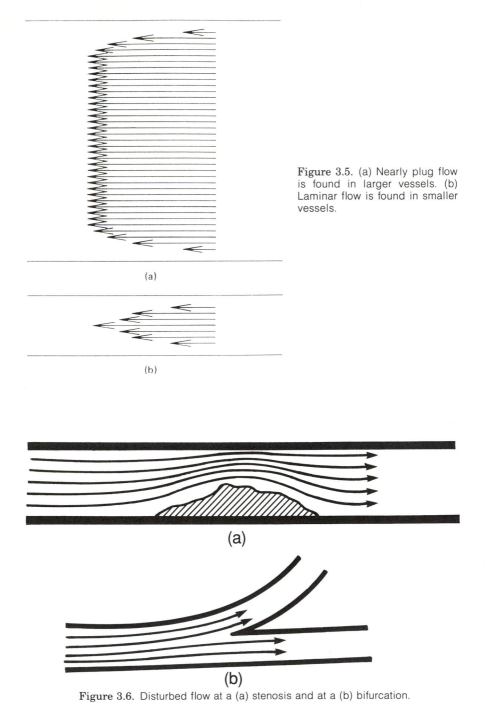

(a)

(b)

Figure 3.5. (a) Nearly plug flow is found in larger vessels. (b) Laminar flow is found in smaller vessels.

(a)

(b)

Figure 3.6. Disturbed flow at a (a) stenosis and at a (b) bifurcation.

the region of stenoses (Section 3.3) or at a bifurcation (splitting of a vessel into two). In disturbed flow, particles of fluid still flow in the forward direction. Parabolic and disturbed flows are forms of laminar flow.

In the final category, turbulent flow, the flow pattern becomes random and chaotic, with particles flowing in all directions, even in circles called eddy currents, yet maintaining a net forward flow (Fig. 3.7). As flow speed increases in a tube, turbulent flow eventually results (Fig. 3.7a). The onset of turbulent flow is predicted by the Reynolds number, which is unitless.

$$\text{Reynolds number} = \frac{\text{average flow speed} \times \text{tube diameter} \times \text{density}}{\text{viscosity}}$$

$$\text{Re} = \frac{V_a \times d \times \rho}{\nu}$$

flow speed $\uparrow$ Reynolds number $\uparrow$
diameter $\uparrow$ Reynolds number $\uparrow$
density $\uparrow$ Reynolds number $\uparrow$
viscosity $\uparrow$ Reynolds number $\downarrow$

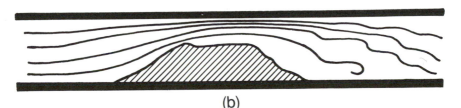

(a)

(b)

Figure 3.7. Turbulent flow in a vessel resulting from (a) high flow speed or (b) an obstruction.

If the Reynolds number exceeds about 2000 to 2500 (depending on the tube's geometry), flow becomes turbulent. This is called the critical Reynolds number. With the exception of the heart and proximal aorta, turbulent flow is not likely in normal human circulation. Turbulent flow can more easily occur beyond an obstruction (Fig. 3.7b), such as a stenosis.

3.3
Stenoses

A narrowing of the lumen of a tube or vessel (stenosis) produces disturbed (Fig. 3.6a) and, possibly, turbulent flow (Fig. 3.7b). The average flow speed in the stenosis must be greater than it is proximal and distal to it so that the volume flow rate is constant throughout the tube.

Examples of increased flow speed at a stenosis and turbulence beyond it are given in Chapter 5. The volume flow rate must be constant for the three regions: proximal to, at, and distal to the stenosis. This is because fluid is neither created nor destroyed as it flows through the tube. This is called the continuity rule. The volume flow rate is equal to the average flow speed multiplied by the cross-sectional area of the flow (tube). Therefore, if the stenosis has an area one half that of the proximal and distal vessel, the average flow speed within the stenosis must be double that proximal and distal to it. An analogy to this is traffic flow on a multilane highway (Fig. 3.8). To maintain volume flow rate (number of vehicles past a point per unit time), the vehicles must travel faster in the narrow region. If a stenosis has a diameter one half that adjacent to it, the area at the stenosis is one fourth that adjacent to it, and the average flow speed in the stenosis must quadruple.

Poiseuille's law converted to an average flow speed rather than a volume flow rate is:

$$\text{average flow speed} = \frac{\text{pressure difference} \times \text{radius}^2}{8 \times \text{length} \times \text{viscosity}}$$

$$v_a = \frac{\Delta P r^2}{8 L \nu}$$

For parabolic flow, the maximum flow speed (at vessel center) is twice the average, i.e., 8 is replaced with 4 in this equation. This form of the pressure-flow relationship is particularly useful because Doppler

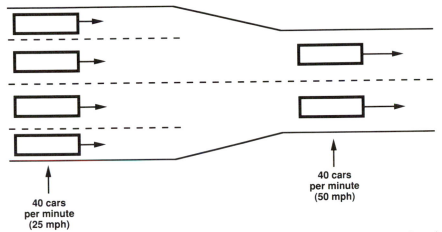

Figure 3.8. Highway traffic flow analogy to fluid volume flow. In the four-lane portion of the highway, 40 cars pass by each minute at a speed of 25 miles per hour. In the two-lane region, to maintain the (volume) flow rate of 40 cars per minute, a speed of 50 miles per hour is required. In this case, the speed times the number of lanes must be constant (100 lane-miles/hour). This is analogous to fluid flow in a tube in which the cross-sectional area times the flow speed must be constant.

shift (Section 4.1) is proportional to flow speed (Section 4.2) not volume flow rate (the volume flow rate must be calculated from the flow speed measurements). We see that flow speed (and, therefore, Doppler shift) increases with tube radius (or diameter) squared. In summary, volume flow rate depends on the radius to the fourth power; flow speed depends on the radius squared.

It is sometimes puzzling to students that Poiseuille's law and the continuity rule for a stenosis (at the beginning of this section) seem contradictory. That is, one says that flow speed is less with smaller diameters (Poiseuille's law), and the other states that flow speed is greater with smaller diameters (continuity rule). How can this be so? The radius in Poiseuille's law is for the entire tube or vessel. The radius in the continuity rule is for a short portion of a vessel (the stenosis). If the radius of the entire vessel is reduced (as in vasoconstriction, the flow speed *is* reduced. If the radius of only a short segment of a vessel is reduced (stenosis), the flow speed in the vessel is unaffected, except at the stenosis, where it is increased. This is because the stenosis has little effect on the flow resistance of the entire vessel if the length of the stenosis is small compared with the vessel's length and if the lumen in the stenosis is not too small (does not approach occlusion). Figure 3.9 shows the situation for a stenosis, indicating that the overall flow resistance for the vessel is the sum of the resistances of the three parts

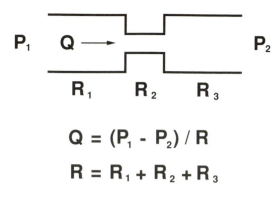

P_1 $Q \longrightarrow$ P_2

R_1 R_2 R_3

$$Q = (P_1 - P_2) / R$$

$$R = R_1 + R_2 + R_3$$

Figure 3.9. The overall flow resistance (R) for a vessel with a stenosis is equal to the sum of the resistances of the three parts (proximal [R_1], stenosis [R_2], and distal [R_3]. The volume flow rate (Q) is equal to the pressure difference at the ends of the vessel divided by the total resistance.

(proximal, stenosis, and distal). If the length of segment two (stenosis) is not too large and its radius is not too small, there is a negligible effect on the overall resistance and, therefore on the proximal and distal flow. However, the flow speed must increase in the stenosis to maintain the continuity of volume flow. These dependencies[15] of volume flow rate and flow speed at the stenosis with increasing stenosis are seen in Figure 3.10.

The maximum normal flow speed in the circulation is about 100 cm/s. However, in stenotic regions, flow speeds can reach several meters per second.

At the stenosis, the pressure is less than it is proximal and distal to it (Fig. 3.11). This is necessary for the fluid to accelerate into the

Figure 3.10. As the diameter of the stenosis is reduced (tighter stenosis), volume flow rate (Q) is unaffected initially because the stenosis does not contribute substantially to the total vessel resistance. As the diameter continues to increase, the vessel's resistance increases, reducing the volume flow rate (eventually to zero at occlusion). As the stenotic diameter decreases, the flow speed increases (because of the flow continuity requirement), reaches a maximum, and then decreases to zero as the increasing flow resistance effect dominates. (From Spencer MP, Reid JM: Quantitation of carotid stenosis with continuous wave (CW) Doppler ultrasound. Stroke *10*:326–330, 1979. Reprinted with permission. Stroke, Copyright 1979 American Heart Association.)

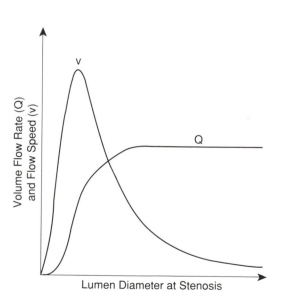

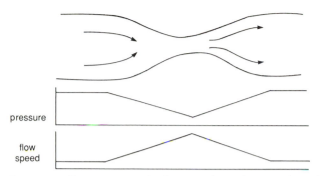

Figure 3.11. To maintain flow continuity, the flow speed must increase through a stenosis. In conjunction with this, the pressure drops (the Bernoulli effect) in the stenosis. (From Kremkau FW: Fluid flow II. J Vasc Technol *17*:153–154, 1993. Reprinted with permission.)

stenosis and decelerate out of it and also to maintain energy balance (the pressure energy is converted to kinetic [flow] energy on entry and then vice versa on exit). This decreased pressure in regions of high flow speed is known as the Bernoulli effect and is described by Bernoulli's equation, which is a description of the constant energy of fluid flow through a stenosis, ignoring viscous losses. As kinetic flow energy increases, the pressure's potential energy decreases. The decrease in pressure that results from the increasing flow speed at the stenosis can be found from a modified form of Bernoulli's equation.

$$\text{presure drop} = \text{¹/₂} \times \text{density} \times (\text{flow speed})^2$$
$$\Delta P = \text{¹/₂} \times \rho \times v^2$$

flow speed ↑ pressure drop ↑

In this equation, the flow speed proximal to the stenosis is assumed to be small enough to be ignored.

The disturbed flow pattern into and out of the stenosis and the increased flow speed within it can cause the onset of turbulent flow. Sounds produced by turbulence (which can be heard with a stethoscope) are called bruits. Ultimate stenosis is called an occlusion. In this case, the vessel is blocked, and there is no flow. Using the garden hose analogy again, we can compress the hose (not near the nozzle) and see little effect on the flow at the nozzle until the hose is compressed to near occlusion (at which point turbulence may occur, and a "bruit" can be felt at the surface of the hose).

Turbulence beyond a significant stenosis results in a distal pressure drop as a result of the loss of energy (associated with pressure or flow) to heat. The result is a drop in the volume flow rate. Doppler ultrasound is good at detecting turbulence. Spectral broadening usually indicates disturbed and turbulent flow. This is discussed in Chapter 5.

For calculating pressure drop across a stenotic heart valve, the following form of the previous equation for the pressure drop is used in Doppler echocardiography:

$$\boxed{P_1 - P_2 = 4\,v_2{}^2}$$

where v_2 is the flow speed in meters per second in the jet. $P_1 - P_2$ in millimeters of mercury is the pressure drop across the valve.

3.4
Pulsatile Flow

Previously, in this chapter, we considered steady flow in which pressures, flow speeds, and flow patterns did not change with time. This is generally the situation on the venous side of the circulatory system, although cardiac pulsations and respiratory cycles can influence venous flow somewhat (e.g., in the inferior vena cava). However, in the arterial circulation, flow is pulsatile, directly experiencing the effects of the beating heart. Superimposed on the net (constant) flow are the pulsatile variations of increasing and decreasing pressure and flow speed. For steady flow, as seen in Section 3.2, the volume flow rate is simply related to the pressure difference and flow resistance. With pulsatile flow, the relationship between the varying pressure and flow rate depends on the flow impedance, which includes the resistance formerly considered and, in addition, the inertia of the fluid as it accelerates and decelerates and the compliance (expansion and contraction) of the nonrigid vessel walls. The mathematic analysis is complicated and is not considered here. Two dominant characteristics of interest in this type of flow are the windkessel effect and flow reversal. When the pressure pulse forces a fluid into a compliant vessel, such as the aorta, it expands, and the volume increases within it. (This is why you can feel your "pulse" on your wrist or neck.) Later in the cycle, when the driving pressure is reduced, the compliant vessel can contract, producing extended flow later in the pressure cycle. This is known as the windkessel effect. In the aorta, it results in continued flow in the forward direction because the aortic valve prevents flow back into the

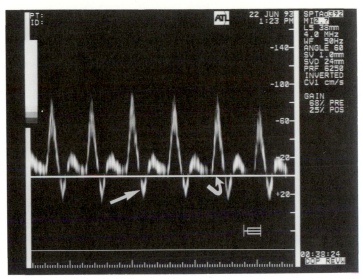

Figure 3.12. Flow reversal (arrow) below the baseline (curved arrow) is seen in the superficial femoral artery in diastole.

heart. In the distal circulation, the expansion of the distensible vessels results in the reversal of flow in diastole as the pressure decreases and the distended vessels contract. Because there are not valves to prevent reverse flow here, flow reversal is observed (Fig. 3.12). The results, therefore, of pulsatile flow in compliant vessels include added forward flow in diastole and flow reversal in diastole, depending on their locations within the arterial circulation. As discussed further in Chapter 5, arterial diastolic flow (absence, presence, direction, and quantity) reveals much concerning the state of downstream arterioles in which flow cannot be directly measured with ultrasound.

3.5
Review

Fluids (gases and liquids) are substances that flow. Blood is a liquid that flows through the vascular system under the influence of pulsatile pressure provided by the beating heart. Volume flow rate is proportional to the pressure difference at the ends of a tube and inversely proportional to the flow resistance. The flow resistance increases with viscosity and the tube's length and decreases (strongly) with an increasing tubular diameter. Seven (two temporal and five spatial) flow classifications include steady, pulsatile, plug, laminar, parabolic, disturbed, and turbulent. In a stenosis, flow speeds up, pressure drops (Bernoulli effect), and flow is disturbed. If the flow speed exceeds a critical value, as described by the Reynolds number, the onset of turbulence occurs. Pulsatile flow is common in the arterial circulation. Diastolic flow and/ or flow reversal occur in some locations within the arterial system. The fluid's inertia and the vessel's compliance are characteristics that are important in determining flow with pulsatile driving pressure.

Definitions of terms discussed in this chapter are listed as follows:

Bernoulli effect. Pressure reduction in a region of high flow speed.
Bruit. Audible sounds (using a stethoscope) originating in vessels with turbulent flow.
Compliance. Distensibility. Nonrigid stretchability of vessels.
Critical Reynolds number. Reynolds number above which turbulence occurs.
Density. Mass divided by volume.
Disturbed flow. Flow that cannot be described by straight, parallel streamlines.
Eddies. See vortices.
Energy. Ability to do work.
Energy, kinetic. Energy of motion.
Energy, potential. Energy of position or state.
Flow. To move in a stream. Volume flow rate.
Flow speed. Rate of motion of a portion of a flowing fluid.
Force. That which changes the state of rest or motion of an object.
Heat. Energy resulting from thermal molecular motion.
Inertia. Resistance to acceleration.
Laminar flow. Flow in which fluid layers slide over each other in a smooth, orderly manner, with no mixing between layers.
Mass. Measurement of an object's resistance to acceleration.
Parabolic flow. Laminar flow with a profile in the shape of a parabola.
Plug flow. Flow with all fluid portions traveling with nearly the same flow speed and direction.
Poise. Unit of viscosity.
Poiseuille's law. The mathemathic description of the dependence of flow rate on pressure, the vessel's length and radius, and fluid viscosity.
Pressure. Force divided by area.
Resistance (flow). Pressure difference divided by volume flow rate for steady flow.
Reynolds number. A number that depends on flow speed and viscosity and predicts the onset of turbulence.

Speed. Displacement divided by time over which displacement occurs.

Stenosis. Narrowing of a vessel.

Stoke. Unit of kinematic viscosity.

Streamline. A line representing the path of motion of a particle of fluid.

Turbulence. Random, chaotic, multidirectional flow of a fluid with mixing between layers. Not laminar.

Turbulent flow. See turbulence.

Velocity. Speed with direction of motion specified.

Viscosity. Resistance of a fluid to flow.

Viscosity, kinematic. Viscosity divided by density.

Volume flow rate. Volume of fluid passing a point per unit time (in seconds or minutes).

Vortices. Regions of circular flow patterns present in turbulence.

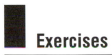

Exercises

3.1 Which of the following are parts of the circulatory system (more than one correct answer)?

a. heart
b. cerebral ventricle
c. artery
d. arterial
e. capillary
f. bile duct
g. venule
h. vein

3.2 The _____ are the tiniest vessels in the circulatory system.

3.3 Doppler ultrasound can measure flow in (more than one correct answer).

a. heart
b. arteries
c. arterioles
d. capillaries
e. venules
f. veins

3.4 Which of the following are fluids?

   a. gas
   b. liquid
   c. solid
   d. a and b
   e. a, b, and c

3.5 Which of the following do (does) not flow?

   a. gas
   b. liquid
   c. solid
   d. a and b
   e. a, b, and c

3.6 To flow is to move in a _____ .

3.7 Blood is made up of _____ , _____ , leukocytes, and platelets. Plasma is primarily _____ .

3.8 A normal hematocrit is about _____ percent.

   a. 10
   b. 20
   c. 30
   d. 40
   e. 50

3.9 Which are the dominant cells in blood?

   a. erythrocytes
   b. lymphocytes
   c. monocytes
   d. leukocytes
   e. platelets

3.10 The mass per unit volume of a fluid is called its

   a. resistance
   b. viscosity
   c. kinematic viscosity
   d. impedance
   e. density

3.11 The characteristic of a fluid that offers resistance to flow is called

    a. resistance
    b. viscosity
    c. kinematic viscosity
    d. impedance
    e. density

3.12 Viscosity divided by density is called

    a. resistance
    b. viscosity
    c. kinematic viscosity
    d. impedance
    e. density

3.13 Poise is a unit of _____ .

3.14 Stoke is a unit of _____ .

3.15 g/mL is a unit of _____ .

3.16 Give the normal values for blood of the following:

    a. density _____
    b. viscosity _____
    c. kinematic viscosity _____

3.17 Pressure is _____ per unit area.

3.18 Pressure is

    a. nondirectional
    b. unidirectional
    c. omnidirectional
    d. all of the above
    e. none of the above

3.19 Flow is a response to pressure _____ or _____ .

3.20 If the pressure is greater at one end of a liquid-filled tube or vessel than it is at the other, the liquid flows from the _____ pressure end to the _____ pressure end.

    a. higher, lower
    b. lower, higher

    c. depends on the liquid
    d. all of the above
    e. none of the above

3.21 A pressure difference can be generated by a _____ .

3.22 Pressure gradient is pressure _____ divided by _____ between the two pressure locations.

3.23 The volume flow rate in a tube is determined by _____ difference and _____ .

3.24 If the following is increased, flow increases.

    a. pressure difference
    b. pressure gradient
    c. resistance
    d. a and b
    e. all of the above

3.25 As flow resistance increases, the volume flow rate _____ .

3.26 If a pressure difference is doubled, the volume flow rate is

    a. unchanged
    b. quartered
    c. halved
    d. doubled
    e. quadrupled

3.27 If flow resistance is doubled, the volume flow rate is

    a. unchanged
    b. quartered
    c. halved
    d. doubled
    e. quadrupled

3.28 Tubes that carry blood in the circulatory system are called _____ .

3.29 The largest vessels are
    a. arteries
    b. veins

   c. arterioles and venules
   d. capillaries
   e. a and b

3.30 The smallest vessels are

   a. arteries
   b. veins
   c. arterioles and venules
   d. capillaries
   e. a and b

3.31 Flow resistance in a vessel depends on

   a. vessel length
   b. vessel radius
   c. blood viscosity
   d. all of the above
   e. none of the above

3.32 Flow resistance decreases with an increase in which of the following?

   a. vessel length
   b. vessel radius
   c. blood viscosity
   d. all of the above
   e. none of the above

3.33 Flow resistance depends most strongly on which of the following?

   a. vessel length
   b. vessel radius
   c. blood viscosity
   d. all of the above
   e. none of the above

3.34 Doubling the radius of a vessel decreases its resistance to _____ of the original value.

   a. one half
   b. one fourth
   c. one eighth
   d. one sixteenth
   e. one thirty-second

3.35 The volume flow rate decreases with an increase in which of the following?

    a. pressure difference
    b. vessel radius
    c. vessel length
    d. blood viscosity
    e. c or d

3.36 When the speed of a fluid is essentially constant across a vessel, the flow is called _____ flow.

    a. volume
    b. parabolic
    c. laminar
    d. viscous
    e. plug

3.37 _____ flow (approximately) is found in larger vessels.

    a. volume
    b. steady
    c. laminar
    d. viscous
    e. plug

3.38 _____ flow is found in smaller vessels.

    a. volume
    b. steady
    c. laminar
    d. viscous
    e. plug

3.39 _____ flow occurs when the parallel streamlines that describe the flow are altered.

3.40 _____ flow involves random and chaotic flow patterns, with particles flowing in all directions.

3.41 Turbulent flow occurs in a vessel when the _____ number exceeds about 2000.

3.42 A narrowing of the lumen of a tube is called a _____ .

3.43 Proximal to, at, and distal to a stenosis _____ must be constant.

   a. laminar flow
   b. disturbed flow
   c. turbulent flow
   d. volume flow rate
   e. none of the above

3.44 For the answer to Exercise 3.43 to be true, flow speed at the stenosis must be _____ that proximal and distal to it.

   a. greater than
   b. less than
   c. less turbulent than
   d. less disturbed than
   e. none of the above

3.45 Poiseuille's equation predicts a(n) _____ in flow speed with a decrease in vessel radius.

3.46 The continuity rule predicts a(n) _____ in flow speed with a localized decrease in vessel diameter (stenosis).

3.47 The volume flow rate out of the heart into the aorta (cardiac output) is about

   a. 1 L/min
   b. 2 L/min
   c. 3 L/min
   d. 4 L/min
   e. 5 L/min

3.48 The normal peak systolic flow speed out of the heart into the aorta is about

   a. 100 cm/s
   b. 200 cm/s
   c. 300 cm/s
   d. 400 cm/s
   e. 500 cm/s

3.49 In a stenosis, the pressure is _____ the proximal and distal values.

    a. less than
    b. equal to
    c. greater than
    d. depends on the fluid
    e. none of the above

3.50 Added forward flow and flow reversal in diastole can occur with _____ flow.

    a. volume
    b. turbulent
    c. laminar
    d. disturbed
    e. pulsatile

3.51 Calculate the flow speed above which turbulent blood flow should occur in the aorta. Assume a diameter of 2 cm and 2000 for the Reynolds number.

3.52 For the stenosis shown in Figure 3.9, the vessel's diameters are $d_1 = 2$ cm, $d_2 = 1$ cm, and $d_3 = 2$ cm. For blood flowing through the stenosis at a rate of 50 mL/s, find the average flow speeds and the Reynolds numbers proximal to, at, and distal to the stenosis.

3.53 Turbulence generally occurs when Reynolds numbers exceed

    a. 100
    b. 200
    c. 1000
    d. 2000
    e. a and b

3.54 As the stenotic diameter decreases, the following pass(es) through a maximum.

    a. flow speed at the stenosis
    b. flow speed proximal to stenosis
    c. volume flow rate
    d. Doppler shift at the stenosis
    e. a and d

Figure 3.13. Proximal to (P), at (S), and distal to (D) a stenosis. (From Kremkau FW: Fluid flow II. J Vasc Technol *17*:153–154, 1993. Reprinted with permission.)

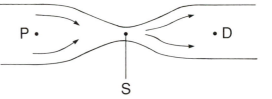

3.55 In Figure 3.13, at which point is pressure lowest?

    a. P
    b. S
    c. D
    d. P and D
    e. none of the above

3.56 In Figure 3.13, at which point is flow speed the lowest?

    a. P
    b. S
    c. D
    d. P and D
    e. none of the above

3.57 In Figure 3.13, at which point is the volume flow rate the lowest?

    a. P
    b. S
    c. D
    d. P and D
    e. none of the above

3.58 In Figure 3.13, at which point is kinetic energy the greatest?

    a. P
    b. S
    c. D
    d. P and D
    e. none of the above

3.59 In Figure 3.13, at which point is pressure energy the greatest?

    a. P
    b. S
    c. D
    d. P and D
    e. none of the above

3.60 In Figure 3.13, at which point is viscosity the greatest?

   a. P
   b. S
   c. D
   d. P and D
   e. none of the above

4 Doppler Effect

The Doppler effect is a change in frequency or wavelength caused by the motion of a wave source, receiver, or reflector. If the source is moving toward the receiver, the receiver is moving toward the source, or the reflector is moving toward the source and receiver, the received wave has a higher frequency than would be experienced without the motion. Conversely, if the motion is away (receding), the received wave has a lower frequency. The amount of increase or decrease in the frequency depends on the speed of motion, the angle between the wave's propagation direction and the direction of motion, and the frequency of the wave emitted by the source. These aspects of the Doppler effect are treated separately in the sections of this chapter.

In this chapter, we consider the following questions: What is the Doppler effect? What is the Doppler shift? How does the Doppler shift for a moving reflector depend on the frequency and reflector motion? The following terms are discussed in this chapter:

Doppler angle
Doppler effect
Doppler equation
Doppler shift
Doppler shift frequency

flow speed
speed
vector
velocity

4.1
Doppler Effect

The Doppler effect occurs for any kind of wave but is commonly experienced in life with sound. This is because speeds of motion experienced commonly can be a significant fraction of the speed of sound (a few percent). With light, this is not true, and only astronomic motions provide speeds great enough to produce a visually observable Doppler effect. This is discussed further in the next section.

A qualitative description of the Doppler effect is presented in the introductory paragraph to this chapter. A quantitative description of the Doppler effect is provided by the Doppler equation. It can be derived, for the three situations previously mentioned, as follows.

For a moving receiver (Fig. 4.1) approaching a stationary source, more cycles of the wave are encountered in 1 second than would occur if the receiver were stationary. The speed of receiver motion divided by the wavelength yields the increase in the number of cycles encountered per second (the increase in received frequency). The wavelength is the propagation speed divided by the frequency so that:

$$\text{received frequency} = \text{emitted frequency} \left[\frac{\text{propagation speed} + \text{receiver speed}}{\text{propagation speed}} \right]$$

$$f_r = f_o \left[\frac{c + v_r}{c} \right]$$

receiver speed ↑   received frequency ↑

The *change* in frequency caused by motion is called the Doppler shift frequency or, commonly, just the Doppler shift. It is equal to the received frequency minus the emitted frequency. In the present case,

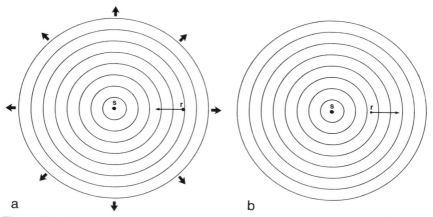

Figure 4.1. (a) A receiver (r) moving toward the source (s) experiences a higher frequency (more cycles per second) than a stationary one would. (b) A receiver moving away from the source experiences a lower frequency than a stationary one would.

it is positive, that is, the received frequency is greater than that without the (approaching) motion.

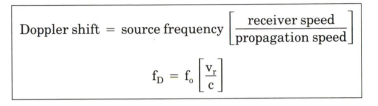

$$\text{Doppler shift } = \text{ source frequency} \left[\frac{\text{receiver speed}}{\text{propagation speed}} \right]$$

$$f_D = f_o \left[\frac{v_r}{c} \right]$$

receiver speed ↑   Doppler shift ↑
source frequency ↑   Doppler shift ↑

If the receiver approaches the source at the speed of sound, the received frequency is twice the source frequency, and the Doppler shift is equal to the source frequency. If the receiver moves away from the source, these equations are the same, except a minus sign appears in place of the plus and the Doppler shift is negative. For a receiver moving away from the source at the speed of the wave, no cycles are experienced by the receiver, and the received frequency is zero. In this case, the (negative) Doppler shift is equal to the source frequency.

For a moving source approaching a stationary receiver, the cycles are compressed in front of the source as it moves into the wave (Fig. 4.2). The source motion causes wave compression or shortening of the wavelength ahead of it. This decreased wavelength results in an increased frequency observed by a stationary receiver in front of the approaching source.

$$\text{emitted frequency } = \text{ source frequency} \left[\frac{\text{propagation speed}}{\text{propagation speed } - \text{ source speed}} \right]$$

$$f_e = f_o \left[\frac{c}{c - v_s} \right]$$

source speed ↑   emitted frequency ↑

The source frequency is the frequency that would be observed by the receiver without a moving source. If the source's speed increases to nearly the wave speed, the emitted frequency approaches infinity. This is known as a shock wave, an example of which is the sonic boom

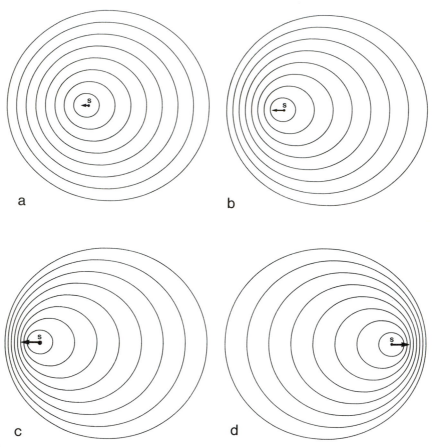

Figure 4.2. A moving source (s) of sound produces a shorter wavelength (higher frequency) ahead of it and a longer wavelength (lower frequency) behind it compared with the wavelengths at the sides, which are the same as for a stationary source: (a) slow speed, (b) medium speed, (c) high speed, and (d) high speed movement in the opposite direction.

received from aircraft traveling at or beyond the speed of sound. For motion away from the receiver, the previous equation applies, except that the minus sign is replaced by a plus sign. For a source speed equal to the wave's speed away from the receiver, the emitted frequency is equal to one half the source frequency.

The Doppler shift for a moving source is as follows:

$$\text{Doppler shift} = \text{source frequency} \left[\frac{\text{source speed}}{\text{propagation speed} - \text{source speed}} \right]$$

$$f_D = f_o \left[\frac{v_s}{c - v_s} \right]$$

> source speed ↑   Doppler shift ↑
> source frequency ↑   Doppler shift ↑

The Doppler shift for the case of a moving receiver is not the same as that for a moving emitter with the same speed of motion (Exercise 4.41). However, there is a negligible difference between the two for low source speeds (compared with the speed of sound).

A moving reflector (Fig. 4.3) or scatterer of a wave is a combination of both a moving receiver and emitter. It is described by a combination of the two Doppler equations presented earlier. The source frequency of the (moving) scatterer is equal to that which it receives (from the stationary source) so that its emitted frequency is as follows:

$$\text{emitted frequency} = \text{source frequency} \left[\frac{\text{propagation speed} + \text{scatterer speed}}{\text{propagation speed} - \text{scatterer speed}} \right]$$

$$f_e = f_o \left[\frac{c + v}{c - v} \right]$$

> scatterer speed ↑   emitted frequency ↑

As an example, let the source frequency be 5 MHz, the scatterer speed be 50 cm/s (0.5 m/s), and the propagation (sound) speed be 1540 m/s. The frequency emitted by the approaching scatterer and thus received by the (stationary) receiver is as follows:

$$f_e = 5 \left[\frac{1540 + 0.5}{1540 - 0.5} \right] = 5.0032$$

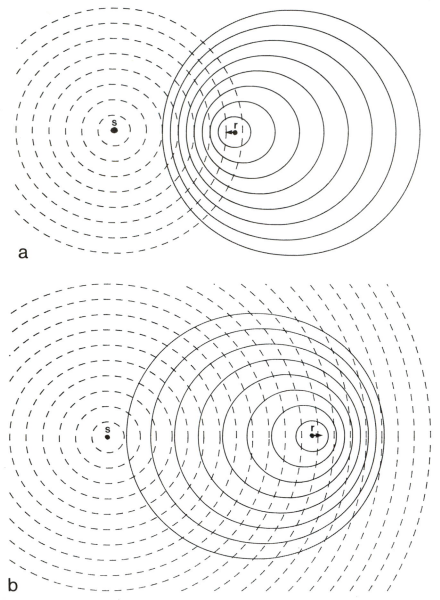

a

b

Figure 4.3. A moving reflector (r) returns a higher frequency echo if it is (a) approaching the source (s) and receiver or a lower frequency echo if it is (b) moving away from the source and receiver.

The received frequency is greater than the source frequency with a positive Doppler shift of 0.0032 MHz or 3.2 kHz. For a scatterer moving away from a receiver, the signs in the equation are reversed (minus in the numerator and plus in the denominator). Other examples using various source frequencies and scatterer speeds are included later in this chapter.

The Doppler shift for a moving scatterer is equal to the emitted (and received) frequency derived above minus the source frequency.

$$\text{Doppler shift} = \text{emitted frequency} - \text{source frequency}$$

$$= \text{source frequency} \left[\frac{2 \times \text{scatterer speed}}{\text{propagation speed} - \text{scatterer speed}} \right]$$

$$f_D = f_e - f_o$$

$$= f_o \left[\frac{2v}{c - v} \right]$$

> scatterer speed ↑   Doppler shift ↑
> source frequency ↑   Doppler shift ↑

The factor of 2 in the Doppler equation, then, is a result of two Doppler shifts for a scatterer as follows: (1) the Doppler shift as a moving receiver (the scatterer) encounters the wave and (2) the Doppler shift as the moving emitter (the scatterer) reradiates the wave. Another way to view the factor of 2 is to consider the transducer to be the source and receiver of sound separated by the round-trip sound path distance that is twice the distance from the transducer to the reflector. As the reflector approaches or recedes from the transducer, this (round-trip) distance is reduced at a rate double the speed of the reflector (Exercises 4.51 and 4.52).

If a reflector approaches the source at the speed of sound, a reflected shock wave is produced. If it recedes at the speed of sound, no echo is generated.

Physiologic blood flow speeds, even in extreme cases, are less than 1 percent of the speed of sound in tissues (1540 m/s). Because the flow speed is small compared with the speed of sound, it may be ignored in the denominator of the Doppler equation above, yielding the forms shown in Figure 4.4, in which the effect of Doppler angle (Section 4.3) is included.

The Doppler shift for a moving scatterer is summarized in symbolic form in Figure 4.4 in which the scatterer speed has been eliminated in the denominator and the Doppler angle has been included. Speed and angle are discussed in more detail later in this chapter. It is the

$$f_D = \frac{2 f_o \, v \cos \theta}{c}$$

$$v = \frac{f_D c}{2 f_o \cos \theta}$$

$$v \,(cm/s) = \frac{77 f_D \,(kHz)}{f_o \,(MHz) \cos \theta}$$

Figure 4.4. Three forms of the Doppler equation for a moving reflector or scatterer of sound.

Doppler shift that the instruments described in Chapters 5 and 6 detect. However, it is the speed of motion or flow of the blood in which we are normally interested. The Doppler equation can be rearranged to place the speed of motion alone on the left side of the equation as follows (see Fig. 4.4):

$$\text{scatterer speed} = \left[\frac{\text{Doppler shift} \times \text{propagation speed}}{2 \times \text{source frequency} \times \text{cosine Doppler angle}} \right]$$

$$v = \left[\frac{f_D c}{2 f_o \cos \theta_D} \right]$$

Substituting the speed of sound in tissues (154,000 cm/s) and using units as indicated for the various quantities yields the equation in the following form (see Fig. 4.4):

$$\text{scatterer speed (cm/s)} = \left[\frac{77 \times \text{Doppler shift (kHz)}}{\text{source frequency (MHz)} \times \text{cosine Doppler angle}} \right]$$

$$v = \left[\frac{77 f_D}{f_o \cos \theta_D} \right]$$

Doppler shift ↑	calculated scatterer speed ↑
source frequency ↑	calculated scatterer speed ↓
cosine Doppler angle ↑	calculated scatterer speed ↓
Doppler angle ↑	calculated scatterer speed ↑

The speed of sound used here is the average speed of sound in soft tissues, 1540 m/s or 1.54 mm/μs. It is tempting to use the speed of sound in blood,[16,17] 1570 to 1575 m/s. However, this may not always be appropriate when considering the interesting clarification given in the next paragraph.

There is a complication in the consideration of the Doppler effect for ultrasound scattered by the cells in circulating blood that has not been considered in the previous discussion. The cells that scatter the ultrasound move along with the surrounding medium (plasma) rather than moving through it, as is the case for an ambulance moving through air (the common illustration of the Doppler effect with the approaching siren). The fact that the scatterers are moving along with the medium means that the Doppler effect does not occur at the scatterer boundary (the boundary between the cell and plasma). Nevertheless, the Doppler effect *is* observed when an ultrasound beam interacts with flowing blood. In fact, the Doppler effect must occur at boundaries where relative motion occurs. For the simplest case (plug flow), this is at the boundary between the stationary tissues (the internal vessel wall or intima) and the flowing blood. As the sound crosses this boundary, it encounters a moving propagation medium (blood), with the result that the wavelength is decreased if the blood is flowing toward the transducer or increased if it is flowing away (Fig. 4.5). In other words, the Doppler shift occurs at the vessel wall and not at the cell membrane.[18–20] The Doppler shift is doubled, as in the previous consideration of a moving scatterer, because, as the reradiated (scattered) wave exits the moving blood and enters the stationary tissue, there is a second positive Doppler shift (or a second negative Doppler shift if the flow is away from the transducer, see Fig. 4.5). This is the most complete and accurate explanation for the factor of 2 in the Doppler equation. For plug flow, the Doppler effect occurs entirely at the intimal surface. For other flow conditions, Doppler shifts are generated at all sights of relative motion (laminae and eddies) in the blood.

4.2
Speed

The fact that the Doppler shift is proportional to the scatterer's speed and, therefore, to blood flow speed explains why the Doppler effect is so useful in medical diagnosis. Doppler instruments measure the Doppler shift. It is the blood flow in which we are interested. The measured shifts are proportional to flow speed, a knowledge of which we desire.

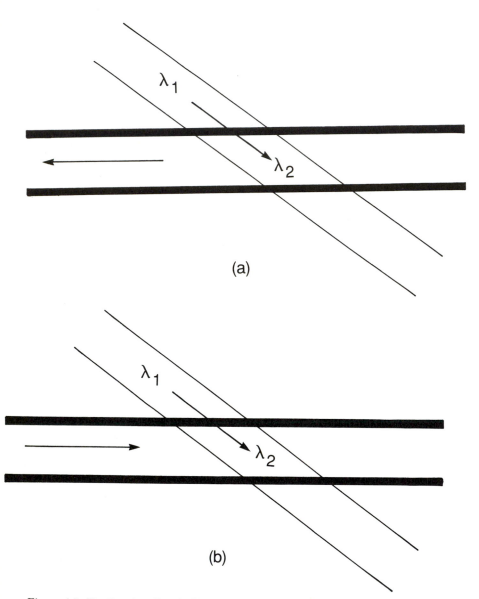

Figure 4.5. The Doppler effect for flowing blood occurs at the vessel wall—blood boundary. (a) As the sound crosses the vessel into approaching blood, the wavelength is shortened. (b) As the sound crosses the vessel into receding blood, the wavelength is lengthened. (c) As sound exits approaching blood, the wavelength is shortened. (d) As sound exits receding blood, the wavelength is lengthened.

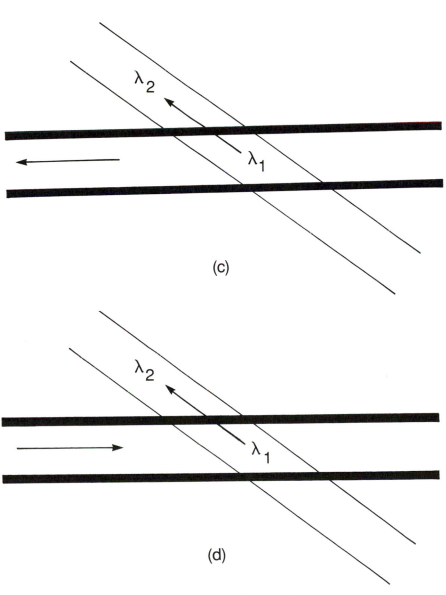

(c)

(d)

Figure 4.5. *Continued*

The approximate Doppler equation (in which the object's speed is small compared with the propagation speed) indicates that the Doppler shift is proportional to the speed of the moving object (source, receiver, or scatterer), and more specifically, it is proportional to the ratio of that speed to the wave propagation speed. This is why, as mentioned in Section 4.1, the Doppler effect with light is not normally experienced in daily life, although it is with sound. The speed of light is about 1 million times that of sound.

If a yellow automobile could travel at 100 million miles/hr (15 percent the speed of light), the positive Doppler shift as it approached would cause it to appear blue, there would be a flash of yellow as it passed by, and then it would appear to be a red vehicle as it receded because of the Doppler downshift (Fig. 4.6, Color Plate III). Fifteen percent of the speed of sound in air is 115 miles/hr. If a vehicle approached at this speed, emitting a tone of 262 Hz (middle C), the tone heard by a stationary observer would be 308 Hz (D# = 311 Hz), and the tone heard after the vehicle passed and was receding would be 228 Hz (A# = 233 Hz). Our human auditory system is capable of detecting frequency changes much smaller than this; therefore, we can hear the Doppler shift occur as a sound-emitting vehicle passes at much lower speeds. The Doppler shift with light has been useful in determining the motion of light-emitting galaxies in the universe. These have red shifts, indicating motion away from us. Furthermore,

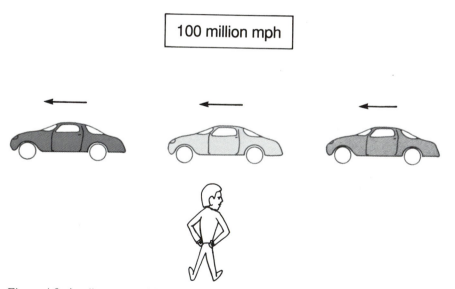

Figure 4.6. A yellow automobile traveling at 15 percent of the speed of light would appear blue as it approached, yellow as it passed by, and red as it receded (see Color Plate III).

the red shifts and calculated speeds of motion are proportional to the distances of these objects from the earth. This indicates that the universe is expanding and that it had its origin at a common location at some point in time long past (the Big Bang Theory). More detailed observations of the motions of nearer objects, such as our sun, have been made possible by Doppler shift measurements of the light from various points located on them. Using light, laser Doppler instruments are available for vascular measurement and monitoring.

Using electromagnetic microwaves, Doppler radar has been applied in weather forecasting and aviation safety. It is also used in the familiar application of police radar detection of vehicle speeds on highways. This is an example of a detected Doppler shift resulting from a reflection from a moving object.

Ultrasonic burglar alarms (Fig. 1.1) and door openers are common in homes and public buildings. These also use the Doppler shift resulting from a moving reflector (person in motion). These systems operate around 25 kHz, emitting ultrasound into and receiving it from the air. A person walking at one step per second generates a Doppler shift of about 65 Hz in such a system.[21]

With diagnostic medical ultrasound, stationary transducers are used to emit and receive the ultrasound. The Doppler effect is a result of the motion of the blood, the flow of which we wish to measure. Physiologic flow speeds, even in highly stenotic jets, do not exceed a few meters per second.

Another long-standing application of Doppler ultrasound in medicine is in monitoring the fetal heartbeat during labor and delivery. Instruments that perform this function can be less sophisticated and less sensitive than are blood flow measurement systems because the echoes from the beating heart are much stronger than those coming from blood. Doppler shifts resulting from typical physiologic flow speeds are given in Table 4.1. Figure 4.7 illustrates the proportional depen-

Table 4–1			
Doppler Frequency Shifts for Various Scatterer Speeds Toward the Sound Source* With a Zero Doppler Angle			
Incident Frequency (MHz)	Scatterer Speed (cm/s)	Reflected Frequency (MHz)	Doppler Shift (kHz)
2	50	2.0013	1.3
5	50	5.0032	3.2
10	50	10.0065	6.5
2	200	2.0052	5.2
5	200	5.013	13.0
10	200	10.026	26.0

* Motion away from the source would yield negative Doppler shifts.

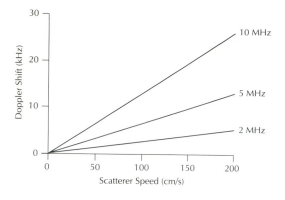

Figure 4.7. Doppler shift as a function of scatterer speed, as determined by the Doppler equation for three incident frequencies (zero Doppler angle).

dence of Doppler shift on scatterer speed. The primary effect of a change in blood flow speed here is a corresponding change in Doppler shift. The strength, intensity, or power of the returning Doppler-shifted echoes is not affected by the flow speed. Such an effect is not predicted by the Doppler equation and has not been found in experimental investigations.[22]

The minimum detectable blood flow speed with Doppler ultrasound is a few millimeters per second. The maximum is determined by aliasing (Section 7.1) with pulsed-Doppler and color-flow (Section 7.2) instruments. In principle, there is no upper limit for continuous-wave instruments.

4.3
Angle

If the direction of sound propagation is exactly opposite the direction of flow, the maximum positive Doppler shift is obtained. If the flow speed and propagation speed directions are the same (parallel), the maximum negative Doppler shift is obtained. If the angle between these two directions (Fig. 4.8) is nonzero, lesser Doppler shifts occur. As seen in the Doppler equation (see Fig. 4.4), the dependence on the Doppler angle is in the form of a cosine. Table 4.2 gives cosine values for various angles. For angles greater than 90 degrees, the cosine is negative, yielding the negative Doppler shift we expect because flow is receding in such a case. The cosine gives the component of the flow velocity vector that is parallel to the sound beam (Fig. 4.9). For a given flow, the greater the Doppler angle is, the lesser the Doppler shift is (Fig. 4.8b and c). Examples of Doppler shifts for various angles are listed in Table 4.3.

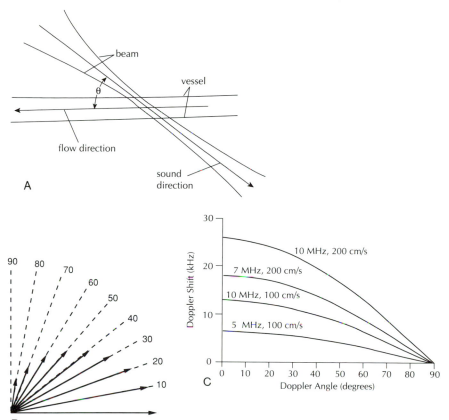

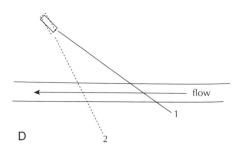

A

B   **Flow**

C

D

Figure 4.8. (A) Doppler angle, θ, is the angle between the direction of flow and the direction of sound propagation. (B) With constant flow, as the Doppler angle increases, the frequency of the echo Doppler shift decreases. The direction of the arrows indicates the beam's direction. The length of the arrows indicates the magnitude of the Doppler shift. (C) Doppler shift is shown as a function of the angle, as determined by the Doppler equation for various incident frequencies and scatterer speeds. (D) The same flow in a vessel, viewed at different angles, yields different Doppler shifts.

Table 4–2

Cosines for Various Angles

Angle A (Degrees)	cos A
0	1.00
5	0.996
10	0.98
15	0.97
20	0.94
25	0.91
30	0.87
35	0.82
40	0.77
45	0.71
50	0.64
55	0.57
60	0.50
65	0.42
70	0.34
75	0.26
80	0.17
85	0.09
90	0.00

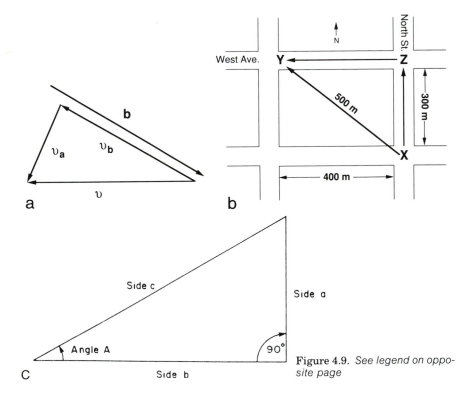

Figure 4.9. *See legend on opposite page*

Table 4–3		

Doppler Frequency Shifts for Various Angles and Scatterer Speeds Toward the Sound Source of Frequency 5 MHz

Scatterer Speed (cm/s)	Angle (Degrees)	Doppler Shift (kHz)
100	0	6.5
100	30	5.6
100	60	3.2
100	90	0.0
300	0	19.0
300	30	17.0
300	60	9.7
300	90	0.0

Flow speed calculations based on Doppler shift measurements can be accomplished correctly only with a knowledge of the Doppler angle involved. They, therefore, are only as good as the accuracy of the measurement or estimate (or guess) of that angle. An estimation of the angle is normally done by orienting a line on the anatomic display such that it is parallel to the presumed direction of flow (parallel to vessel walls for a straight vessel with no flow obstruction). This is a subjective operation performed by the operator of the instrument. Error in this estimation of the Doppler angle is more critical at large angles than at small ones. Table 4.4 gives error values for various angles. Figure 4.10 shows how the error in calculated flow speed increases with the angle. For this reason and because Doppler shifts become very small at large angles, reducing the system's sensitivity, Doppler measurements (and particularly calculated flow speeds) are not reliably achieved at Doppler angles greater than 60 to 70 degrees. Normally, the ultrasound beam does not travel directly down the vessel (because

---

Figure 4.9. (a) The flow velocity vector (v) can be broken into two components, one (v_b) that is parallel to the sound beam's direction (**b**) and one (v_a) that is perpendicular to the sound beam's direction. Only the component parallel to the beam contributes to the Doppler effect. (b) An analogy to the vector components in (A), using a city block example. To get from X to Y, an individual could walk diagonally across the block, a distance of 500 m. However, if buildings prevented this path, an alternate route would be 300 m north on North Street and then 400 m west on West Avenue. The 500-m northwest vector from X to Y is equivalent to a 300-m north vector plus a 400-m west vector (i.e., the result is the same: depart from X and arrive at Y). In this example, the component of the XY vector parallel to North Street is the XZ vector and the component parallel to West Avenue is the ZY vector. (c) With the sides and angles of a right triangle (one in which one of the angles equals 90 degrees) labeled as in this example, the cosine of angle A (cos A) is equal to the length of side b divided by the length of side c.

Table 4–4

Cosine Error for 2- and 5-Degree Angle Errors

True Angle (Degrees)	Percent Cosine Error for +2-Degree Angle Error	Percent Cosine Error for +5-Degree Angle Error
0	0.1	0.4
10	0.7	1.9
20	1.3	3.6
30	2.1	5.4
40	3.0	7.7
50	4.2	10.8
60	6.1	15.5
70	9.6	24.3
80	19.9	49.8

the transducer is offset from the vessel axis; see Fig. 4.8a); therefore, the Doppler angle is dependent on the direction in which the beam is pointed. In principle, if everything is done correctly, the calculated flow speed in the vessel should be the same regardless of the Doppler angle. That is, if the vessel is straight and of uniform diameter and has uniform flow within it, the same flow speed should be found no matter how (at what angle) the beam intersects the vessel (Table 4.5). Because this is commonly not found to be the case, inaccuracies in angle estimation are probably being observed. Also, flow is probably not uniform in direction, even in unobstructed vessels.[10–14] Correct handling of the Doppler angle is an important topic in Chapters 5 and 6.

Because the propagation speed of sound is not the same in blood as it is in soft tissues (it is slightly greater in blood), refraction occurs as the sound crosses the boundary from the vessel wall into the blood. This introduces an error in the estimated angle. However, the error in the calculated flow speed is (surprisingly) independent of the angle and is equal to the percent difference in propagation speeds.[23] It is important to know that a critical angle is reached at about 25 degrees, at which the sound no longer enters the blood at all but is totally reflected at the wall-blood boundary. The increase in reflected intensity (and therefore the decrease in transmitted intensity) at this boundary with decreasing Doppler angle causes the effectiveness of Doppler measurements to be reduced at Doppler angles less than about 30 degrees. However, in Doppler echocardiography, Doppler angles of nearly zero are achieved, and zero is commonly assumed (i.e., the angle correction is not attempted as it is in vascular work). Here, the angle between the beam and the heart wall is large, thus avoiding the critical angle problem.

Because the Doppler measurement is angle dependent (i.e., the Doppler method measures only the component of the flow vector that

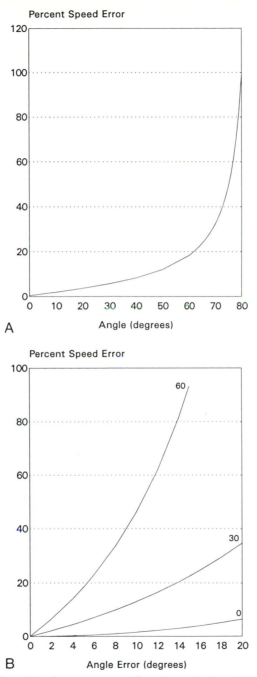

Figure 4.10. (A) Percent cosine error versus Doppler angle for a 5-degree angle error. (B) Percent cosine error versus angle error for three values (0, 30, and 60 degrees) of the correct Doppler angle.

107

Table 4–5

Doppler Shifts (for 4 MHz) at Various Doppler Angles for the Same Flow Ideally Yield a Consistent Calculated Flow Speed

Doppler Shift (kHz)	Angle (Degrees)	Calculated Flow Speed (cm/s)
2.25	30	50
1.99	40	50
1.84	45	50
1.67	50	50
1.30	60	50

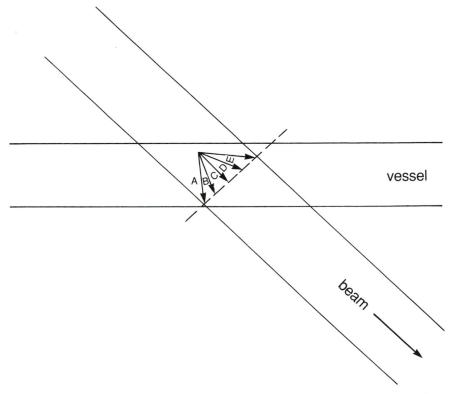

Figure 4.11. Flow velocity vectors A, B, C, D, and E each have the same component along the beam axis (therefore yielding the same Doppler shift frequency). (From Phillips DJ, Beach KW, Primozich J, et al: Should results of ultrasound Doppler studies be reported in units of frequency or velocity? Ultrasound Med Biol 15:205–212, 1989. Reprinted with permission from Elsevier Science Ltd, The Boulevard, Longford Lane, Kidlington OX5 1GB, UK.)

is parallel to the sound beam), a single Doppler measurement can correspond to many different flow velocities (speeds and directions, Fig. 4.11). If two measurements of the same flow are made at two different angles, the correct flow speed and direction (velocity) can be determined.

Figures 6.18f and g in Chapter 6 give a color-flow example of zero Doppler shift that could be interpreted as an occluded vessel. However, a 90-degree Doppler angle is the cause. When a different angle is achieved, flow (color) appears in the vessel.

The primary effect of a change in Doppler angle is a change in Doppler shift. The strength, intensity, or power of the returning Doppler-shifted echoes is not affected by the angle.

In conclusion, we emphasize that, to proceed from a measurement of Doppler-shift frequency to a calculation of flow speed, the Doppler angle must be known or correctly assumed. Otherwise, an incorrect flow speed calculation results.

We have only considered in this discussion the Doppler angle in the scan plane. The flow may not be parallel to the imaging scan plane, which includes the Doppler beam; therefore, there may be a component of Doppler angle between the flow direction and the scan plane. Thus, the three-dimensional character of the components involved in the process (vessel anatomy, flow, and ultrasound image) must be kept in mind.

4.4
Frequency

For a given flow in a vessel, the Doppler shift measured by an instrument is proportional to the operating frequency of the instrument (Fig. 4.12). Table 4.1 gives Doppler shifts for various frequencies. Thus, the measurement of Doppler shifts from flow in the same vessel by using two different transducers operating at 2 and 4 MHz would yield two different Doppler shifts, with the higher frequency transducer having a Doppler shift double that of the lower frequency transducer. When comparing Doppler shifts, therefore, the frequency of the devices must be considered.[24] In the calculation of flow speed, the operating frequency is incorporated. Thus, comparisons of flow speeds between different instruments have taken this variable into account. However, recall that such calculations depend on the accuracy of the angle estimation.

Thus far, we have assumed that, for a given frequency ultrasound beam, the only thing that produces a frequency shift in the returning echoes is the motion associated with blood flow. In truth, other factors

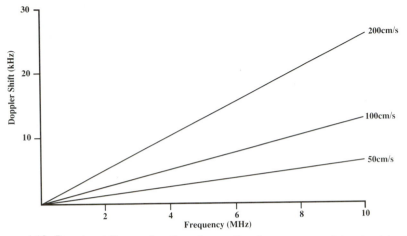

Figure 4.12. Doppler shift as a function of operating frequency, as determined by the Doppler equation for various flow speeds (zero Doppler angle).

produce a frequency shift also, four of which are mentioned here. Erythrocytes are small compared with the wavelengths of ultrasound used. The echo intensity from such small objects is proportional to the frequency to the fourth power. Because ultrasound pulses involve a range of frequencies (described by the bandwidth[1]), the higher frequencies are scattered more strongly, and the lower are scattered less strongly. This produces a positive frequency shift (not a Doppler shift) in the returning echoes. By contrast, the attenuation of ultrasound in tissues increases with frequency. Therefore, as the sound travels out and the echoes travel back, the higher frequencies within the bandwidth are attenuated more than the lower ones are. This causes a downshift in the mean frequency of the returning echoes. The nonlinear characteristics of the tissue as a sound propagation medium cause higher harmonic frequencies to be generated as the sound wave converts from a sinusoidal form to a saw-toothed form. This produces an increase in the mean frequency of the sound as it travels. Finally, the electrical properties of the transducer cause it to treat various frequencies more or less efficiently than others. This can result in an increase or decrease in the mean frequency. The net result of these up- and downshifts is almost impossible to predict but, apparently, has a negligible effect on the Doppler shifts encountered physiologically.

The frequency dependencies of scattering and attenuation mentioned in the previous paragraph compete in the sense that scattering characteristics produce stronger echoes with higher frequencies, although attenuation reduces the strength of higher frequency echoes received at the transducer. Attenuation has the dominant effect; therefore, higher frequencies do not penetrate as effectively as lower ones do. In practice, frequencies comparable to those used for sonography are used for Doppler measurements (i.e., 2 to 10 MHz). Doppler frequencies for given-depth applications are, in practice, slightly less than those used for anatomic imaging at that depth.

4.5
Review

The Doppler effect is a change in the frequency or wavelength that results from motion. In most medical ultrasound applications, the motion is that of blood flow in the circulation. The change in frequency of the returning echoes with respect to the emitted frequency is called the Doppler shift. For flow toward the transducer, it is positive; for flow away, it is negative. The Doppler shift depends on the speed of the scatterers of sound, the angle between their flow direction and that of the sound propagation, and the operating frequency of the Doppler system. Thus, reporting a Doppler shift frequency without specifying the operating frequency and Doppler angle is incomplete. A moving scatterer of sound produces a double Doppler shift. Greater flow speeds and smaller Doppler angles produce larger Doppler shifts but not stronger echoes. Higher operating frequencies produce larger Doppler shifts. Typical ranges of flow speeds (10 to 100 cm/s), Doppler angles (30 to 60 degrees), and operating frequencies (2 to 10 MHz) yield Doppler shifts in the range 100 Hz to 11 kHz for vascular studies. In Doppler echocardiography, in which angles of 0 to 20 degrees and speeds of a few meters per second are encountered, Doppler shifts can be as high as 30 kHz. Table 4.6 gives Doppler shifts for various frequencies, angles, and speeds.

The definitions of terms used in this chapter are listed below:

Doppler angle. The angle between the sound beam and the direction of flow.
Doppler effect. Frequency change of the reflected sound wave as a result of the reflector's motion relative to the transducer.
Doppler equation. The mathematic description of the relationship between Doppler shift, frequency, Doppler angle, propagation speed, and reflector speed.

Table 4–6

Doppler Shifts for Various Frequencies, Angles, and Speeds

Frequency (MHz)	Angle (Degrees)	Speed (cm/s)	Shift (kHz)
2	0	10	0.26
2	0	50	1.30
2	0	100	2.60
2	30	10	0.22
2	30	50	1.12
2	30	100	2.25
2	45	10	0.18
2	45	50	0.92
2	45	100	1.84
2	60	10	0.13
2	60	50	0.65
2	60	100	1.30
5	0	10	0.65
5	0	50	3.25
5	0	100	6.49
5	30	10	0.56
5	30	50	2.81
5	30	100	5.62
5	45	10	0.46
5	45	50	2.30
5	45	100	4.59
5	60	10	0.32
5	60	50	1.62
5	60	100	3.25
10	0	10	1.30
10	0	50	6.49
10	0	100	13.0
10	30	10	1.12
10	30	50	5.62
10	30	100	11.2
10	45	10	0.92
10	45	50	4.59
10	45	100	9.18
10	60	10	0.65
10	60	50	3.25
10	60	100	6.49

Doppler shift. Reflected frequency minus incident frequency. Change in frequency caused by motion.

Doppler shift frequency. Doppler shift.

Flow speed. Rate of motion of a portion of a flowing fluid.

Speed. Displacement (distance moved) divided by the time over which displacement occurs.

Vector. A quantity with magnitude and direction.

Velocity. Speed with the direction of motion specified. Velocity is a vector.

Exercises

4.1 The _____ effect is used to detect and measure _____ in vessels.

4.2 Motion of an echo-generating structure causes an echo to have a different _____ than the emitted pulse.

4.3 The Doppler effect is a change in reflected _____ caused by reflector _____.

4.4 If the reflector is moving toward the source, the reflected frequency is _____ than the incident frequency.

4.5 If the reflector is moving away from the source, the reflected frequency is _____ than the incident frequency.

4.6 If the reflector is stationary with respect to the source, the reflected frequency is _____ _____ the incident frequency.

4.7 Measurement of Doppler shift yields information about reflector _____.

4.8 If the incident frequency is 1 MHz, the propagation speed is 1600 m/s, and the reflector speed is 16 m/s toward the source, the Doppler shift is _____ MHz, and the reflected frequency is _____ MHz.

4.9 If 2-MHz ultrasound is reflected from a soft tissue boundary moving at 10 m/s toward the source, the Doppler shift is _____ MHz.

4.10 If 2-MHz ultrasound is reflected from a soft tissue boundary moving at 10 m/s away from the source, the Doppler shift is _____ MHz.

4.11 Doppler shift is the difference between _____ and _____ frequencies.

4.12 When the incident sound direction and reflector motion are not parallel, the calculation of the reflected frequency involves the _____ of the angle between these directions.

4.13 If the angle between the incident sound's direction and the reflector's motion is 60 degrees, the Doppler shift and reflected frequency in Exercise 4.8 are _____ MHz and _____ MHz.

4.14 If the angle between the incident sound's direction and the reflector's motion is 90 degrees, the cosine of the angle is _____, and the reflected frequency in Exercise 4.8 is _____ MHz.

4.15 A policeman in a (Doppler) radar-equipped patrol car detects the speed of an automobile to be 55 mph. If the angle between the radar beam and the direction of the automobile is 60 degrees, the actual speed of the automobile is _____ mph.

4.16 Fill in the missing values in the table.

f (MHz)	v (cm/s)	θ (degrees)	f_D (kHz)
2.5	50	0	(a) ___
5	50	(b) ___	3.25
7.5	(c) ___	0	4.87
(d) ___	100	0	3.25
5	100	0	(e) ___
7.5	100	(f) ___	9.74
2.5	(g) ___	0	4.87
(h) ___	150	0	9.74
7.5	150	0	(i) ___
5	50	30	(j) ___
5	50	(k) ___	1.62
5	50	(l) ___	0
5	(m) ___	30	5.62
5	100	60	(n) ___
5	(o) ___	90	0
5	150	(p) ___	8.44
(q) ___	150	60	4.87
5	150	90	(r) ___

4.17 The maximum normal flow speed encountered in the circulatory system is approximately

a. 1 mm/s
b. 1 cm/s
c. 100 cm/s
d. 100 m/s
e. 1 km/s

4.18 For operating frequency 2 MHz, flow speed 10 cm/s, and Doppler angle 0, calculate the Doppler shift.

4.19 For operating frequency 4 MHz, flow speed 10 cm/s, and Doppler angle 30 degrees, calculate the Doppler shift.

4.20 For operating frequency 6 MHz, flow speed 50 cm/s, and Doppler angle 60 degrees, calculate the Doppler shift.

4.21 For operating frequency 5 MHz, Doppler angle 45 degrees, and Doppler shift 4.60 kHz, calculate the flow speed.

4.22 For operating frequency 6 MHz, Doppler angle 60 degrees, and Doppler shift 1.95 kHz, calculate the flow speed.

4.23 If the propagation speed in blood is greater than that in the surrounding tissue, is the effect of refraction to increase or decrease the Doppler angle?

4.24 Does the result in Exercise 4.23 increase or decrease the Doppler-shift frequency?

4.25 What is the Doppler shift if a receiver is moving toward a 5-MHz source at the speed of sound?

4.26 If a receiver is moving away from a 5-MHz source at the speed of sound, what is the Doppler shift?

4.27 In Exercise 4.26, what frequency does the receiver detect?

4.28 If a 5-MHz source moves toward a receiver at the speed of sound, what frequency is received?

4.29 If a 5-MHz source moves away from a receiver at the speed of sound, what frequency is received?

4.30 The Doppler shifts for a moving source, a moving receiver, and a moving reflector (all moving at the same speed) produce the same Doppler shifts. True or false?

4.31 For blood flowing in a vessel with a plug flow profile, where does the Doppler shift occur?

4.32 In view of the answer to Exercise 4.31, are blood cells necessary for using Doppler ultrasound? Why or why not?

4.33 Physiologic flow speeds can be as much as _____ percent of the propagation speed in soft tissues.

    a. 0.01
    b. 0.3
    c. 5
    d. 10
    e. 50

4.34 Which Doppler angle gives the greatest Doppler shift?

    a. -90
    b. -45
    c. 0
    d. 45
    e. 90

4.35 To proceed from a measurement of Doppler shift frequency to a calculation of flow speed, _____ _____ must be known or correctly assumed.

4.36 The intensity of returning Doppler-shifted echoes is not affected by _____ or _____.

4.37 The Doppler-shift frequency is not dependent on

    a. amplitude
    b. flow speed
    c. operating frequency
    d. Doppler angle
    e. propagation speed

4.38 If the operating frequency is doubled, the Doppler shift is _____.

4.39 If the flow speed is doubled, the Doppler shift is _____.

4.40 If the Doppler angle is doubled, the Doppler shift is _____.

4.41 Calculate the 5-MHz Doppler shifts (a) for a receiver moving at 100 m/s, (b) for a source moving at 100 m/s, and (c) for a reflector moving at 100 m/s.

4.42 In Figure 4.7, what are the operating frequencies, assuming a 60-degree angle?

4.43 In Figure 4.12, what is the Doppler angle if the flow speeds are 282, 141, 70?

4.44 A 4-MHz, 500-cm/s curve would be identical to which curve in Figure 4.8c.

4.45 A 2-MHz, 250-cm/s curve would be identical to which curve in Figure 4.8c.

4.46 For a Doppler angle of 60 degrees, a flow speed of 1.5 m/s, and an operating frequency of 5 MHz, the Doppler shift is ——————— kHz, which is ——————— percent of the operating frequency.

4.47 In Figure 4.13, which angle is the incidence angle? Which angle is the Doppler angle? Which angle is the transmission angle? If there is no refraction, which angle is equal to the transmission angle? With no refraction, which angle is equal to the Doppler angle? The incidence angle plus the Doppler angle (no refraction) equals what?

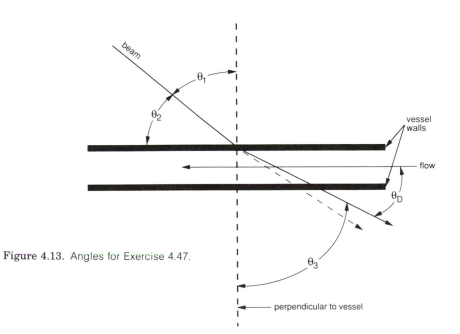

Figure 4.13. Angles for Exercise 4.47.

4.48 The cosine of an angle can be no greater than

    a. π
    b. 1
    c. 0
    d. -1
    e. $-\pi$

4.49 The cosine of an angle can be no less than

    a. 10
    b. 1
    c. 0
    d. -1
    e. -10

4.50 The difference between the Doppler shift for a moving receiver and a moving source is negligible if the speed of movement is _____ enough.

4.51 As a reflector approaches a transducer at 50 cm/s, the round-trip distance between them is reduced at the rate _____ cm/s.

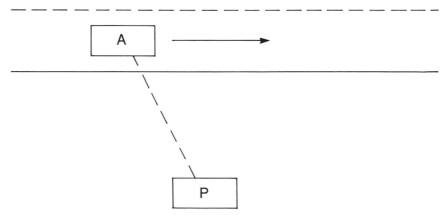

Figure 4.14. A police radar unit (P) and motorist (A). Illustration for Exercise 4.54.

4.52 As a reflector recedes from a transducer at 50 cm/s, the round-trip distance between them is increased at the rate _____ cm/s.

4.53 Exercises 4.51 and 4.52 present one reason why there is a factor of _____ in the Doppler equation for a reflector.

4.54 Figure 4.14 shows police radar unit (P) that uses the Doppler effect to determine the speed of an automobile (A). What happens to the Doppler shift as the vehicle travels down the highway at a constant speed?

4.55 In Figure 4.8d, which viewing angle (1 or 2) gives the greatest Doppler angle? Which gives the greatest Doppler shift?

5 Spectral Instruments

Three types of instruments are used for Doppler detection of flow in the heart, arteries, and veins: continuous-wave and pulsed-wave spectral instruments and color-flow instruments. The continuous-wave instrument detects Doppler-shifted echoes in the region of the overlap between the beams of the transmitting transducer and the receiving transducer elements. Transducers are discussed in Section 2.2. The primary difference between transducers designed for imaging and those designed exclusively for continuous-wave Doppler use is that the latter are not damped and are, therefore, more efficient.

The pulsed-wave Doppler instrument emits ultrasound pulses and receives echoes using a single element or array transducer. Because of the required Doppler-frequency–shift detection, the pulses are longer than those for imaging. Through range gating, pulsed-wave Doppler provides the ability to select information from a particular location (depth) within the anatomy (along the beam). To use the pulsed-wave Doppler effectively, it is commonly combined with real-time sonography in one instrument. Such instruments are called duplex scanners because of their dual functions (anatomic imaging and flow measurement). Continuous- and pulsed-wave instruments present Doppler-shift information in audible form and as a visual (usually spectral) display.

Color-flow instruments provide two-dimensional, cross-sectional, real-time, color-coded Doppler-shift or time-shift information superimposed on the real-time, gray-scale anatomic display. The color coding provides two-dimensional information regarding the presence of flow and its direction, speed, and character. Spectral instruments are described in this chapter. Color-flow instruments are described in Chapter 6.

In this chapter, we consider the following questions. In what ways is Doppler information presented? How is flow detection localized to a specific site in the tissue? What is meant by spectral analysis? What are the differences between continuous- and pulsed-wave Doppler spectral instruments? The following terms are discussed in this chapter:

bidirectional	pulsed wave
clutter	range gating
continuous wave	receiver gate
Doppler angle	sample volume
duplex instrument	signal
fast Fourier transform	spectral analysis
Fourier analysis	spectral broadening
Fourier transform	spectral display
frequency spectrum	spectral width
generator gate	spectrum
pulse repetition frequency	spectrum analyzer
pulsed Doppler	wall filter
pulsed mode	window
pulsed ultrasound	zero-crossing detector

5.1
Continuous Wave

Doppler ultrasound instruments provide continuous or pulsed voltages to the transducer and convert voltages received from the transducer to audible or visual information corresponding to reflector or scatterer motion. If an instrument can distinguish between positive and negative Doppler shifts, it is said to be bidirectional. Continuous-wave Doppler instruments include a continuous-wave voltage generator and a receiver that detects the change in frequency (Doppler shift) that results from reflector or scatterer motion for presentation as an audible sound and as a visual presentation corresponding to the motion of the objects.

A diagram of the components of a continuous-wave Doppler system is given in Figure 5.1. The voltage generator (oscillator) produces a continuously alternating voltage of a frequency in the range of 2 to 10 MHz, which is applied to the source transducer element. The ultrasound frequency is determined by the voltage generator. It is set to

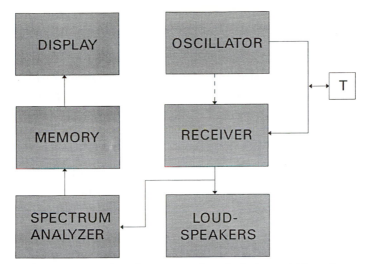

Figure 5.1. Block diagram of continuous-wave Doppler instrument. The voltage generator (oscillator) produces a continuously alternating voltage that drives the source transducer (T). The receiving transducer (T) produces a continuous voltage in response to the echoes it continuously receives. The receiver detects differences in frequency between the voltages produced by the oscillator and by the receiving transducer. The Doppler shifts produce voltages that drive loudspeakers in the audible range and through a spectrum analyzer and memory, a visual display. The frequency of the audible sound is equal to the Doppler shift. It is proportional to the reflector speed and to the cosine of the angle between the sound propagation direction and the boundary motion. T represents the dual source and receiving transducer assembly. There are usually separate loudspeakers for positive and negative Doppler shifts.

equal the operating frequency of the transducer (Section 2.2). In the transducer assembly, there is a separate receiving transducer element that produces voltages with frequencies equal to the frequencies of the returning echoes. If there were reflector motion, the reflected ultrasound and the ultrasound produced by the source transducer would have different frequencies. The receiver detects the difference between these two frequencies (the Doppler shift) and drives a loudspeaker at this difference frequency. Doppler shifts are typically one thousandth of the source frequency, which puts them in the audible range. The Doppler shifts are also commonly sent to a spectral display for visual observation and evaluation. This is discussed in Sections 5.3 and 5.4.

The receiver (Fig. 5.2) amplifies the echo voltages it receives from the receiving transducer, acquires (demodulates) the Doppler shift information in the returning echoes and usually determines the direction of motion (positive or negative Doppler shift). Doppler shifts are determined by mixing the returning voltages with the continuous-wave voltage from the voltage generator (see Fig. 5.1, dashed path). This produces the sum and difference of the voltage generator and echo frequencies (see Fig. 5.2). The difference is the desired Doppler shift. The sum is a much higher frequency (approximately double the operating frequency) and is easily filtered out. The difference is zero for echoes returning from stationary structures. For echoes from moving structures or flowing blood, this difference is the Doppler shift that provides information about motion and flow.

Positive and negative shifts indicate motion toward and away from the transducer, respectively. The receiver shown in Figure 5.2 does not provide this directional information. Determining direction (positive versus negative Doppler shifts) and separating Doppler shift voltages into separate forward and reverse channels is commonly accomplished by the phase quadrature detector (Fig. 5.3). Two voltages from the voltage generator (one delayed by one quarter of a cycle [Fig. 5.4], i.e., the "quad") are mixed with the returning echo voltages, yielding the difference (Doppler shifts). The echo voltages contain the Doppler shifts that represent flow toward and away from the transducer. The filter outputs of the direct channel and the delayed (quadrature) channel are the Doppler shifts from the echo voltage input.

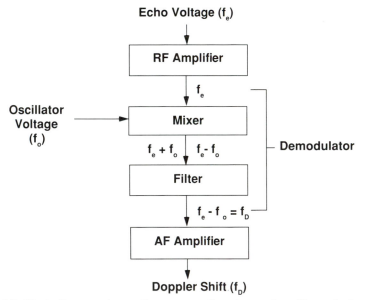

Doppler Shift (f_D)

Figure 5.2. Block diagram of a continuous-wave Doppler receiver. The radio frequency (RF) amplifier increases the echo voltage amplitude. The frequency of the echo voltage is f_e. In the mixer, it is combined with the oscillator (voltage generator) voltage the frequency of which is f_o. The mixer yields the sum and difference of these two frequency inputs ($f_e + f_o$ and $f_e - f_o$). The low-pass (high-frequency rejection) filter removes $f_e + f_o$, leaving $f_e - f_o$, which is the Doppler shift frequency (f_D). It is then strengthened in the audio frequency (AF) amplifier. The mixer and filter together constitute the Doppler demodulator.

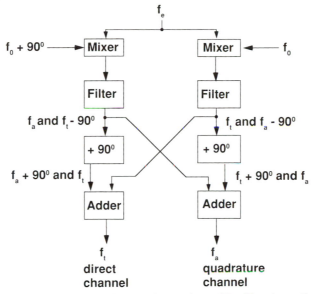

Figure 5.3. The phase quadrature detector detects the positive (f_t) and negative (f_a) Doppler shifts contained in the incoming echo voltage (f_e) and separates them into two channels for delivery to loudspeakers and visual display. These channels are called direct and quadrature (on the left and right, respectively). Detection proceeds as follows. The echo voltage is mixed with the oscillator voltage (f_o) in two mixers. The oscillator voltage in the direct channel leads that in the quadrature channel by one quarter cycle (90 degrees; see Fig. 5.4). The frequency sum ($f_e + f_o$) is filtered out, as in Figure 5.2, yielding the Doppler shift f_D, which is $f_e - f_o$. The Doppler shift may be positive (f_t, for flow toward the transducer) or negative (f_a, for flow away from the transducer). Because of the oscillator-voltage phase difference ($f_o + 90°$ versus f_o), the two filter outputs are different. Positive shifts in the direct channel lag behind those in the quadrature channel by 90 degrees (Fig. 5.5A). Negative shifts in the quadrature channel lag behind those in the direct channel by 90 degrees (Fig. 5.5B). Next, a further 90-degree phase shift results in the separation of the positive and negative shifts into separate channels, direct and quadrature, respectively, as follows. The phase-shifted positive Doppler shifts in the direct channel are now in phase with the unshifted ones in the quadrature channel (Fig. 5.5C); the negative shifts are 180 degrees out of phase (Fig. 5.5D). When added together, the negative shifts cancel (Figs. 5.4B and C), yielding positive shifts as the output voltage in the direct channel. A similar process in the quadrature channel yields the negative shifts as output.

If the Doppler shift is positive (flow toward the transducer), the shift in the direct channel lags behind that in the quadrature channel by one quarter of a cycle (90 degrees). If the Doppler shift is negative (receding flow), the shift in the quadrature channel lags behind that in the direct channel by one quarter of a cycle. The Doppler shifts in each of these channels are then shifted by one quarter of a cycle. A negative shift in the direct channel now leads the one in the quadrature channel (prior to the additional 90-degree shift) by one half of a cycle.

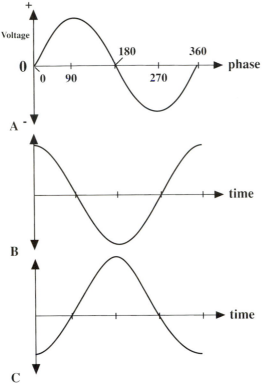

Figure 5.4. (A) One complete variation (cycle) of alternating voltage may be thought of as traveling around a 360-degree circle. One quarter of a cycle is 90 degrees of the phase angle. Phase is a description of the progression through a cycle (analogous to phases of the moon). One quarter of a cycle is 90 degrees, and one half is 180 degrees. At 360 degrees, the cycle is completed, but this is also the 0-degree phase of the next cycle. (B) This voltage leads (A) by 90 degrees (one-quarter cycle). (C) This voltage lags (A) by 90 degrees and lags (B) by 180 degrees. If (B) and (C) are added together, a zero voltage results (i.e., the two voltages are equal and opposite; therefore, they cancel each other when summed).

When added, these two voltages cancel (Figure 5.5), yielding no output. Positive shifts in these two channels are in phase (no lead or lag), yielding output from the direct channel adder. Positive shifts in the quadrature channel lead those in the direct channel by one half of a cycle; negative shifts in the two channels are in phase. Thus, the output of the quadrature channel adder is negative shifts.

The outputs of the two adders can be sent to separate loudspeakers so that forward and reverse sounds (shifts) may be heard separately. The outputs can also be sent to a visual display to show positive and negative shifts above and below the display's (zero Doppler shift) baseline.

Simpler instruments, such as the hand-held, nondirectional device, yield only the audible output. Analog zero-crossing detector devices (Fig. 5.6) provide an average Doppler shift that changes with time.

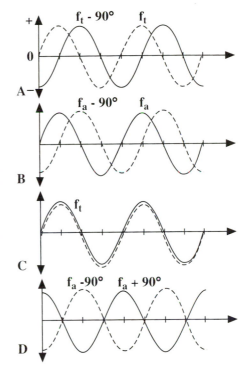

Figure 5.5. Solid curves refer to the direct channel; dashed curves refer to quadrature. The vertical axis is voltage; the horizontal axis is time. (A) Positive Doppler shifts (f_t) at the output of the direct channel filter lag those in the quadrature channel by 90 degrees. (B) Negative Doppler shifts (f_a) at the output of the quadrature channel lag those in the direct channel by 90 degrees. (C) Positive Doppler shifts at the input to the direct channel adder are in phase (0-degree phase difference), yielding an f_t output. (D) Negative Doppler shifts at the input to the direct channel adder are 180 degrees out of phase, yielding a zero f_a output.

This is fed to a strip chart recorder that produces hard copy of the average Doppler shift versus time. The zero-crossing detector counts how often the Doppler shift voltage changes from negative to positive or vice versa. The higher the count is, the higher the frequency is. This count is presented on the vertical axis of a two-dimensional graph in which the horizontal axis represents time (see Fig.5.6c). More sophisticated systems have spectral displays, as discussed in Sections 5.3 and 5.4. The average Doppler shift yielded by the zero-crossing approach favors lower frequencies because the higher ones often do not cross the baseline (see Fig. 5.6a).

Doppler receivers often have a reject or threshold function for the elimination of noise and weaker Doppler signals. Thus, the Doppler receiver has some of the functions of the imaging receiver described in Section 2.3 with the addition of the detection of Doppler shift.

A continuous-wave instrument detects flow that occurs anywhere within the intersection of the transmitting and receiving beams of the dual-transducer assembly (Fig. 5.7). The Doppler sample volume (the region from which Doppler-shifted echoes return and are presented

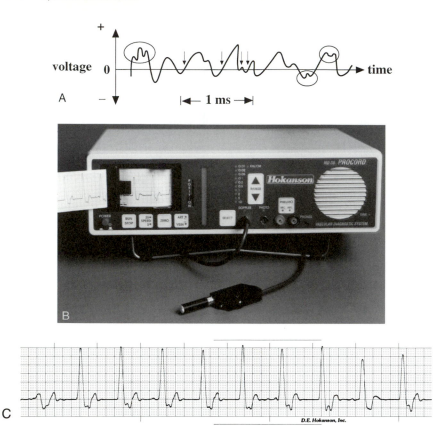

Figure 5.6. (A) A zero-crossing detector counts the number of zero crossings per second in the positive or negative direction. In the 1-ms period shown, four zero crossings (negative to positive) occurred (arrows), corresponding to a mean frequency of 4 kHz. Higher frequencies that are missed by the zero-crossing technique are circled. (B) A zero-crossing continuous-wave Doppler instrument. (C) Chart output from a zero-crossing instrument.

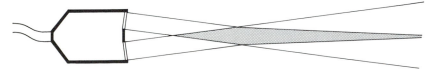

Figure 5.7. Continuous-wave Doppler systems have dual-element transducer assemblies: one for transmitting and one for receiving. The region over which Doppler information can be acquired (Doppler sample volume) is the region of transmitting and receiving beam overlap (shaded region).

audibly or visually) is the overlapping region of the transmitting and receiving beams.

Because the sample volume is large, continuous-wave Doppler systems can give complicated and confusing presentations if reflectors or scatterers with different motions or flows are included in the sound beams (e.g., two blood vessels being viewed simultaneously). Pulsed-Doppler systems (Section 5.2) solve this problem by detecting motion or flow at selected distances or depths with relatively small sample volumes. On the other hand, the large sample volume of a continuous-wave system is helpful when searching for a Doppler maximum, such as when the pressure drop in a stenotic cardiac valve is calculated using the Bernoulli equation (Section 3.3).

Because a distribution of flow velocities is encountered by the sound as it traverses a vessel (see Fig. 3.3 and Section 3.2), a distribution of many Doppler-shifted frequencies returns to the transducer and the instrument (except in the case of pure plug flow). In the arterial circulation or in the heart, these Doppler shifts are continually changing over the cardiac cycle and can be displayed as a function of time with appropriate real-time frequency-spectrum processing (Fig. 5.8 and Sec-

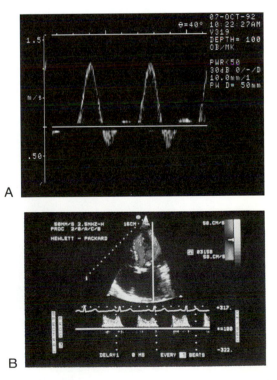

Figure 5.8. (A) Display of Doppler shift frequencies as a function of time (spectral display). (B) Continuous-wave Doppler spectral display from the heart.

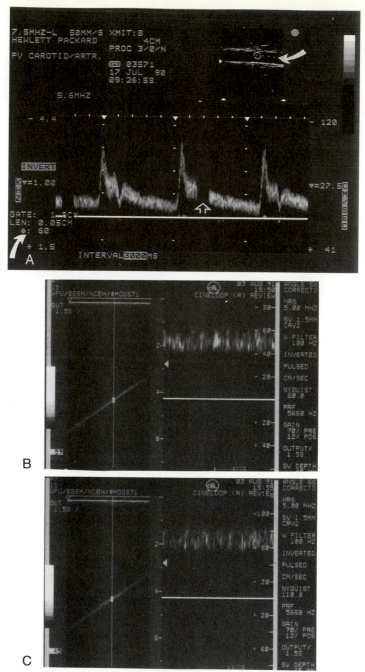

Figure 5.9. (A) Spectral display with Doppler-shift (in kilohertz) calibration of the vertical axis on the left and flow speed (in centimeters per second) calibration on the right. Conversion from the former to the latter requires angle correction (curved arrows). The Doppler angle in this example is 60 degrees. The gap of missing Doppler information (open arrow) occurs when the instrument takes time to generate a frame of the anatomic image (upper right). In (B) and (C), a moving-string test object is imaged and the Doppler spectrum shown. (B) With proper angle correction (56 degrees), the 50-cm/s string speed is correctly shown. (C) With improper angle correction (66 degrees), an incorrect string speed of 70 cm/s is shown. This a 40 percent error.

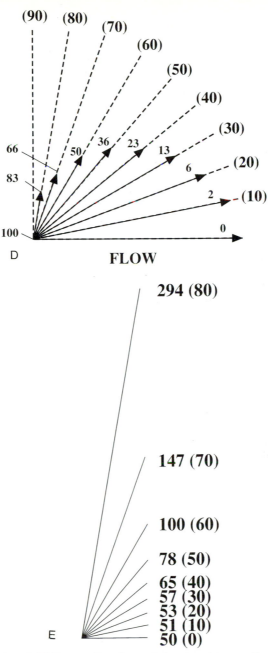

Figure 5.9. *Continued* (D) If a zero Doppler angle is assumed correctly, there is zero error in the calculated flow speed. However, if the angle is actually nonzero, error enters. It increases as the angle error increases. For example, if the Doppler angle is 10 degrees but is assumed to be zero, the calculated flow speed will be 2 percent less than the correct value. At 60 and 80 degrees, the errors are 50 and 83 percent, respectively. At 90 degrees, there is zero Doppler shift. The calculated flow speed is zero (100 percent error). (E) If the Doppler angle is zero but is assumed to be some other value, the calculated flow speeds are too large. Here the value is 50 cm/s. The error increases with angle (in parentheses). For example, at 60 and 80 degrees, the values are 100 and 294 cm/s, respectively. (Parts B and C from Kremkau FW: Doppler principles. Semin Roentgenol 27:6–16, 1992. Reprinted with permission.)

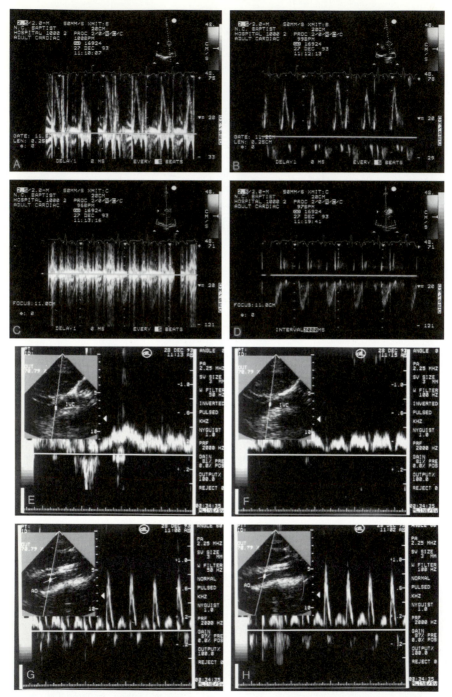

Figure 5.10. *See legend on opposite page*

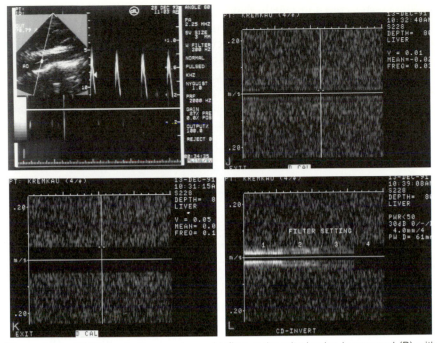

Figure 5.10. (A) Clutter in the spectrum of inflow at the mitral valve is removed (B) with a higher wall-filter setting. (C) Clutter in the spectrum of the left-ventricular outflow tract is removed (D) with higher wall-filter setting. (E) Clutter in the inferior vena caval (IVC) flow is removed with a wall filter (F). (G) Clutter in aortic (AO) flow is removed with a wall filter (H). (I) The wall filter is set too high (200 Hz), eliminating all but the peak systolic portion of the spectrum. (J) Using Doppler receiver noise on the spectrum (with a high Doppler gain), a low wall-filter setting is seen to eliminate Doppler shifts, corresponding to flow speeds less than 1 cm/s. (K) A higher setting eliminates speeds less than 5 cm/s. (L) Four wall-filter settings reduce or eliminate frequencies, as shown.

tions 5.3 and 5.4). These displays provide quantitative data for evaluating Doppler-shifted echoes otherwise presented audibly. The display device is a cathode ray tube, as discussed in Section 2.3. The displayed Doppler information is normally stored in a digital memory (Section 2.3) before display.

To convert a display correctly from Doppler shift versus time to flow speed versus time (see Fig. 5.8), the Doppler angle must be accurately incorporated into the calculation process (Fig. 5.9). Figures 5.9B and C illustrate the importance of accurate angle correction. This is discussed in Section 4.3. Figures 5.9D and E show errors encountered when the Doppler angle is incorrectly handled.

To eliminate the high-intensity, low-frequency Doppler-shift echoes (clutter) resulting from the motion of the heart or vessel wall and cardiac valves with pulsatile flow, a high-pass wall filter (which rejects frequencies below an adjustable value) is utilized (Fig. 5.10). Sometimes called a wall-thump filter, it rejects these strong echoes that would overwhelm the weaker echoes from the blood. These strong echoes have low Doppler-shift frequencies because the walls do not move as fast as the blood does. The upper limit of the filter is adjustable over a range of about 50 to 3200 Hz. Caution should be used with the filter because it can alter conclusions regarding diastolic flow and distal flow resistance (discussed in Section 5.4).

5.2
Pulsed Wave

A diagram of the components of a pulsed-Doppler (pulsed-wave) instrument is given in Figure 5.11A. The voltage generator (oscillator) is similar to that in Figure 5.1. The oscillator gate allows pulses of several cycles of voltage to pass on to the transducer where the ultrasound pulses are produced. As discussed in Chapter 2, imaging pulses are two or three cycles long. The pulses used in pulsed Doppler instruments, however, have minimum pulse lengths of about five cycles. This is necessary to determine the Doppler shifts of returning echoes properly. The pulses may be as long as 25 or 30 cycles. The transducer assembly need only contain one transducer element, which functions as both the source and receiving transducer, although most transducers are arrays, as described in Section 2.2. The voltage pulses resulting

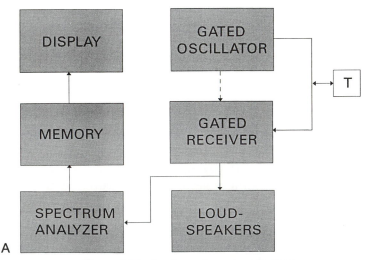

Figure 5.11. *See legend on opposite page*

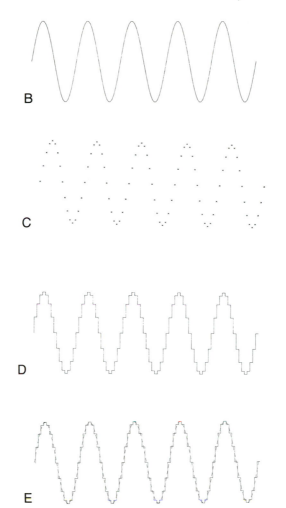

Figure 5.11. (A) Block diagram of pulsed-Doppler instrument. The voltage generator (oscillator) produces a continuously alternating voltage. The generator gate converts this continuous voltage to voltage pulses of several cycles each that drive the transducer (T). Received pulses (echoes) are delivered to the receiver where their frequencies are compared with the oscillator frequency. The difference (Doppler shift) is sent to the loudspeakers and display. The receiver also contains a gate that selects echoes from a given depth, according to their arrival time, and thus gives motion information from a selected depth. (B) Five cycles of a 500-Hz Doppler shift frequency occurring in 10 ms. (C) In a pulsed-Doppler instrument, each pulse yields echoes from the sample volume. These echoes, after Doppler detection, yield samples (x) of the Doppler shift from the sample volume. Here, 80 samples are determined in a 10-ms period. Therefore, pulse repetition frequency of the instrument is 8 kHz (each pulse yielding one sample of the Doppler shift). (D) The pulsed-Doppler receiver gate is also called a sample-and-hold amplifier. It samples the returning stream of echoes (resulting from one emitted pulse of ultrasound) at the appropriate time for the desired depth (see Table 5.1) and holds the value until the next pulse and sample are accomplished. (E) Low-pass filtering (that removes higher frequencies) smooths the sampled result (solid line), yielding the desired Doppler shift waveform (dashed line) comparable to (B).

from received echoes are processed in the receiver. There they are amplified, their frequency is compared with the frequency of the voltage generator, and the Doppler shift's magnitude and sign are derived. The Doppler shifts are sent to loudspeakers for an audible output and to the display for visual observation. Based on their arrival time (see 13 μs/cm rule in Section 2.1), echoes coming from reflectors at a given depth may be selected by the receiver gate; thus, motion information may be obtained from a specific depth. The receiver's gate length and location (depth into tissue) are controllable by the operator. There is no need for time gain (attenuation) compensation in pulsed Doppler instruments.

A continuous-wave Doppler instrument detects the Doppler-shift frequencies, as described in Section 5.1 (phase quadrature detection). A pulsed-Doppler instrument does not detect the complete Doppler shift but rather yields samples of it. The Doppler shifts are determined as described in Section 5.1, except that the mixer does not receive a continuous input echo voltage but one in a pulsed form. Echoes arrive from the sample volume depth in pulsed form at a rate determined by (equal to) the pulse repetition frequency. Each of these returning echoes yields a sample of the Doppler shift from the Doppler detector. These samples are connected and smoothed (filtered) to yield the sampled waveform (Fig. 5.11b to e).

There is an upper limit to Doppler shifts that can be detected by pulsed instruments, which is one half of the pulse repetition frequency (in the range of 5 to 30 kHz). When this limit (sometimes called the Nyquist limit) is exceeded, aliasing occurs (Section 7.1). Improper Doppler-shift information (improper direction and improper value) results. An analogous optical form of aliasing occurs in motion pictures when wagon wheels appear to rotate at various speeds and in a reverse direction. Higher pulse repetition frequencies permit higher Doppler shifts to be detected but also increase the chance of a range ambiguity artifact (Section 7.1). Continuous-wave Doppler instruments do not have this limitation (but neither do they provide any depth localization capability).

The receiver gate selects one listening region (sample volume) from which returning Doppler-shifted echoes are accepted (Table 5.1 and Figs. 5.12 to 5.14). The width of the sample volume is equal to the width of the beam. The gate has some length (depth range) over which it permits reception (Table 5.2). For example (using the rule of a 13-μs round-trip travel time per centimeter of depth [Section 2.1]), a gate that passes echoes arriving from 13 to 15 μs after pulse generation is effectively listening over a depth range of 10.0 to 11.5 mm. In this case, the gate is located at a depth of 10.8 mm with a length (depth range) of $\pm$ 0.8 mm. Generally, larger gate lengths (e.g., 10 mm) are

Table 5–1	

Echo Arrival Time (t) for Various Reflector Depths (Gate Locations)

Depth (mm)	Time (μs)
10	13
20	26
30	39
40	52
50	65
60	78
70	91
80	104
90	117
100	130
150	195
200	260

used when searching for the desired vessel and flow location, with shorter gate lengths (e.g., 2 mm) for spectral analysis (Sections 5.3 and 5.4) and evaluation. The shorter gate length improves the signal-to-noise ratio and the quality of the spectral trace. A single gate allows only one depth and length selection (from which all Doppler-shifted echoes are accepted in combination) at any time.

The Doppler sample volume (the region from which Doppler-shifted echoes return and are presented audibly or visually) is determined by the width of the beam, the receiver gate's length, and the emitted pulse's length. One half of the pulse length is added to the gate length to yield the effective sample volume length (Table 5.3). Thus, the pulse length must shorten as the gate length is reduced. The sample volume width is equal to the beam width at the sample volume depth.

The volume flow rate (in milliliters per second) can be calculated from the mean flow speed multiplied by the vessel's cross-sectional area. To do this correctly, the various Doppler shifts representing the cells moving at various speeds must be averaged properly, the angle properly accounted for to convert mean Doppler shift to mean speed, and the vessel cross-sectional area correctly determined. Several things can go wrong in this process, yielding faulty results.[25]

Combinations of instruments discussed in Sections 2.3, 5.1, and 5.2 are available commercially. Pulsed- and continuous-wave Doppler are often available in the same instrument. Real-time, cross-sectional ultrasound imaging (sonography) instruments are available with pulsed Doppler or both continuous- and pulsed-wave Doppler. These provide the ability to image anatomic structures and analyze motion and flow at a known point in the anatomic field (see Fig. 5.9a). Imaging allows intelligent positioning of the gate and angle correction in a

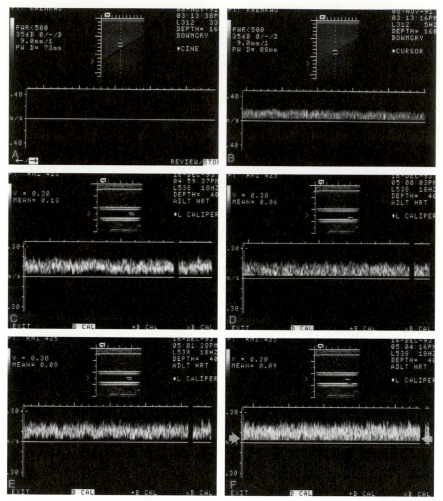

Figure 5.12. (A) The pulse-Doppler sample volume is located at a 73-mm depth (95-μs arrival time). No Doppler shift is seen on the lower display because the Doppler-shifted echoes from within the tube arrive at about 114 μs. (B) When the gate is open later (corresponding to an 88-mm depth), the Doppler shifts are received and displayed (constant flow rate in the tube). (C) The gate is located in the center of the tube. (D) The gate is located near the tube wall. The mean flow speed is 6 cm/s compared with the 13-cm/s flow speed in Part C. This is the expected result with laminar flow. (E) The gate is again located at the center of the tube. (F) The gate length is extended to include the flow from the center out to the tube wall. Note the strengthening of the lower flow speeds (Doppler shifts) (arrows) compared with those in Part E in which the slower flow is not included in the sample volume.

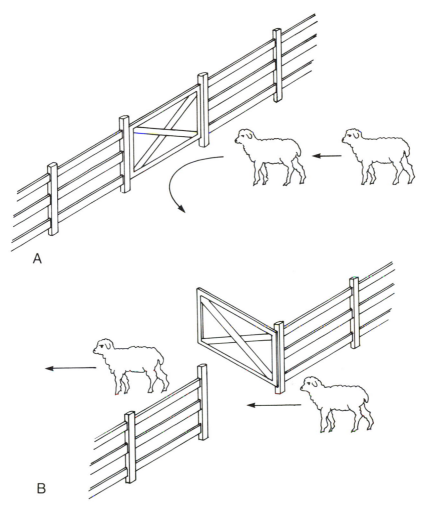

Figure 5.13. (A) Two sheep arrive at a closed gate and are not received into the pen. (B) Two sheep arrive later at the gate when it is open and are received. In a Doppler receiver, the gate accepts and rejects echoes in a similar manner.

pulsed-wave Doppler system. The availability of continuous- and pulsed-wave Doppler in the same system is useful because difficulty is encountered in a pulsed system if the flow rates become so high that the Doppler shift exceeds one half of the pulse repetition frequency (aliasing occurs) (Section 7.1). At that point, the ability to shift to the continuous-wave system (even though it means giving up depth localization) is advantageous. Continuous-wave Doppler is also useful

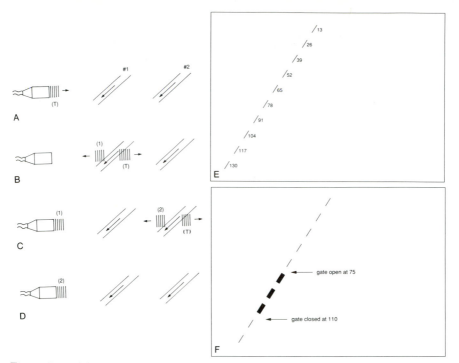

Figure 5.14. (A) A pulse (T) leaves the transducer. (B) An echo (1) is generated in vessel 1. (C) Echo 1 arrives at the transducer. At the same time, another echo (2) is generated at vessel 2. (D) Echo 2 arrives at the transducer after echo 1 did (C). These echoes will be processed by the instrument if the receiver gate is open when they arrive. (E) Echoes from 1-, 2-, 3-, 4-, 5-, 6-, 7-, 8-, 9-, and 10-cm depths arrive at the times (in microseconds) indicated. (F) If the gate is open from 75 to 100 μs after pulse emission, only the echoes in (E) arriving at 78, 91, and 104 μs are accepted. The others are rejected.

Table 5–2

Spatial Gate Length for Various Temporal Gate Lengths

Length (mm)	Time (μs)
1	1.3
2	2.6
3	3.9
4	5.2
5	6.5
10	13.0
15	19.5
20	26.0

Table 5–3		
Amount Added to Effective Gate Length by Pulse Length for Various Cycles per Pulse and Frequencies		
Added (mm)	Cycles	Frequencies (MHz)
1.9	5	2
3.8	10	2
7.7	20	2
0.8	5	5
1.5	10	5
3.1	20	5
0.4	5	10
0.8	10	10
1.5	20	10

when searching for a maximum Doppler shift, such as when the pressure drop (using the Bernoulli equation) across a stenotic cardiac valve is determined.

Duplex systems must be time shared. That is, imaging and Doppler-flow measurements cannot be done simultaneously. Systems using mechanical transducers (Fig. 2.25) must stop the transducer movement to perform the Doppler function. The anatomic image is frozen on the display during Doppler acquisition. Electronic scanning with arrays (Figs. 2.26 to 2.29) permits rapid switching between imaging and Doppler functions (several times per second), allowing what can appear to be simultaneous acquisition of real-time image and Doppler-flow information (see Fig. 5.9a to c). Imaging frame rates are slowed to allow for the acquisition of Doppler information between frames.

5.3
Spectral Analysis

The demodulated (Doppler shift) voltage from the receiver in Figure 5.1 does not go directly to the display but undergoes further processing. Otherwise, it would look like Figure 5.15a. This is what a listener hears from the loudspeaker. Spectral analysis provides a more meaningful and useful way to present the Doppler information visually.

"Spectral" means relating to a spectrum. A spectrum is an array of the components of a wave separated and arranged in the order of increasing wavelength or frequency. "Analysis" comes from a Greek word meaning to break up (i.e., to take apart). Thus, spectral analysis

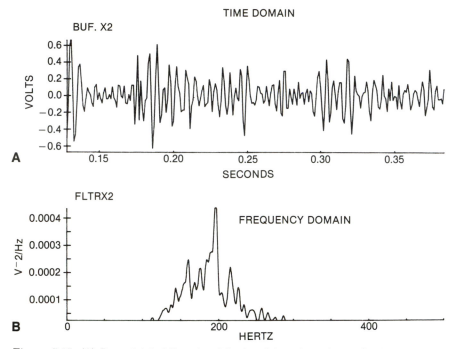

Figure 5.15. (A) Demodulated Doppler-shift signal for microspheres flowing at nearly uniform speed. When applied to a loudspeaker, a mix of many frequencies is heard. Approximately 10 cycles occur over the period 0.20 to 0.25 seconds. Thus, the fundamental period of this signal is about 5 ms, yielding a fundamental frequency of 200 Hz. (B) After the Fourier transform is applied, a frequency spectrum is obtained. The center frequency is approximately 200 Hz. This is what was predicted in Part A. (From Burns PN: The physical principles of Doppler and spectral analysis. J Clin Ultrasound *15*:567–590, 1987. Copyright © 1987. Reprinted by permission of John Wiley & Sons, Inc.)

is the breaking up of the components of a complex wave or signal and spreading them out in frequency order.

A prism does this for light. When white light passes through a prism, it is separated into a sequence of the various colors that make up the white appearance. White light is a combination of the full range of frequencies (colors) visible to the human eye. Frequency is interpreted as color by the brain, with red being the lowest frequency and violet being the highest. The prism breaks up these frequency components and spreads them out so that the various colors are seen in what is called a color spectrum. A similar process is performed electronically for the returning echoes in a Doppler system.

The human auditory system does this for sound. The ear and brain break down the complex sounds we receive into the component frequencies contained in the sounds. Thus, we can listen to a Doppler signal and recognize normal and abnormal flow sounds. A visual presentation of these sounds provides the additional capacity to recognize flow characteristics and diagnose disease.

In Chapter 3, flow profiles in vessels were described. The character of the flow profiles was determined by the size of the vessel and the uniformity of its wall. Changes in size, turns, and abnormalities, such as the presence of plaques and stenoses, alter the character of the flow. Flow can be characterized as plug, laminar, parabolic, disturbed, and turbulent. Except for pure plug flow, portions of the flowing fluid within a vessel are moving at different speeds (even for normal steady flow) and, sometimes, in different directions. Thus, as the ultrasound beam intersects this flow and echoes are produced, many different Doppler shifts are received from the vessel by the system (even from a small sample volume). If all the blood cells were moving at the same speed and in the same direction, a single Doppler shift would result. However, this is not the case. The extent of the range of generated Doppler-shift frequencies depends on the character of the flow. For near-plug flow (normal flow in a large vessel), a narrow range of Doppler-shift frequencies is received. In smaller vessels, and in disturbed and turbulent flow, much broader ranges of Doppler-shift frequencies can be received. Other vessels can have an intermediate-flow character called blunted parabolic flow.

The fast Fourier transform (FFT) is the mathematic technique[26-28] that the instrument uses to derive the Doppler spectrum from the returning echoes of various frequencies (Figs. 5.15 and 5.16). The FFT displays can show spectral broadening, which is the widening of the Doppler-shift spectrum, i.e., the increase of the range of Doppler-shift frequencies present, as a result of a broader range of flow speeds and directions encountered by the sound beam. This occurs for normal flow in smaller vessels and for disturbed and turbulent flow in any vessel.

The FFT process includes sampling the complicated (containing many frequencies) Doppler signal, typically, 25,600 times per second (25.6-kHz sampling rate). A 10-ms period (yielding 256 samples) is sufficient to provide a useful spectrum. Thus, 100 spectra per second can be produced. Each spectrum can include the amplitudes of 128 frequencies, the lowest of which is equal to the number of FFTs per second (100 Hz here) and the highest being one half of the sampling rate (12.8 kHz here). This rapid sequence of FFT-generated spectra can be displayed visually, as described in the following section.

5.4

Spectral Displays

The received Doppler signal is a combination of many Doppler-shift frequencies, yielding a complicated waveform (see Figs. 5.15a and 5.16b). Using the FFT discussed in the previous section, these frequencies are separated into a spectrum that can be presented on a two-dimensional display as the Doppler-shift frequency on the horizontal axis and the power or amplitude of each frequency component on the vertical axis (see Figs. 5.15b and 5.16a). For venous flow, such a spectral display would commonly be rather constant. However, for the pulsatile flow in the arterial circulation, such a presentation would be continually changing, shifting to the right in systole as the blood accelerates and Doppler shifts increase, shifting to the left in diastole, and changing in power or amplitude over the cardiac cycle.

The interpretation of this changing presentation is difficult, and indeed, the character of the changes over the cardiac cycle could be important. Therefore, a presentation of this changing spectrum as a

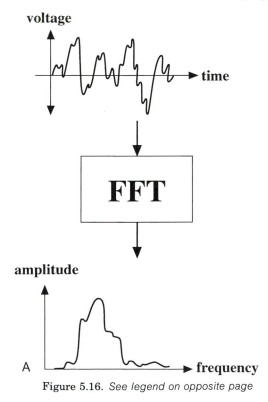

Figure 5.16. *See legend on opposite page*

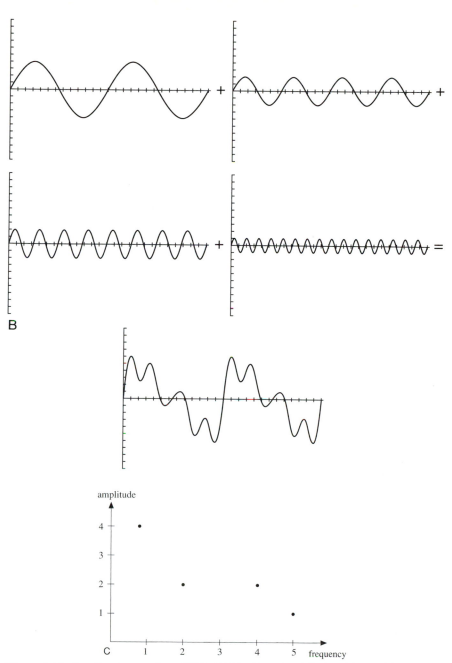

Figure 5.16. Fast Fourier transform (FFT). (A) The Doppler-shift signal (containing many frequencies) is transformed by the FFT into a spectrum. [Figure 5.15 shows an example of the Doppler signal (A) before and (B) after FFT processing.] (B) Four voltages of different frequencies are combined to give the complicated result. (C) FFT analysis of this combined voltage would yield this spectrum.

145

function of time is valuable and useful. Such a trace is shown in Figures 5.17 and 5.18. The two-display dimensions are used in this presentation as follows. The vertical axis represents the Doppler-shift frequency, and the horizontal axis represents time (Fig. 5.19). The amplitude or power of each Doppler-shift frequency component at any instant (vertical axis in Fig. 5.15b) is now presented as brightness (gray scale) (see Fig. 5.8a) or color (see Fig. 1.3b, Color Plate I). Doppler signal power is proportional to blood cell density (number of cells per unit volume).

Usually, a bright spot on a spectral display means that a strong Doppler-shift frequency component at that instant of time was received

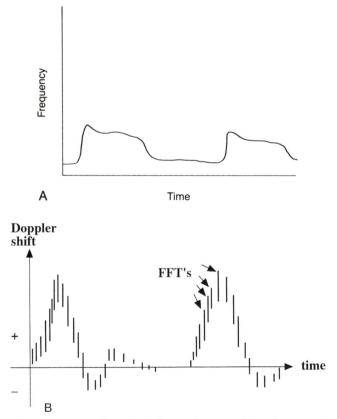

Figure 5.17. (A) A display of Doppler shift as a function of time for pure plug flow. The Doppler shift frequency is on the vertical axis. The amplitude of the Doppler-shift frequency at each instant of time is represented by gray level or color. In this example, there is only a single shift frequency at each instant of time (i.e., no spectrum). (B) A spectral display for nonplug flow is composed of several FFT spectra arranged vertically next to each other across the time (horizontal) axis.

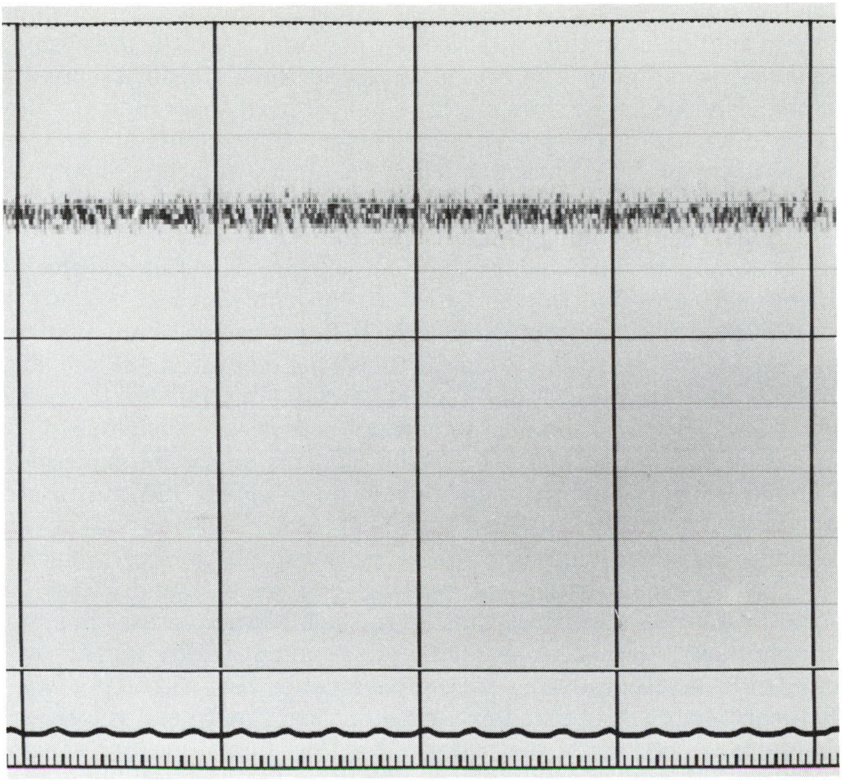

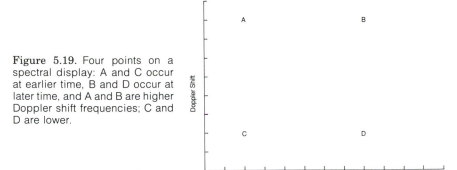

Figure 5.18. A spectral display of the signal shown in Figure 5.15. The flow is constant, yielding Doppler shift frequencies around 200 Hz (horizontal markers represent 100 Hz). (From Burns PN: The physical principles of Doppler and spectral analysis. J Clin Ultrasound *15*:567–590, 1987. Copyright © 1987. Reprinted by permission of John Wiley & Sons, Inc.)

Figure 5.19. Four points on a spectral display: A and C occur at earlier time, B and D occur at later time, and A and B are higher Doppler shift frequencies; C and D are lower.

A   B

Doppler Shift

C   D

Time

(see Fig. 5.8). A dark spot means that a Doppler-shift frequency component at that point in time was weak or nonexistent. If the gray scale is reversed, as in Figure 5.18, bright represents weak and dark represents strong. Intermediate values of gray shade or brightness indicate intermediate amplitudes or powers of frequency components at the given times. A strong signal at a particular frequency and time means that there are many scattering blood cells moving at velocities (speeds and directions) corresponding to that Doppler shift. A weak frequency (usually presented as dark) means that few cells are traveling at velocities corresponding to that Doppler shift at that point in time.

Spectral trace presentations provide information about flow that can be used to discern conditions at the site of measurement and distal to it.[29,30] Peak flow speeds and spectral broadening indicate the degree of stenosis. Spectral broadening means a vertical thickening of the spectral trace (Fig. 5.20). If all the cells were moving at the same speed, a single Doppler-shift frequency would be received, and the spectral trace would be a thin line (see Fig. 5.17a). As described in the previous section, this is not found in practice. However, narrow spectra can be observed, particularly in large vessels (see Figs. 3.12 and 5.21a). The apparent narrowing of the spectrum as the blood accelerates in systole can be misinterpreted. A spectrum of consistent width appears to be thinner in a steeply rising portion of a curve (Fig. 5.22). As flow is disturbed or becomes turbulent, greater variation in the velocities of the various portions of the flowing blood produce a greater range of Doppler-shift frequencies. This results in a broader spectrum being presented on the spectral display (see Fig. 5.20A to D). Thus, spectral broadening indicates disturbed or turbulent flow and can be related to pathologic conditions. However, spectral broadening can be artificially produced by excessive Doppler receiver gain (see Fig. 5.20E and F).

Another term related to spectral broadening is "window." This refers to the dark (or light for white-background displays) anechoic area in the lower portion of the spectral trace, particularly in systole for normal flow (see Figs. 5.20A and 5.21a). As flow is disturbed or becomes turbulent, spectral broadening occurs, and the window is diminished or eliminated (see Fig. 5.20). Therefore, spectral broadening and window reduction or loss are equivalent terms.

Narrow spectra are expected in large vessels, broad spectra in small vessels, and intermediate spectra in medium-sized vessels. This is shown in Figure 5.21. Using pulsed-wave Doppler to monitor flow at various sites inside a vessel, a narrow spectrum would be expected near the center of the vessel (where the cells are moving the fastest), and a broader spectrum would be expected near the walls where viscous drag is slowing the flow. This is shown in Figures 5.12C to F and 5.23.

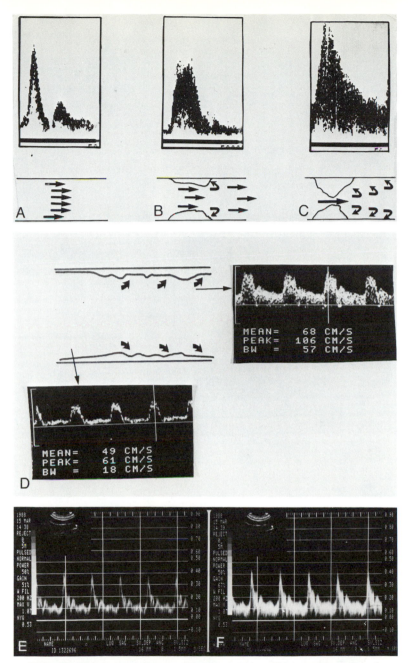

Figure 5.20. (A) With normal flow and a plug or blunt flow speed profile, there is a narrow spectrum. (B) Disturbed flow produces spectral broadening. (C) Significant stenosis produces much spectral broadening and an altered waveform shape (Parts A to C from Burns PN: The physical principles of Doppler and spectral analysis. J Clin Ultrasound *15*:567–590, 1987. Copyright © 1987. Reprinted by permission of John Wiley & Sons, Inc.) (D) Spectral broadening produced by an atheroma. (E) Correct Doppler receiver gain setting. (F) Apparent spectral broadening caused by excessive gain. (Parts D to F from Taylor KJW, Holland S: State-of-the-art Doppler ultrasound I. Basic principles, instrumentation and pitfalls. Radiology *174*:297–307, 1990. Reprinted with permission.)

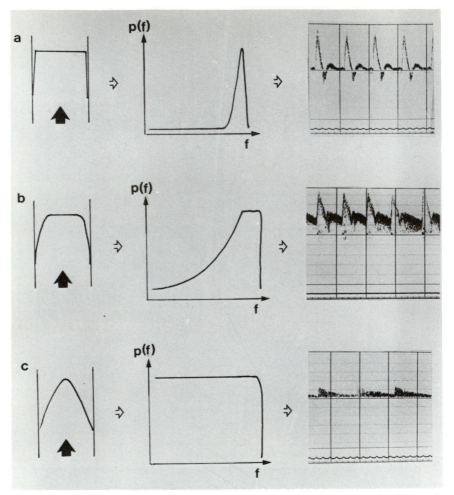

Figure 5.21. Flow-speed profiles (left), Doppler spectra (power versus frequency) (center), and spectral displays (right) for (a) nearly plug flow in the aorta, (b) blunted parabolic flow in the celiac trunk, and (c) parabolic flow in the ovarian artery. (From Burns PN: The physical principles of Doppler and spectral analysis. J Clin Ultrasound *15*:567–590, 1987. Copyright © 1987. Reprinted by permission of John Wiley & Sons, Inc.)

Complicated flow (for example, in the vicinity of the carotid bulb and flow divider) is not as easily predicted but is different at various sites (Fig. 5.24). Turbulent flow may occur during short portions of the cardiac cycle when high enough flow speeds are achieved. Spectral broadening does not necessarily indicate turbulence. Figure 5.25 shows a broad spectrum that is probably not caused by disturbed or turbulent flow but simply by complicated geometry, i.e., a tortuous vessel causing

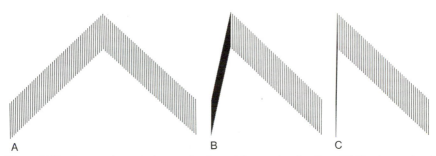

Figure 5.22. Apparent spectral narrowing in rapidly accelerating flow. (A) Slowly accelerating and decelerating flow shows that the spectral widths (bandwidths) are all equal. In (B) and (C), as the acceleration phase becomes steeper, it appears to have a narrower bandwidth. However, the vertical lines representing bandwidth in all cases are the same.

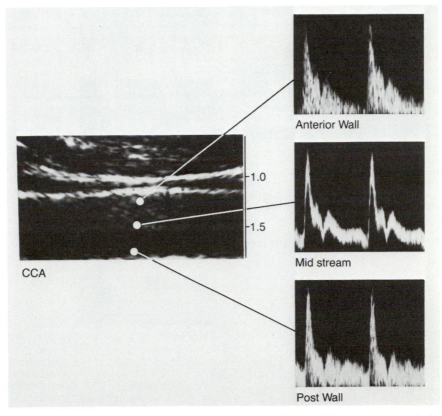

Figure 5.23. Spectral traces showing increased spectral bandwidth near vessel walls in the common carotid artery (CCA). As expected, a narrower bandwidth is found at midstream. (From Taylor DC, Strandness DE: Carotid artery duplex scanning. J Clin Ultrasound 15:635–644, 1987. Copyright © 1987. Reprinted by permission of John Wiley & Sons, Inc.)

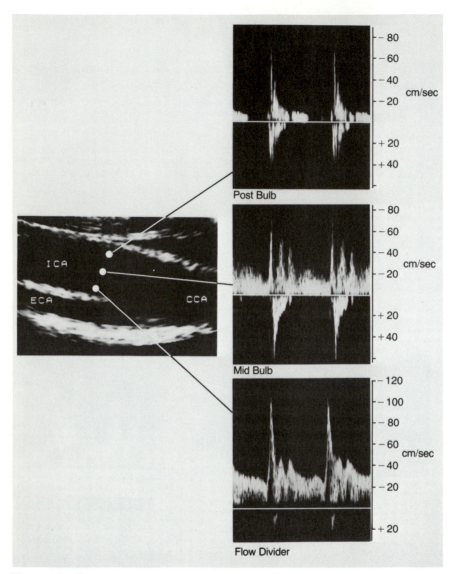

Figure 5.24. Spectral waveforms show laminar flow with mild spectral broadening adjacent to the carotid bifurcation and areas of increasing turbulence and boundary layer separation along the outer aspect of the carotid bulb. ICA, internal carotid artery; ECA, external carotid artery; CCA, common carotid artery. (From Taylor DC, Strandness DE: Carotid artery duplex scanning. J Clin Ultrasound 15:635–644, 1987. Copyright © 1987. Reprinted by permission of John Wiley & Sons, Inc.)

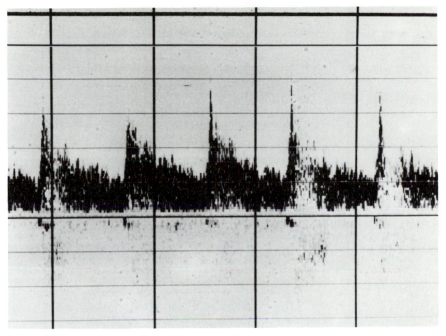

Figure 5.25. Spectral trace from the splenic artery showing spectral broadening probably caused by the tortuous character of the vessel. (From Burns PN: The physical principles of Doppler and spectral analysis. J Clin Ultrasound *15*:567–590, 1987. Copyright © 1987. Reprinted by permission of John Wiley & Sons, Inc.)

a variety of Doppler angles and therefore a broad range (spectrum) of Doppler-shift frequencies. A broad spectrum can be found, even in large vessels, if the sample volume length covers a large portion of the vessel diameter (see Figs. 5.12F and 5.26).

As mentioned at the beginning of this section, Doppler-flow measurements can yield information regarding downstream (distal) conditions. Flow reversal in early diastole and lack of flow in late diastole (see Figs. 3.12 and 5.21a) indicate high resistance to flow downstream (e.g., because of vasoconstriction of the arterioles).[9] If flow resistance is reduced because of vasodilation, impressive differences in the spectral display are observed (Fig. 5.27). A comparison between low- and high-resistance flow spectra is given in Figures 1.4 and 5.28.

Normal vessels can be occluded in diastole when the pressure drops below the critical value for flow.[9] When this happens, no diastolic Doppler shift is detected. Various quantitative indices have been developed to describe such differences in spectral traces that indicate downstream conditions (Fig. 5.29 and Table 5.4). The differences in spectral-trace shapes for high- and low-resistance flow and for high- and

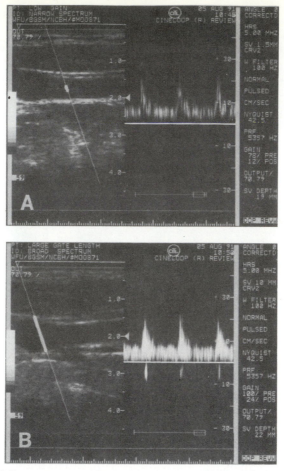

Figure 5.26. (A) Narrow spectrum from a common carotid artery using a small (1.5-mm) sample gate. (B) Spectral broadening resulting from the inclusion of all the flow across the vessel with a large gate (10 mm). (From Kremkau FW: Doppler principles. Semin Roentgenol 27:6–16, 1992. Reprinted with permission.)

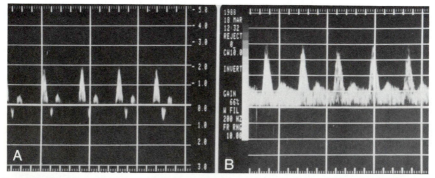

Figure 5.27. (A) High-resistance flow in the popliteal artery with the leg at rest. (B) Low-resistance flow after minimal exercise. (From Taylor KJW, Holland S: Doppler ultrasound I. Basic principles, instrumentation and pitfalls. Radiology 174:297–307, 1990. Reprinted with permission.)

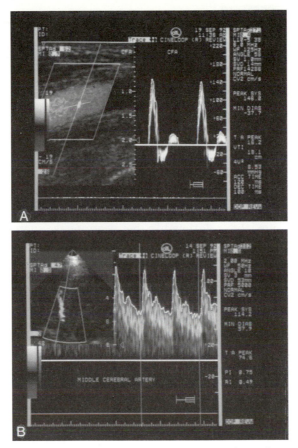

Figure 5.28. (A) High-resistance flow is seen in the common femoral artery of the resting lower limb. (B) Low-resistance flow is seen in the middle cerebral artery. Although these spectral displays are very different, they are both normal for the locations and conditions given.

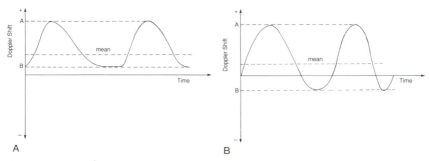

Figure 5.29. Spectral display of peak Doppler shift as a function of time. A represents the maximum value at peak systole, and B represents the minimum value at end diastole. (A) Unidirectional flow. (B) Reverse flow in diastole.

Table 5–4		
Spectral Display Indices		
Name	**Abbreviation**	**Expression***
Pulsatility index	PI	$\dfrac{A - B}{\text{mean}}$
Resistance Index	RI	$\dfrac{A - B}{A}$
Systolic to diastolic ratio	SDR	$\dfrac{A}{B}$
B/A ratio	BAR	$\dfrac{B}{A}$

* See Figure 5.29 for the meaning of A and B.

low-angle measurements are shown in Figure 5.30. Changing the angle does not change the relationship between peak systolic and end-diastolic flows, but changing the distal resistance does (see Figs. 5.27 and 5.30). The pulsatility-index approach works because flow resistance is not constant over the cardiac cycle with distensible vessels and pulsatile pressures. That is, resistance is not constant but is greater at lower pressures and smaller at higher pressures. For rigid pipes, resistance does not depend on pressure (Poiseuille's law, Section 3.2). Care must be exercised in the use of the wall filter because it can affect the pulsatility index (Fig. 5.31 and 5.10I).

The interpretation of spectral-trace information can be easily oversimplified. In Figure 5.32, it may appear that A represents the fastest blood flow. It is true that A represents the largest Doppler shift on this spectral display, but laminar flow is necessary for the largest spectral Doppler shift to correspond to the largest flow speed. In Figure 5.33, for example, the arrows indicate that the highest Doppler shifts correspond to the fastest flow and the lowest, to the slowest. This simplified approach is true only for undisturbed and nonturbulent flow in which all portions of fluid are flowing parallel to each other with a common Doppler angle.

The correlation of high flow speed with high Doppler shift, as shown in Figure 5.33, seems straightforward. However, this is only true if all portions of the fluid are moving parallel so that they all have the same Doppler angle with the ultrasound beam. If flow is disturbed or turbulent (see Fig. 5.20), if the vessel is tortuous (see Fig. 5.25), or if flow is helical, as claimed for the carotid artery,[13,14] this assumption is not valid. Then the simple interpretation is incorrect. The peak Doppler shifts do not necessarily represent the fastest flow but, possibly, slow flow that is moving directly toward the transducer (a small Doppler angle and a high Doppler shift). Likewise, the lowest Doppler shifts do not necessarily represent the slowest flow but, possibly, fast flow

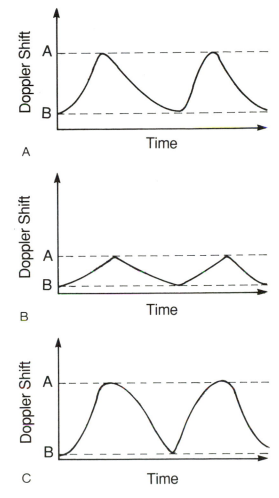

Figure 5.30. (A) Spectral trace for low-resistance, low-angle flow. (B) Spectral trace for low-resistance, high-angle flow. All portions of the Doppler shift are proportionally reduced. (C) Spectral trace for high-resistance, low-angle flow. Diastolic portions of the flow are reduced more than are the systolic portions. This would yield a larger pulsatility index, indicating higher distal flow resistance.

that is moving nearly perpendicular to the beam (a large Doppler angle and a low Doppler shift). Spectral traces that have their vertical axes calibrated in speed units (meter or centimeter per second) are correct presentations only if the Doppler angle correction is proper (Sections 4.3 and 5.1) *and* straight parallel laminar undisturbed flow is being measured.

Flow velocity is a vector, i.e., it has speed and direction. A Doppler instrument detects a Doppler shift that is proportional to speed of flow along the direction of the sound beam (the magnitude of the component of the velocity vector parallel to the beam, see Fig. 4.9a). Thus, if the flow is not straight (parallel), large Doppler shifts do not necessarily

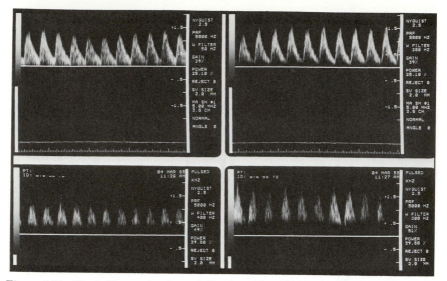

Figure 5.31. Effect of increasing the wall filter from 50 to 800 Hz simulates the appearance of a high-resistance flow and can lead to a misdiagnosis. (From Taylor KJW, Holland S: State-of-the-art Doppler ultrasound I. Basic principles, instrumentation and pitfalls. Radiology *174*:297–307, 1990. Reprinted with permission.)

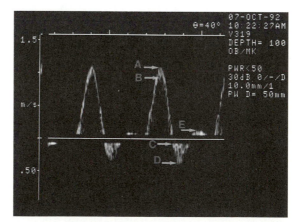

Figure 5.32. Pulsatile Doppler spectrum from a Doppler flow phantom. A is maximum and B is minimum Doppler shift at peak systole. C and D are minimum and maximum shifts in early diastole. E is maximum shift in late diastole. (From Kremkau FW: Fluid flow III. J Vasc Technol *17*:321–322, 1993. Reprinted with permission.)

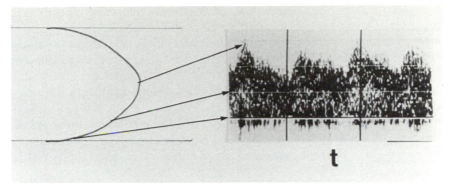

Figure 5.33. Broad spectrum of parabolic flow in a small vessel. The arrows suggest that the highest Doppler shifts correspond to the fastest flow and the lowest, to the slowest. This simplified approach is true only for undisturbed and nonturbulent flow in which all portions of fluid are flowing parallel to each other (common Doppler angle). (From Taylor KJW, Holland S: Doppler ultrasound I. Basic principles, instrumentation and pitfalls. Radiology *174*:297–307, 1990. Reprinted with permission.)

correspond to the fastest flow, and small ones do not necessarily correspond to the slowest flow (Fig. 5.34).

5.5
Review

Doppler instruments make use of the Doppler shift to yield information regarding motion and flow. Continuous-wave systems provide motion and flow information without depth selection capability. Pulsed-Doppler systems provide the ability to select the depth from which the Doppler information is received. Spectral analysis provides visual information on the distribution of received Doppler-shift frequencies

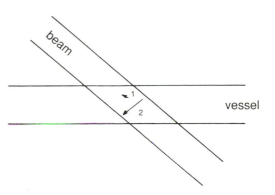

Figure 5.34. A large flow vector can produce a smaller Doppler shift than a small one if they are not parallel. This small flow vector (1) has a larger component along the beam than the large vector (2) that is nearly perpendicular to the beam. (From Kremkau FW: Fluid flow III. J Vasc Technol *17*:321–322, 1993. Reprinted with permission.)

that result from the distribution of scatterer velocities (speeds and directions) encountered. In addition to audible output, the imaging of flow spectra is possible in Doppler systems. Combined (duplex) systems that use dynamic sonography and continuous- and pulsed-wave Doppler are available commercially (Fig. 5.35A) The color-flow capability discussed in Chapter 6 can also be included. The Doppler controls discussed in this chapter are illustrated in Figure 5.35.

The Doppler spectrum is generated by the range of scatterer velocities encountered by the ultrasound beam. It is derived electronically by using the FFT and presented on the display as the Doppler shift

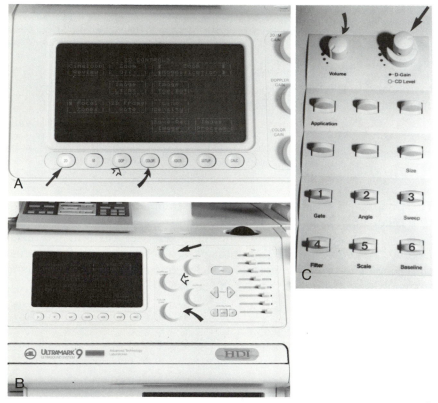

Figure 5.35. (A) This instrument provides push-button selection of gray-scale anatomic imaging (arrow), spectral Doppler (open arrow), color-flow (curved arrow), or combinations of these operating modes. (B) Gray-scale gain (arrow), spectral Doppler gain (open arrow), and color-flow gain controls (curved arrow) are indicated. (C) Doppler controls include gain (arrow), loudspeaker volume (curved arrow), gate length (1), Doppler angle correction (2), spectral display time (horizontal) axis sweep speed (3), wall filter setting (4), spectral display vertical axis scale setting (Nyquist limit and pulse repetition frequency control) (5), and baseline shift control (6). (D and E) Software panel controls for Doppler functions.

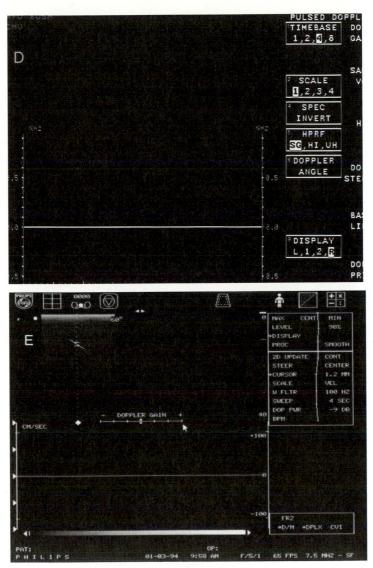

Figure 5.35. *Continued*

versus time, with brightness indicating power. Flow conditions at the site of measurement are indicated by the width of the spectrum, with spectral broadening and loss of window indicating disturbed and turbulent flow. Flow conditions downstream, particularly distal flow resistance, are indicated by the relationship between peak systolic and end-diastolic flow speeds. Various indices for quantitatively presenting this information have been developed. Overly simplistic interpretation of spectral traces should be avoided.

The definitions of terms used in this chapter are listed next.

Bidirectional. Indicating Doppler instruments capable of distinguishing between positive and negative Doppler shifts (forward and reverse flow).

Clutter. Noise in the Doppler signal generally caused by high-amplitude, Doppler-shifted echoes from moving heart or vessel walls.

Continuous wave. A wave in which cycles repeat indefinitely. Not pulsed.

Doppler angle. The angle between the sound beam and the flow direction.

Duplex instrument. An ultrasound instrument that combines gray-scale sonography with pulsed Doppler and possibly continuous-wave Doppler.

Fast Fourier transform (FFT). Digital computer implementation of the Fourier transform.

Fourier analysis. The application of the Fourier transform to determine the frequency components present.

Fourier transform. A mathematic technique for obtaining a Doppler spectrum.

Frequency spectrum. The range of frequencies present. In a Doppler instrument, the range of Doppler-shift frequencies present in the returning echoes.

Generator gate. The electronic portion of a pulsed-Doppler system that converts the continuous voltage of the voltage generator to a pulsed voltage.

Pulse repetition frequency. The number of pulses per unit time. Sometimes called the pulse repetition rate.

Pulsed Doppler. A Doppler device or procedure that uses pulsed-wave ultrasound.

Pulsed mode. The mode of operation in which pulsed ultrasound is used.

Pulsed ultrasound. Ultrasound produced in pulse form by applying electric pulses or voltages of a few cycles to the transducer.

Pulsed wave. A wave consisting of a series of pulses each containing a few cycles of ultrasound. Not continuous.

Range gating. Selecting the depth from which echoes are accepted based on the echo's arrival time.

Receiver gate. A device that allows only echoes from a selected depth (arrival time) to pass.

Sample volume. The region from which Doppler shifts are acquired.

Signal. Information-bearing voltages in an electric circuit. An acoustic, visual, electric, or other conveyance of information.

Spectral analysis. Separating frequencies in a Doppler signal for display as a Doppler spectrum.

Spectral broadening. The widening of the Doppler-shift spectrum, i.e., the increase of the range of Doppler-shift frequencies present because of a broader range of flow velocities encountered by the sound beam. Occurs for normal flow in smaller vessels and for turbulent flow in any vessel.

Spectral display. The visual display of a Doppler spectrum.

Spectral width. The range of Doppler shifts or flow speeds present at a given point in time.

Spectrum. A range of frequencies.

Spectrum analyzer. A device that derives a frequency spectrum from a complex signal.

Wall filter. An electric filter that passes frequencies above a set level and eliminates strong low-frequency Doppler shifts (clutter) from the pulsating heart or vessel walls.

Window. An anechoic region underneath a region of echo frequencies presented on a Doppler spectral display.

Zero-crossing detector. A simple analog detector that yields the mean Doppler shift as a function of time.

Exercises

5.1 All Doppler instruments distinguish between positive and negative Doppler shifts. True or false?

5.2 Instruments that distinguish between positive and negative Doppler shifts yield motion _____ information and are called _____.

5.3 Continuous-wave Doppler instruments use single-element transducers similar to those used in imaging. True or false?

5.4 The components of a continuous-wave Doppler system include _____, _____, _____, _____, _____ _____, _____, and _____.

5.5 Quantitative information about the frequencies contained in returning Doppler-shifted echoes can be displayed on an _____ versus _____ plot that is continuously changing with time.

5.6 To display the pattern of time change of a Doppler spectrum, a display of _____ versus _____ can be used.

5.7 In Exercise 5.6, the amplitude of each frequency component is represented by _____ level or _____.

5.8 The received frequency spectrum exists (rather than a single frequency) because of the distribution of _____ _____ encountered by the ultrasound.

5.9 Because velocity is speed and direction, variations in either of these in the flow region monitored by the Doppler instrument contribute to the received frequency spectrum. True or false?

5.10 The components of a pulsed-Doppler instrument are the same as those for a continuous-wave instrument, except for the addition of two _____.

5.11 The purpose of the generator gate is to convert a _____ voltage to a _____ voltage.

5.12 The purpose of the receiver gate is to allow the selection of Doppler-shifted echoes from specific _____, according to _____ _____.

5.13 Pulsed-Doppler instruments require a two-element transducer assembly. True or false?

5.14. An increased gate-open time increases the length of the sample volume. True or false?

5.15. A later receiver gate corresponds to a deeper gate location. True or false?

5.16 There is no problem with aliasing as long as the Doppler shifts are _____ half the pulse repetition frequency.

    a. less than
    b. equal to
    c. greater than
    d. all of the above
    e. a or b

5.17 Pulsed-Doppler instruments use the _____ _____ _____ technique to present Doppler shift spectra as a function of time.

5.18 The abbreviation for the technique referred to in Exercise 5.17 is _____.

5.19 In Figure 5.9A, is the instrument a pulsed- or a continuous-wave device?

5.20 In Figure 5.36, is the instrument a pulsed- or a continuous-wave device?

5.21 If a sheep leaves its pen and runs to another pen 25 m distant at a speed of 50 cm/s, when must the gate to the second pen open to allow the sheep to pass through when it arrives?

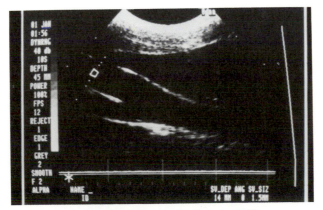

Figure 5.36. Display for Exercise 5.20.

5.22 If a sheep leaves its pen and travels to a brook, at which point it turns around and returns to the pen, when must the gate to its pen open to allow the sheep to pass through when it returns? (The distance to the brook is 25 m, and the sheep travels at 50 cm/s.)

5.23 Transducers designed for Doppler use are sometimes not _____. This is because they emit _____ pulses than those used in imaging. Undamped transducers are more _____ than damped ones.

5.24 For a 5-MHz instrument and 60-degree Doppler angle, a 100-Hz filter eliminates flow speeds below

a. 1 cm/s
b. 2 cm/s
c. 3 cm/s
d. 4 cm/s
e. 5 cm/s

5.25 For a 2.5-MHz instrument and zero-degree Doppler angle, a 100-Hz filter eliminates flow speeds below

a. 1 cm/s
b. 2 cm/s
c. 3 cm/s
d. 4 cm/s
e. 5 cm/s

5.26 The functions of a Doppler receiver include which of the following?

a. amplification
b. phase quadrature detection
c. demodulation
d. rejection
e. all of the above

5.27 An earlier receiver gate time means a _____ sample volume depth.

a. later
b. shallower
c. deeper
d. stronger
e. none of the above

5.28 Name the two types of instruments used for Doppler spectral display.

5.29 Name the Doppler instrument the sample volume of which is the region in which the transmitting and receiving transducer beams overlap.

5.30 Name the instrument the sample volume of which is determined by the receiver gate.

5.31 Name the instrument that combines the pulsed-Doppler technique with imaging.

5.32 Name the instrument that offers depth selectivity.

5.33 The _____ detects the difference between the frequencies of the emitted and received ultrasound.

5.34 The Doppler shift is typically _____ of the source frequency.
 a. one thousandth
 b. one hundredth
 c. one tenth
 d. 10 times
 e. 100 times

5.35 To convert a spectral display correctly from Doppler shift to flow speed, the _____ _____ must be accurately incorporated.

5.36 The Doppler spectrum is visually presented on a _____ _____ tube.

5.37 The high-pass filter in the receiver is called a _____ filter or _____-_____ filter.

5.38 Pulsed-Doppler instruments produce pulses that are about _____ to _____ cycles long. The length of the sample volume in a pulsed-Doppler instrument is determined by the receiver _____ length and the emitted _____ length.

5.39 The Doppler shift upper limit to avoid aliasing is sometimes called the _____ limit.

5.40 If aliasing is avoided by increasing the pulse repetition frequency, name the other artifact that may be encountered.

5.41 Which type of Doppler instrument is most likely to be used in measuring extremely high flow rates?

5.42 All pulsed instruments have anatomic imaging capability to allow intelligent positioning of the gate. True or false?

5.43 Continuous- and pulsed-wave Doppler capabilities are never provided in the same instrument. True or false?

5.44 Which type of duplex system cannot image while Doppler information is being acquired?

5.45 Two- or three-cycle pulses are used for

    a. pulsed Doppler
    b. continuous-wave Doppler
    c. imaging
    d. color-flow Doppler
    e. all of the above

5.46 Spectral analysis is the breaking up of the _____ of a complex wave or signal and spreading them out in _____.

5.47 Which of the following is a spectrum analyzer for light?

    a. mirror
    b. filter
    c. prism
    d. window
    e. reflector

5.48 Spectral analysis is performed in a Doppler instrument _____.

    a. electronically
    b. mathematically
    c. acoustically

d. mechanically

e. more than one of the above

5.49 A Doppler spectrum is produced because many different Doppler _____ are received from the flow.

5.50 The statement in Exercise 5.49 is true because portions of the flowing fluid within the heart or a vessel are moving at different _____ and, sometimes, in different _____.

5.51 If all the blood cells in a vessel were moving in the same direction at the same speed (plug flow), a _____ Doppler shift would result at any instant in time.

5.52 For normal flow in a large vessel, a _____ range of Doppler shift frequencies is received.

a. narrow

b. broad

c. steady

d. disturbed

e. all of the above.

5.53 The type of flow in Exercise 5.52 is called _____ flow.

a. turbulent

b. disturbed

c. laminar

d. steady

e. plug

5.54 The Doppler spectrum can be presented in two ways, as a display of _____ or _____ versus Doppler shift frequency or Doppler shift frequency versus _____. The latter is the common presentation in spectral Doppler instruments.

5.55 For pulsatile flow, in Exercise 5.54, which form of presentation is preferable, the first or the second?

5.56 Doppler-shift versus time presentations indicate the amplitude or power of each frequency component by _____ or _____   _____.

5.57 The Doppler signal's power is proportional to

   a. volume flow
   b. flow speed
   c. Doppler angle
   d. cell density
   e. more than one of the above

5.58 In Figure 5.19, A represents

   a. early time and high Doppler shift
   b. early time and low Doppler shift
   c. late time and high Doppler shift
   d. late time and low Doppler shift
   e. none of the above

5.59 In Figure 5.19, B represents

   a. early time and high Doppler shift
   b. early time and low Doppler shift
   c. late time and high Doppler shift
   d. late time and low Doppler shift
   e. none of the above

5.60 In Figure 5.19, C represents

   a. early time and high Doppler shift
   b. early time and low Doppler shift
   c. late time and high Doppler shift
   d. late time and low Doppler shift
   e. none of the above

5.61 In Figure 5.19, D represents

   a. early time and high Doppler shift
   b. early time and low Doppler shift
   c. late time and high Doppler shift
   d. late time and low Doppler shift
   e. none of the above

5.62 In Figure 5.19 with a dark background, if A is bright, many cells are moving in such a way that a large Doppler shift occurs at early time. True or false?

5.63 In Figure 5.19 with a dark background, if D is dark, many cells are moving in such a way that they produce low Doppler shifts at late time. True or false?

5.64 In the previous six exercises, the highest Doppler shift necessarily means the highest flow speed only if _____ flow is assumed.

5.65 For disturbed or turbulent flow in Figure 5.19, A could represent

    a. high speed and large Doppler angle
    b. high speed and small Doppler angle
    c. low speed and small Doppler angle
    d. low speed and large Doppler angle
    e. more than one of the above

5.66 For disturbed or turbulent flow in Figure 5.19, C could represent

    a. high speed and large Doppler angle
    b. high speed and small Doppler angle
    c. low speed and small Doppler angle
    d. low speed and large Doppler angle
    e. more than one of the above

5.67 Doppler ultrasound provides information about flow conditions only at the site of measurement. True or false?

5.68 Stenosis affects

    a. peak systolic flow speed
    b. end-diastolic flow speed
    c. spectral broadening
    d. window
    e. all of the above

5.69 Spectral broadening is a _____ of the spectral trace.

    a. vertical thickening
    b. horizontal thickening
    c. brightening
    d. darkening
    e. horizontal shift

5.70 If all cells in a vessel were moving at the same constant velocity, the spectral trace would be a _____ line.

    a. thin horizontal
    b. thin vertical
    c. thick horizontal
    d. thick vertical
    e. none of the above

5.71 In Figure 5.22C, in which part of the flow cycle is spectral broadening (bandwidth) the least?

    a. acceleration
    b. deceleration
    c. neither

5.72 Disturbed flow produces a narrower spectrum. True or false?

5.73 Turbulent flow produces a narrower spectrum. True or false?

5.74 As stenosis is increased, which of the following increase(s)?

    a. luminal diameter
    b. systolic Doppler shift
    c. diastolic Doppler shift
    d. spectral broadening
    e. more than one of the above

5.75 Higher flow speed always produces a higher Doppler shift on a spectral display. True or false?

5.76 Spectral broadening _____ the window.

    a. increases
    b. decreases
    c. brightens
    d. does not affect

5.77 Flow reversal in diastole indicates

    a. stenosis
    b. aneurysm
    c. high distal resistance
    d. low distal resistance
    e. more than one of the above

5.78 Decreased distal resistance normally causes end-diastolic flow to

    a. increase
    b. decrease
    c. be disturbed
    d. become turbulent
    e. more than one of the above

5.79 Match the following.

    _____ **a.** narrow spectra   **1.** small vessels
    _____ **b.** broad spectra   **2.** large vessels
    _____ **c.** intermediate   **3.** medium vessels
             spectra

5.80 Which is expected at the center of a vessel? Narrow or broad spectrum?

5.81 Which is expected at the center of a vessel? Higher or lower flow speeds?

5.82 Spectral broadening always indicates turbulence. True or false?

5.83 Increasing distal resistance and increasing Doppler angle have the same effect on the spectral display. True or false?

5.84 Which normally has the smallest end-diastolic flow?

    a. common carotid artery
    b. internal carotid artery
    c. external carotid artery

5.85 Zero and reverse flow in late diastole are normal findings in some locations in the circulation. True or false?

5.86 The pulsatility-index approach works because flow resistance _____ over cardiac cycle. This is because the vessels are _____. In this case, resistance is _____ at lower pressures and _____ at higher pressures.

5.87 Under what condition can a relatively high Doppler shift come from a relatively slowly moving flow?

5.88 Under what condition can a relatively low Doppler shift come from a relatively rapidly moving flow?

5.89 When the spectral trace is calibrated in flow speed (in centimeters per second), the highest flow speed shown always represents the fastest cells in the vessel. True or false?

5.90 If the flow speed is less than 125 cm/s and the Doppler shift is less than 4 kHz, both indicating normal carotid artery flow, what operating frequency is being used if the Doppler angle is 60 degrees?

   a. 1 MHz
   b. 2 MHz
   c. 3 MHz
   d. 4 MHz
   e. 5 MHz

5.91 In Figure 5.37, if the sample volume is placed as shown and the plaque (P) is not visualized, the operator would probably place the angle correction indicator (dashed line) parallel to the vessel walls. This would result in a _____ flow speed indication.

   a. correct
   b. high
   c. low

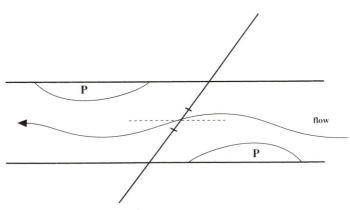

Figure 5.37. Illustration for Exercise 5.91.

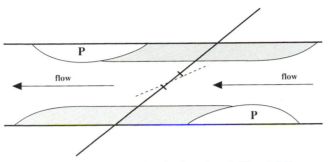

Figure 5.38. Illustration for Exercises 5.92 and 5.93.

5.92 In Figure 5.38, if plaque P were visualized, but the remainder (shaded) were not, the operator would probably place the angle correction indicator (dashed line) as shown. This would result in a _____ flow speed indication.

a. correct
b. high
c. low

5.93 In Figure 5.38, if the angle correction indicator (dashed line) is placed parallel to the vessel walls, rather than as shown, the Doppler shift is _____, and the indicated flow speed is _____.

a. increased, unchanged
b. increased, increased
c. decreased, unchanged
d. decreased, decreased
e. unchanged, increased

6 Color-Flow Instruments

Color-flow imaging presents two-dimensional, cross-sectional blood flow information in real time in conjunction with two-dimensional, cross-sectional, gray-scale anatomic imaging.[7,8,31–39] Two-dimensional, real-time presentations of flow information allow the observer to readily locate regions of abnormal flow for further evaluation (spectral analysis). The direction of flow is readily appreciated, and disturbed or turbulent flow is presented dramatically in a two-dimensional form. Color-flow instruments present pulse-echo, gray-scale anatomic information in the conventional form, but also include circuitry that allows the rapid detection of the Doppler frequency or echo arrival time shifts at several locations along each scan line and presentations of these in color at the appropriate locations in the cross-sectional image. The color-flow imaging instrument is therefore a combined pulse-echo, gray-scale imaging instrument and pulse-Doppler or time-shift multigate instrument. Conventional continuous-wave and pulse-Doppler spectral analysis capabilities are commonly included in these instruments.

In this chapter, we consider the following questions: What techniques are used to rapidly determine two-dimensional flow information? How is the two-dimensional flow information color encoded on a sonographic display? What types of flow information are presented on such displays? The following terms are discussed in this chapter:

autocorrelation	cross correlation
clutter	ensemble length
color flow	frame rate

hue	saturation
luminance	variance
priority	wall filter

6.1
Color-Flow Principle

Color-flow imaging extends the use of the pulse-echo imaging principle (Chapter 2). A pulse of ultrasound is emitted from a transducer, which then receives the returning echoes from the tissues. Echoes returning from stationary tissues are detected and presented in gray scale in appropriate locations along the scan line. The depth is determined by the echo's arrival time, and the brightness is determined by the echo's amplitude. If a returning echo has a different frequency than what was emitted, a Doppler shift (frequency change) has occurred because the echo-generating object was moving (Chapter 4). If the motion is toward or away from the transducer, the Doppler shift is

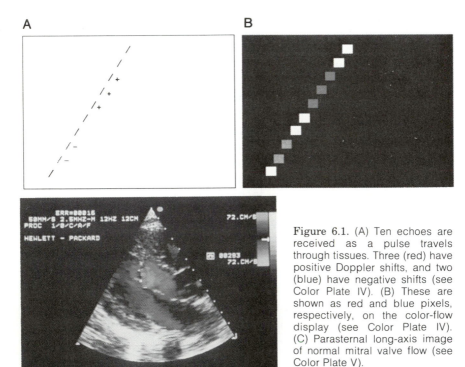

Figure 6.1. (A) Ten echoes are received as a pulse travels through tissues. Three (red) have positive Doppler shifts, and two (blue) have negative shifts (see Color Plate IV). (B) These are shown as red and blue pixels, respectively, on the color-flow display (see Color Plate IV). (C) Parasternal long-axis image of normal mitral valve flow (see Color Plate V).

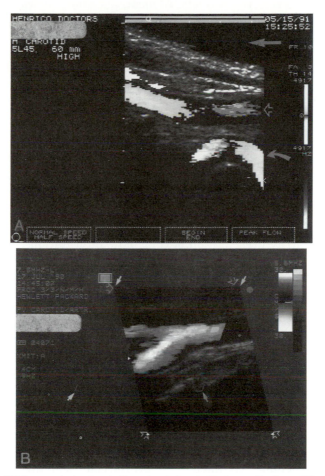

Figure 6.2. (A) An anechoic stand-off wedge is located between the face of the transducer and the skin line (straight arrow). This causes the pulse paths (and therefore the scan lines) to be nonperpendicular to the flow of a vessel that runs parallel to the skin. This figure also shows the change of the sign of the Doppler shift (and therefore the color) that results from vessel curvature. On the right side of the carotid artery (open arrow), flow is slightly away from the transducer; on the left side, it is directed toward the transducer. The opposite situation is seen in the vertebral artery (curved arrow). Flow in both arteries is from right to left on this image (see Color Plate VI). (B) A perpendicular Doppler angle is avoided in this image by electronically steering the color-producing Doppler pulses to the left of vertical. The corners of the resulting parallelogram in which color can be displayed are shown by the solid arrows. Note that, on this instrument, the gray-scale anatomic imaging pulses can also be steered (in this case to the right of vertical). The corners of the resulting parallelogram are shown with open arrows (see Color Plate VII). (Reprinted from Kremkau FW: Principles and pitfalls of real-time color-flow imaging. In Bernstein EF (ed): Vascular Diagnosis, 4th edition. St. Louis, Mosby-Year Book, 1993. Reprinted with permission).

positive or negative, respectively. At locations along the scan line where Doppler shifts have been detected, their sign, the magnitude of the mean, and sometimes, the variance are recorded. These pieces of information are used to determine the appropriate hue, saturation, and luminance (discussed in Section 6.2) of each color pixel at its location on the display. Doppler-shifted echoes can be recorded and presented at many locations along each scan line (Fig. 6.1, Color Plates IV and V). As in all sonography, many such scan lines make up one cross-sectional image (Figs. 1.5, 2.2, 2.4, and 6.1C, Color Plate V). Several of these images are presented each second, yielding what is commonly called real-time sonography. Color-flow images can also be produced without using the Doppler effect. Instead, the change in echo arrival time as the blood cells move closer to or farther away from the transducer is used to determine their speed of motion. This is discussed further in Section 6.3.

Linear-array presentation of color-flow information is sometimes inadequate when the vessel runs parallel to the skin's surface.[38] This is because the pulses (and scan lines) run perpendicular to the transducer's surface (and, therefore, to the skin's surface) resulting in a 90-degree angle where the pulses intersect the flow in the vessel. This would yield no Doppler or time shift and, therefore, no color within the vessel if the flow is parallel to the vessel walls. Two approaches have been used to avoid this situation (Fig. 6.2, Color Plate VI and VII). A standoff wedge can be placed between the transducer surface and the skin, causing the emitted pulses to travel at an angle other than perpendicular to the skin and, therefore, yielding an angle less than 90 degrees for vessels parallel to the skin. Another approach is to use phasing (Section 2.2) to steer each emitted pulse from a linear-sequenced array in a given direction (for example 20 degrees away from perpendicular). All the color pulses and color scan lines are steered at this angle, resulting in a parallelogram presentation of color-flow information on the display.

6.2
Principles of Color Vision

The three components of a color, as seen on a display, include hue, saturation, and luminance.[32,38,39] Hue is the color perceived. It represents the frequency of the light (an electromagnetic wave), with the range of frequencies detectable by the human eye ranging from the lowest (red) to the highest (violet) with increasing intermediate frequency progression through orange, yellow, green, and blue. This frequency range is about 400 to 800 million MHz. Saturation is the amount of hue present in a mix with white (which is a combination of all visible hues). This is similar to mixing a deep color paint with white to produce a pale color (e.g., red mixed with white yields pink). The less white present, the greater the saturation. The more white present, the less the saturation. Luminance is the brightness of the hue and saturation presented.

In conventional gray-scale anatomic imaging, the saturation is zero (there is no hue), and the luminance represents the echo amplitude. This yields gray-scale imaging, ranging from black to white through various shades of gray.

In color-flow imaging, various combinations of hue, saturation, and luminance are used to indicate the sign, magnitude of the mean, and sometimes, the magnitude of the variance of the Doppler or time shifts found at each location. The mean and variance are encountered because Doppler or time shift (representing flow within each sample volume) is not the result of a single moving reflector (erythrocyte) but the result of millions of moving cells which, even in normal flow, are not all moving at the same velocity (speed and direction) (Sections 5.3 and 5.4). The instrument detects the mean of these many Doppler or time shifts at each location and, in some cases, the variance (which is a measure of the spread around the mean [spectral broadening] and, therefore, an indicator of the extent of flow disturbance or turbulence).

Red, green, and blue are known as primary additive colors because various combinations of them can produce virtually any color desired. Color video displays produce various colors by using red, green, and blue phosphor dots (Section 6.4). Red and green, mixed equally, produce yellow. Green and blue produce cyan, the technical term for aqua. Red and blue produce magenta (not used in color-flow displays). Red, green, and blue, equally mixed, produce white (or gray, depending on luminance).

6.3
Instruments

The color-flow instrument (Fig. 6.3) consists of a pulser, a beam former, a receiver, a memory, and a display. The displays are discussed in Section 6.4. The pulser produces the electric voltages that drive the transducer array. The beam former provides appropriate sequencing and phasing to scan electronically and focus the sound beam in a rectangular, parallelogram, or sector format through the tissue cross section. The control of output intensity is accomplished through the pulser.

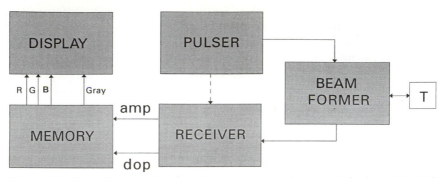

Figure 6.3. Block diagram of a color Doppler imaging instrument. As in a gray-scale (amplitude [amp] path) imaging instrument, pulser, beam former, receiver, memory, and display are included. However, the receiver is capable of detecting Doppler or arrival time shifts throughout the scanning field. Information regarding flow is stored in the memory through the Doppler (dop) path at appropriate locations. The display shows the color-flow information superimposed on the gray-scale anatomic image. T, transducer; R, red; G, green; B, blue. (Modified from Kremkau FW: Principles of color flow imaging. J Vasc Technol *15*:104–111, 1991. Reprinted with permission.)

Color-flow images are produced by linear and convex sequenced arrays and phased sector arrays. The receiver receives the voltages from the transducer that represent the echoes returning from the tissue as a pulse travels. Non–Doppler-shifted echoes are processed conventionally, as in any sonography instrument (Section 2.3). This includes amplification, attenuation compensation, dynamic range compression, radio frequency to video demodulation, and threshold (rejection). The echoes then exit the receiver in the form of voltages representing echo amplitudes that are then stored in the memory at appropriate locations in digital form with numbers representing amplitudes.

Doppler-shifted echoes are detected in the receiver by using an autocorrelation technique that rapidly determines the mean and variance of the Doppler-shift signal at each location along the scan line (at each selected echo arrival time during pulse travel). The autocorrelation technique[40] is a mathematic process that yields the mean Doppler shift and spread around the mean (variance) for each sample time (and corresponding depth) following pulse emission. The Doppler detector yields, for each location, the mean Doppler shift magnitude, sign (positive or negative), and variance (Fig. 6.4). These three quantities are stored at appropriate locations in the memory that correspond to anatomic sites where Doppler shifts have been found. There are approximately 100 to 400 Doppler samples (locations) per scan line on a color-flow display. Depending on the depth and width of the color presentation, approximately 5 to 50 frames per second can be shown. Multiple pulses are involved in the autocorrelation process. One pair

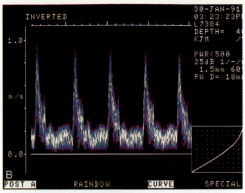

PLATE I

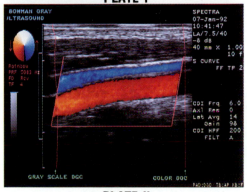

PLATE II

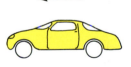

100 million mph

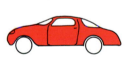
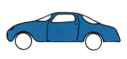
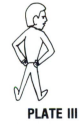

PLATE III

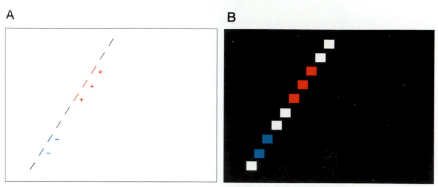

PLATE IV

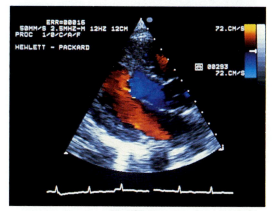

PLATE V

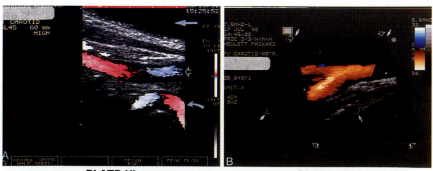

PLATE VI   **PLATE VII**

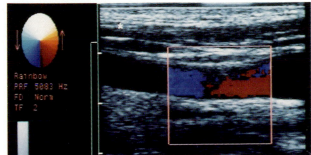

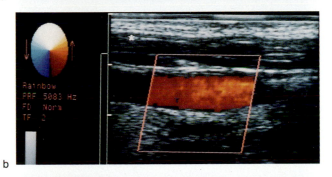

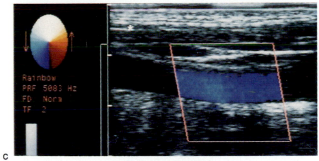

PLATE VIII PART 1

PLATE VIII PART 2

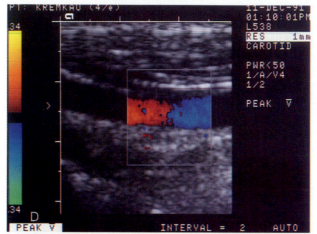

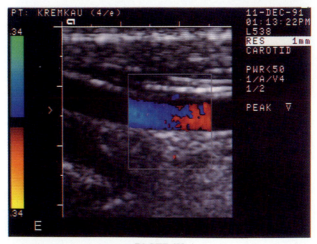

PLATE IX

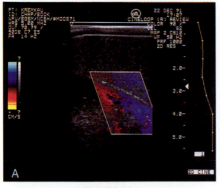

PLATE X

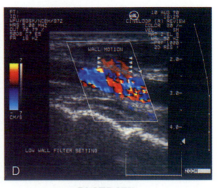

PLATE XIII

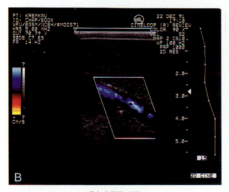

PLATE XI

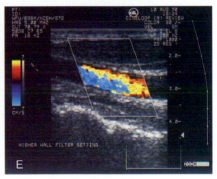

PLATE XIV

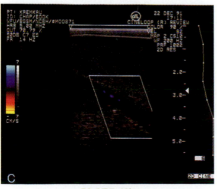

PLATE XII

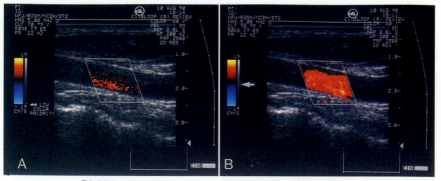

PLATE XV

PLATE XVI

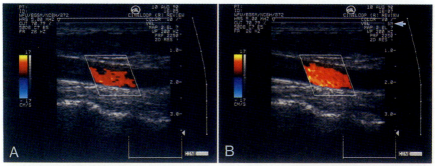

PLATE XVII

PLATE XVIII

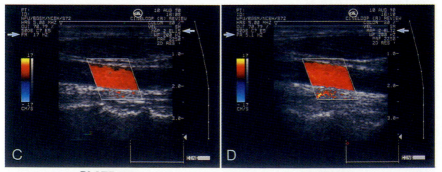

PLATE XIX

PLATE XX

PLATE XXI

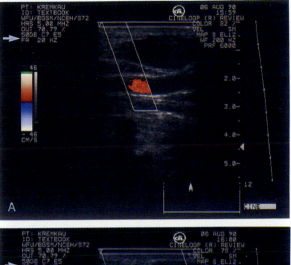

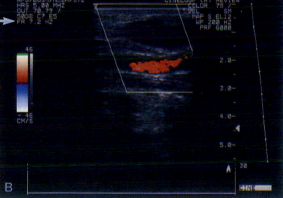

PLATE XXII

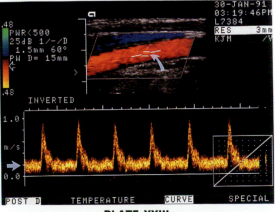

PLATE XXIII

PLATE XXIV

PLATE XXV

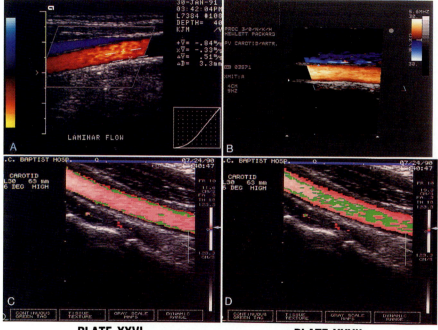

PLATE XXVI

PLATE XXVII

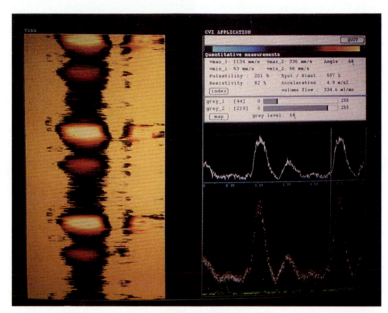

PLATE XVIII

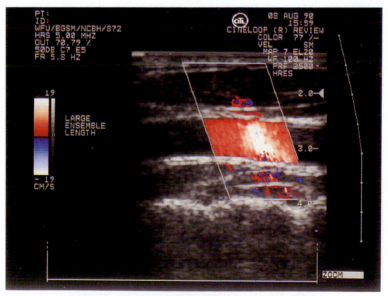

PLATE XXIX

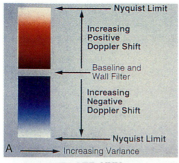

PLATE XXX

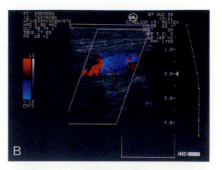

PLATE XXXI

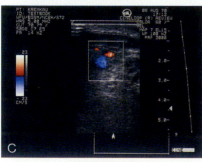

PLATE XXXII

PLATE XXXIII

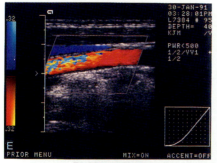

PLATE XXXIV

PLATE XXXV

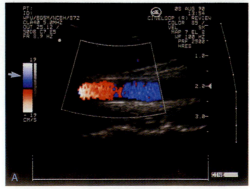

PLATE XXXVI

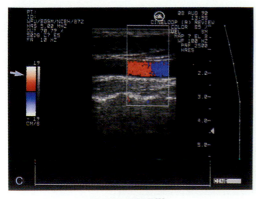

PLATE XXXVII

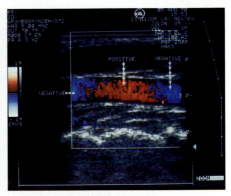

PLATE XXXVIII

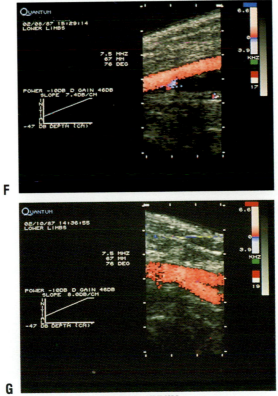

PLATE XXXIX

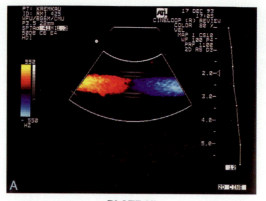

PLATE XL

PLATE XLI

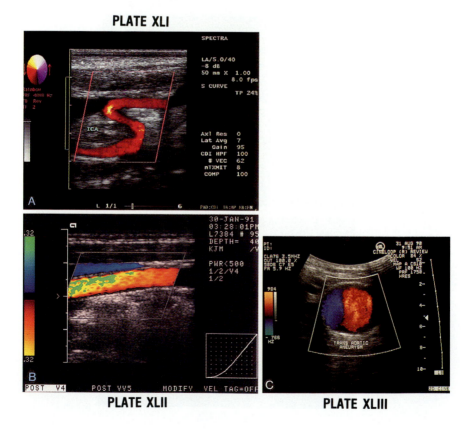

PLATE XLII

PLATE XLIII

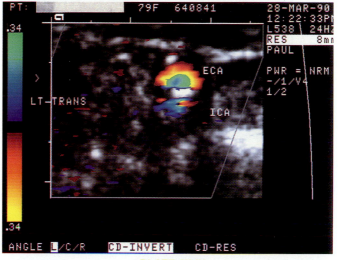

PLATE XLIV

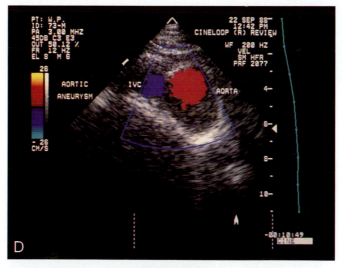

PLATE XLV

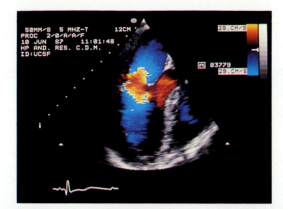

PLATE XLVI

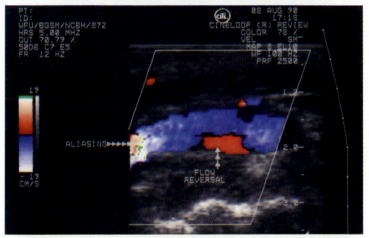

PLATE XLVII

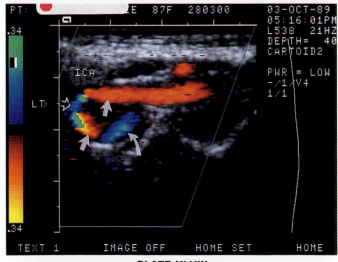

PLATE XLVIII

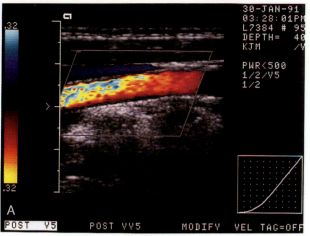

PLATE XLIX

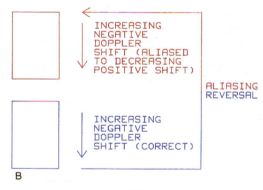

PLATE L

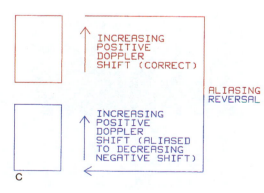

PLATE LI

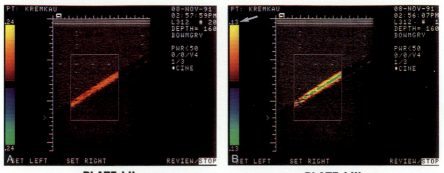

PLATE LII   **PLATE LIII**

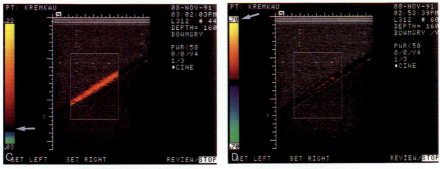

PLATE LIV   **PLATE LV**

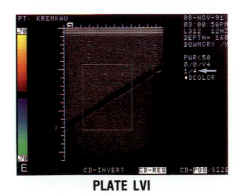

PLATE LVI

PLATE LVII

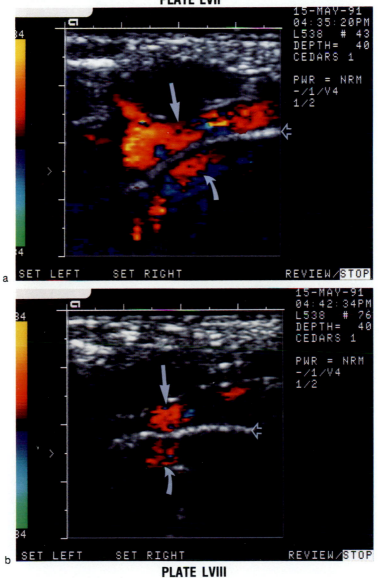

PLATE LVIII

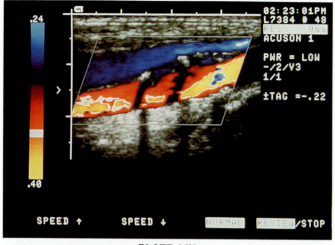

PLATE LIX

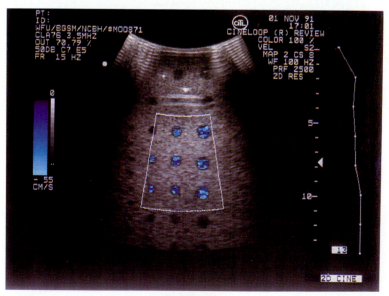

PLATE LX

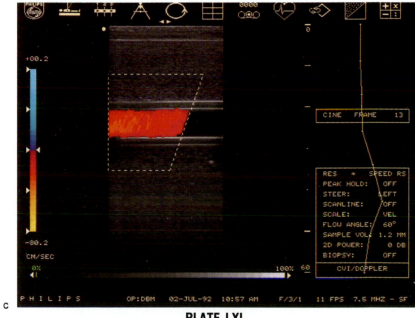

PLATE LXI

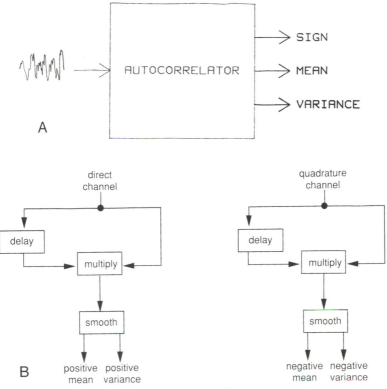

Figure 6.4. (A) The autocorrelator rapidly performs Doppler demodulation on the complicated echo signal (entering at left). The autocorrelator yields the sign of the mean Doppler shift, the magnitude of the mean Doppler shift, and the magnitude of the Doppler shift variance at each location in the scanned cross section. These three pieces of information are stored in each pixel location in the memory. Color assignments are appropriately made to indicate these three pieces of information two dimensionally on the display. (From Kremkau FW: Principles of color flow imaging. J Vasc Technol *15*:104–111, 1991. Reprinted with permission.) (B) Outputs from direct and quadrature channels of the phase quadrature detector (see Fig. 5.3) are fed to the autocorrelator inputs. In each channel, the signal is multiplied by a version of itself delayed by one pulse-repetition period. High-frequency variations are filtered out (smoothed) to yield the mean and variance of the Doppler shifts.

of pulses yields a phase-difference determination. Two-phase determinations yield a Doppler-shift (flow speed) estimate. Therefore, a three-pulse minimum is required for one speed estimate. More are required for improved accuracy of the estimates or for variance determinations.

Rather than using Doppler shift to identify and quantify the speed of flowing blood, another approach can be used.[41,42] In Figure 6.5, a group of blood cells is shown at some location in the vessel at time t_1. At a later time (t_2), this group of cells has moved to a new position,

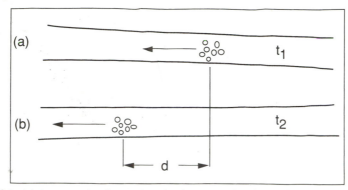

Figure 6.5. (a) A group of cells at a location in a vessel at time t_1. (b) At a later time (t_2), the group has moved a distance d to a new location. (From Tegeler CH, Kremkau FW, Hitchings LP: Color velocity imaging: introduction to a new ultrasound technology. J Neuro-imaging *1*:85–90, 1991. Reprinted with permission.)

separated from the old position by a distance d. If all the cells move together at the same velocity, the speed (v) is equal to d/T, where T is the difference between the two times ($t_2 - t_1$). When ultrasound pulses are sent into the vessel in a path parallel to the vessel walls from left to right, the echo arrival times for the two times shown in Figure 6.5 are as illustrated in Figure 6.6. A longer time is required for the pulse round-trip travel at time t_1 compared with that for time t_2. The difference between the two times is Δt. To determine flow speed, the instrument measures this difference in echo arrival times (Δt) observed at two different times (t_1 and t_2). From this echo-arrival difference, the flow speed is calculated as follows. The average speed of sound in soft tissues is 1.54 mm/μs, yielding the round-trip travel time rule of 13 μs/cm. When the round-trip travel time is divided by this number, the result is the distance to the group of cells that are producing the received echo. The difference in echo arrival time, Δt, between the two times, t_1 and t_2, divided by 13 μs/cm yields the distance, d, that the group of cells traveled during time T. The time T between two subsequent pulses, is equal to the pulse repetition period, which is one divided by the pulse repetition frequency (PRF). The distance d divided by the time difference T (or multiplied by PRF) yields the speed v of the cell group (i.e., blood flow speed). Combining the mathematic steps described here yields the following expression:

$$v = \frac{\Delta t \times PRF}{13}$$

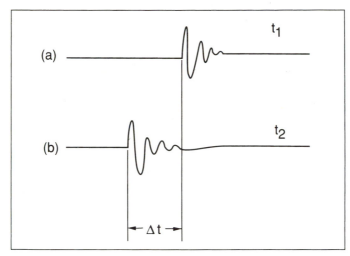

Figure 6.6. (a) Echo from the group of cells in Figure 6.5A. (b) Echo from the group of cells in Figure 6.5B arrives a time Δt earlier than the echo in Part A. (From Tegeler CH, Kremkau FW, Hitchings LP: Color velocity imaging: introduction to a new ultrasound technology. J Neuroimaging *1*:85–90, 1991. Reprinted with permission.)

where Δt is in microseconds, PRF in hertz, and v in centimeters per second. If the sound beam is not parallel to the flow direction, as is common in clinical practice, the calculated flow speed will be less than the actual flow speed, with the factor being the cosine of the angle between the sound and flow directions. This angular dependence is identical to that in the Doppler equation. Thus, although the two techniques are different, they have the same angle dependence. Incorporating the angle correction yields the equation:

$$v \text{ (cm/s)} = \frac{\Delta t \text{ } (\mu s) \text{ PRF (Hz)}}{13 \cos \theta}$$

The time-domain, color-flow instrument must determine the echo arrival time shift between subsequent pulses that is caused by the blood flow movement between pulses. This is accomplished by a mathematic technique called cross correlation. In this technique, two waveforms from subsequent pulses (see Fig. 6.6) are stored, and the second is delayed a sufficient amount of time so that the two waveforms have maximum correlation (i.e., their overlapping similarity is maximum). At that point, the delay time is equal to Δt. The component of flow velocity parallel to the sound beam can then be calculated and color assignment can be made at the appropriate pixel location on the display.

This is done at many (sample or gate) locations along each scan line, resulting in a two-dimensional color representation of flow speed on the instrument display. A positive time shift indicates approaching flow; a negative shift indicates receding flow.

Color controls[38] (Fig. 6.7) include the color window's (rectangle or sector) width and depth, gain and depth gain compensation, steering angle, color inversion, wall filter, priority, baseline shift, velocity range (PRF), color map selection, variance, smoothing, and ensemble length. Steering angle control permits the avoidance of 90-degree angles (Fig. 6.8, Color Plates VIII and IX). Color inversion alternates the color assignments above and below the baseline on the color map (Fig. 6.8, Color Plates VIII and IX). The wall filter allows the elimination of clutter caused by tissue and wall motion (Fig. 6.9, Color Plates X to XIV). However, care must be taken not to set the wall filter too high, or slower blood flow signals will be removed (Fig. 6.9c, Color Plate XII). The color velocity range sets the PRF and Nyquist limit at the color bar extremes. Decreasing the value permits the observation of slower flows (smaller Doppler shifts) but increases the probability of aliasing for faster flows. This is discussed further in Section 7.2. Priority selects the gray-scale echo strength below which color will be shown, instead of the gray level at each pixel location (Fig. 6.10, Color Plates XV and XVI). Baseline control allows shifting up or down to scroll in a manner similar to that done in spectral displays to eliminate aliasing (Section 7.2). Smoothing (also called persistence) provides frame-to-frame averaging to fill in missing pixels and provide a smoother image (Fig. 6.11, Color Plates XVII to XX). Ensemble length is the number

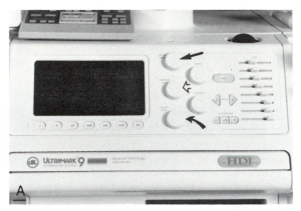

Figure 6.7. (A) Color Doppler gain control (curved arrow). Gray-scale (arrow) and spectral Doppler (open arrow) gain controls are also indicated. Software panel controls for color Doppler (B) and color-time-shift (C) functions.

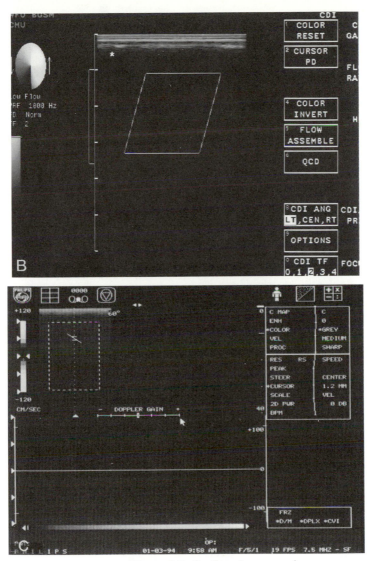

Figure 6.7. *Continued*

of pulses required for each color scan line. The minimum is three, with values of 8 to 20 being common. Larger ensemble lengths provide a better detection of slow flows and complete representation of flow within a vessel (Fig. 6.11, Color Plates XVII to XX) but at the expense of longer time and, therefore, lower frame rates. Wider color windows (viewing areas) reduce frame rates also because more pulses (i.e., scan

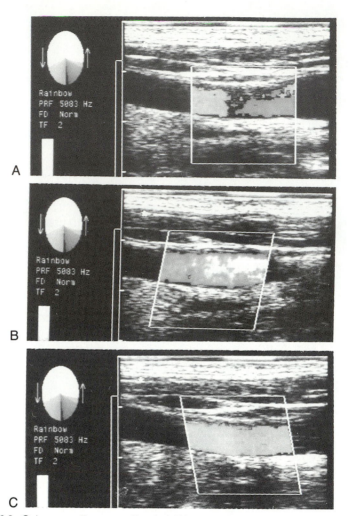

Figure 6.8. Color scan lines are directed (A) vertically, (B) to the left of vertical, and (C) to the right of vertical. Flow is from left to right, producing positive and negative Doppler shifts, depending on the relationship between scan lines and flow. (From Kremkau FW: Doppler principles. Semin Roentgenol 27:6–16, 1992. Reprinted with permission.) (D) In this hue map, red and blue are assigned to positive and negative Doppler shifts, respectively, progressing to yellow and cyan (by addition of green) at the Nyquist limits (see Color Plate VIII). (E) In this map, the color assignments are reversed from (D), i.e., blue and red are assigned to positive and negative Doppler shifts, respectively. Note the color change occurring within the color window. This is caused by vessel curvature as in Figure 6.2A (see Color Plate IX). (From Kremkau FW: Principles and pitfalls of real-time color-flow imaging. In Bernstein EF (ed): Vascular Diagnosis, 4th edition, St. Louis, Mosby-Year Book, 1993. Reprinted with permission.)

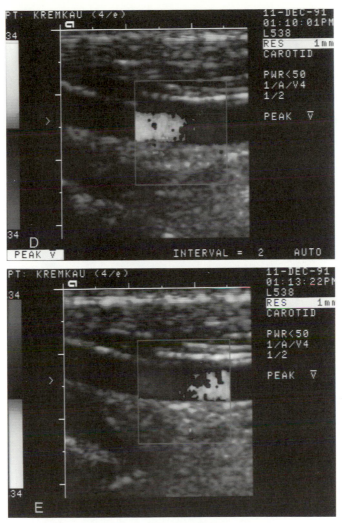

Figure 6.8. *Continued*

lines) per frame are required (Fig. 6.12, Color Plates XXI and XXII). Figure 1.5, Color Plate II, shows a color-flow image that involves color depth or time gain compensation.

Several aspects of color-flow imaging are limiting in their character. These include a lack of complete spectral information, angle dependence (Section 6.4), and lower frame rates. Spectral Doppler presents the entire range of Doppler-shift frequencies received as they change over the cardiac cycle (Fig. 6.13, Color Plate XXIII). Color Doppler displays can only present a statistical representation of the complete

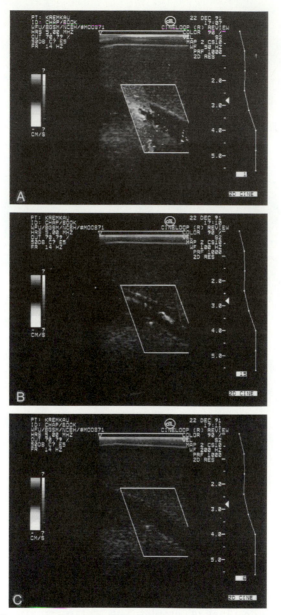

Figure 6.9. (A) Tissue motion causes clutter, obscuring the flow in the vessel and clouding the gray-scale tissue with color Doppler information (see Color Plate X). (B) The wall filter has been increased to 100 Hz, eliminating the color clutter (see Color Plate XI). (C) The wall filter has been increased (too much) to 200 Hz, eliminating virtually all of the color-flow information in the vessel (see Color Plate XII). (D) With a low wall-filter setting

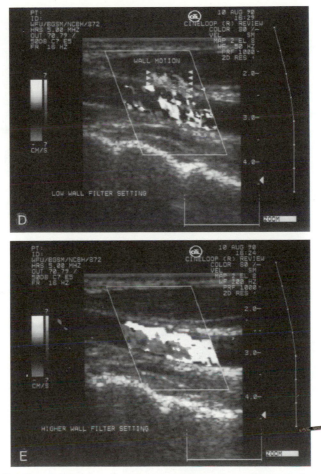

Figure 6.9. *Continued* (50 Hz), wall motion appears in color on the image (see Color Plate XIII). (E) With a higher wall-filter setting (200 Hz), this motion no longer appears in color (see Color Plate XIV). (Parts A to C from Kremkau FW: Principles and pitfalls of real-time color-flow imaging. In Bernstein EF (ed): Vascular Diagnosis, 4th edition. St. Louis, Mosby-Year Book, 1993. Parts D and E from Kremkau FW: Principles and instrumentation. In Merritt CRB (ed): Doppler Color Imaging. New York, Churchill Livingstone, 1992. Reprinted with permission.)

spectrum at each pixel location on the display. The sign, mean value, and possibly, the variance of the spectrum are color coded into combinations of hue, saturation, and luminance presented at each display pixel location. Some Doppler instruments have the ability to read out the quantitative digital values for the mean Doppler shift (sometimes converted to angle-corrected equivalent flow speed) at chosen pixel locations (Fig. 6.14, Color Plates XXIV to XXVII). It is important to realize

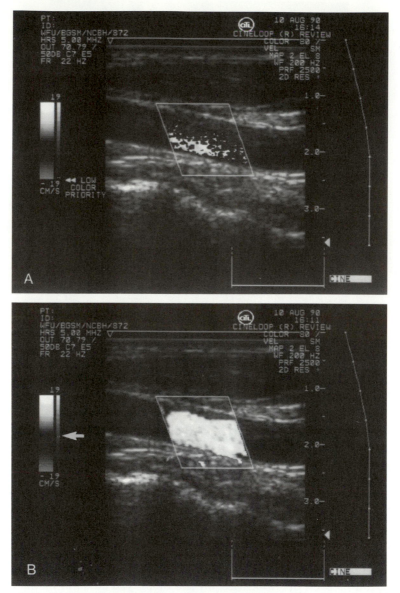

Figure 6.10. (A) With the color priority set low (at the bottom of the gray bar), weak non-Doppler–shifted reverberation and off-axis echoes within the vessel take precedence over the Doppler-shifted echoes, and little color is displayed (see Color Plate XV). (B) With a higher priority, halfway up the gray bar (arrow), the Doppler-shifted echoes (color) take precedence over the weaker gray-scale echoes (see Color Plate XVI) (From Kremkau FW: Principles and instrumentation. In Merritt CRB (ed): Doppler Color Imaging. New York, Churchill Livingstone, 1992. Reprinted with permission.)

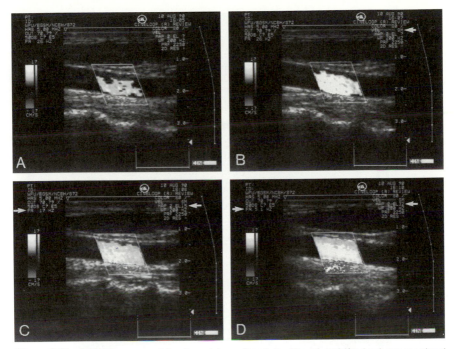

Figure 6.11. (A) With no smoothing (persistence), only the Doppler-shifted echoes received from the pulses generating an individual frame are shown (see Color Plate XVII). (B) With smoothing, consecutive frames are averaged, filling gaps in the presentation and presenting a smoother but less detailed representation of flow (see Color Plate XVIII). (C and D) More accurate and complete detection of flow information is obtained with increasing ensemble lengths (see Color Plates XIX and XX). The ensemble lengths shown are (B) 7, (C) 15, and (D) 32. Note the decrease in frame rate from 26 to 17 to 5.1 frames per second. (From Kremkau FW: Principles and instrumentation. In Merritt CRB (ed): Doppler Color Imaging. New York, Churchill Livingstone, 1992. Reprinted with permission.)

that these are mean values that must be compared with care to the peak systolic values that are commonly used in evaluating spectral displays (Fig. 6.13, Color Plate XXIII). The implication of this, in the case of the detection of a stenosis in the presence of turbulence, is that the turbulence causes increasing weighting of lower Doppler shifts, thus reducing the mean Doppler shift. The peak is unchanged in the presence of turbulence, as observed on a spectral display. However, in the color-flow display, the mean would be reduced in the presence of turbulence. Time-domain techniques do provide peak and spectral information, which can be shown on conventional flow speed versus time plots (Fig. 6.15, Color Plate XXVIII). These can be converted through calculation to volume flow rate versus time plots.[41,42]

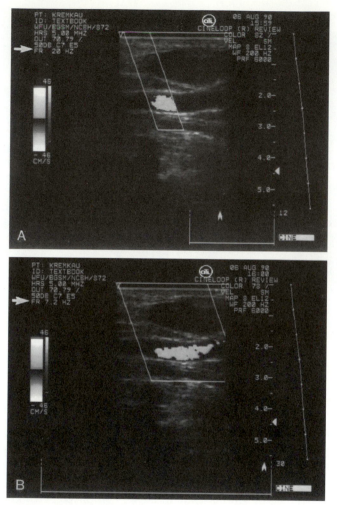

Figure 6.12. Tripling the color window width decreases the frame rate from (A) 20 Hz (see Color Plate XXI) to (B) 7.2 Hz (see Color Plate XXII). (From Kremkau FW: Principles and instrumentation. In Merritt CRB (ed): Doppler Color Imaging. New York, Churchill Livingstone, 1992. Reprinted with permission.)

Because color-flow techniques require several pulses per scan line (as opposed to one pulse per scan line for single-focus, gray-scale anatomic imaging [Chapter 2]), frame rates are generally lower than those for comparable-depth, gray-scale anatomic imaging. If the frame rate is low enough, as in Figure 6.16 (Color Plate XXIX), a significant portion of the cardiac cycle is represented across the color image from left to right. In this figure, the time across the color window represents about 20 percent of the cardiac cycle. The bright portion represents

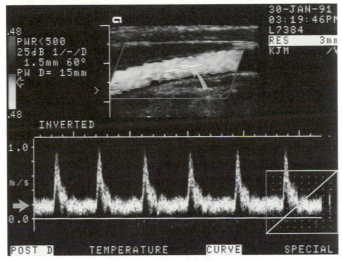

Figure 6.13. Color-flow display of the common carotid artery, including a color-coded pulsed-Doppler spectrum. The colors are assigned to the spectrum according to Doppler shift amplitudes. From the dark red color in the sample volume (curved arrow), we can estimate from the color map (open arrow) a flow speed of about 10 cm/s. How would this compare with values on the spectrum? Three important considerations enter here: mean versus peak, angle correction, and cardiac cycle. The color-flow frame was generated during diastole. From the diastolic portion of the spectrum, we can estimate the mean value to be about 20 cm/s (arrow). Angle correction was not applied to the color-flow display. Had it been, the 60-degree angle would have doubled the extreme color bar values to 96 cm/s, and our estimate would become approximately 20 cm/s, in agreement with the spectrum (see Color Plate XXIII). (From Kremkau FW: Principles and pitfalls of real-time color-flow imaging. In Bernstein EF (ed): Vascular Diagnosis, 4th edition. St. Louis, Mosby-Year Book, 1993. Reprinted with permission.)

the largest Doppler shifts, but these are not a result of a region in which the Doppler angle is the smallest (the Doppler angle is approximately constant across the color window in this example) or there is vessel narrowing (there is none in this example). Here, the bright region represents the largest Doppler shifts at peak systole, with the darker red to the left representing late diastole and early systole and that on the right representing early diastole. In such a case, it would be a mistake to consider the single frame being viewed as a representation of the flow at an instant in time. In fact, the representation is of flow at various instants in time over a significant portion of the cardiac cycle with time progressing from left to right across the color window.

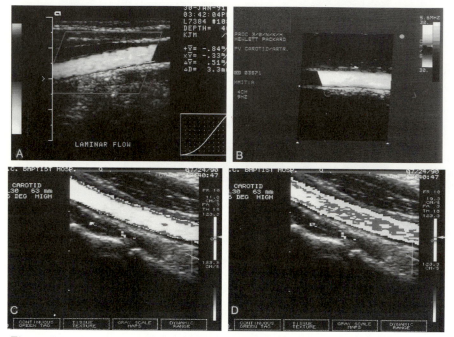

Figure 6.14. (A) Digital readout of stored mean Doppler shift (converted to mean flow speed) at specific pixel locations. The conversion to speed requires an angle correction, just as in spectral Doppler techniques. The value at the vessel center (84 cm/s) is greater than at the edge (33 cm/s), as expected for laminar flow (see Color Plate XXIV). (B) Laminar flow. The color bar used in this scan progresses from dark red and dark blue to bright white (decreasing saturation and increasing luminance). This presentation nicely shows laminar flow. The regions near the vessel wall are dark, with progressive brightening and decreasing saturation to white at the center left. This corresponds to the low-flow speeds at the vessel wall and high-flow speeds at the vessel center, which are characteristic of laminar flow (see Color Plate XXV). (C) The green tag is set at a specific level (arrow) on an angle-corrected calibrated color bar. The green region on the display, therefore, indicates areas where that specific flow speed exists (see Color Plate XXVI). The green tag is set at 11.6 and (D) 19.3 (see Color Plate XXVII). As the set flow speed value increases, the indicated region (green) moves to the center, where higher speeds are expected (Part A from Kremkau FW: Principles and pitfalls of real-time color-flow imaging. In Bernstein EF (ed): Vascular Diagnosis, 4th edition. St. Louis, Mosby-Year Book, 1993. Parts B to D from Kremkau FW: Principles and instrumentation. In Merritt CRB (ed): Doppler Color Imaging. New York, Churchill Livingstone, 1992. Reprinted with permission.)

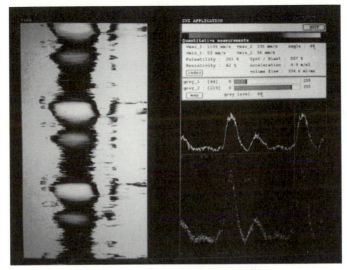

Figure 6.15. Peak, spectral, and volume flow rate information derived from time-domain color-flow information (see Color Plate XXVIII). (From Kremkau FW: Principles and pitfalls of real-time color-flow imaging. In Bernstein EF (ed): Vascular Diagnosis, 4th edition. St. Louis, Mosby-Year Book, 1993. Reprinted with permission.)

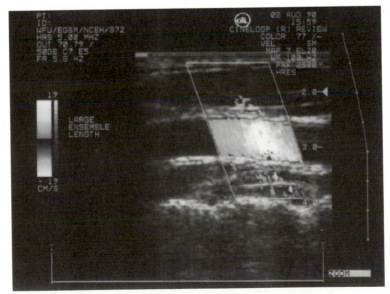

Figure 6.16. In this scan, a large ensemble length (20 pulses per color scan line) is used. This yields accurate Doppler shift determination at each location with color filling in to the vessel walls in the region of slow flow. This is done at the expense of frame rate, which in this example is less than 6 Hz (see Color Plate XXIX). (From Kremkau FW: Principles of color flow imaging. J Vasc Technol *15:*104–111, 1991. Reprinted with permission.)

6.4

Displays

The display is a color video monitor that includes three electron guns that correspond to thousands of triple groups of tiny color phosphor dots (red, green, and blue) on the inside face of the tube. At each pixel location on the display, a gray level (brightness) appropriate to the stored number in memory is shown for each non–Doppler-shifted echo stored. Where Doppler- or time-shifted echoes have been stored, hue, saturation, and luminance appropriate to the shift information are presented according to a choice of schemes, each of which is presented on the display as a color map (color bar or color wheel) (Fig. 6.17, Color Plates XXX to XXXV). The map allows the observer to interpret what the hue, saturation, and luminance mean at each location in terms of sign, magnitude, and variance of the Doppler shifts. Hue indicates sign. Changes in hue, saturation, or luminance up and down the map indicate increasing magnitude. Changes in hue across the map (from left to right) indicate increasing variance (if it is being used).

As with any Doppler-shift (or time-shift) technique, the angle is important. Figures 6.8A to C show perpendicular, upstream, and down-stream views of flow in a vessel. Figure 6.18 (Color Plates XXXVI to XXXIX) shows convex-array and linear-array views of vascular flow. Note that the images in parts A and C are similar in appearance, with red on the left and blue on the right. However, the color bars are inverted. How is this inconsistency explained? In fact, why does the color change at all in Figure 6.18C (Color Plate XXXVII)? The color changes in Figure 6.18A (Color Plate XXXVI) because, with a sector format, pulses (and scan lines) travel in different directions (see Fig. 2.4). They thus have different Doppler angles with flow in a straight vessel. Some view the flow upstream and some, downstream (Fig. 6.18B). At a 90-degree Doppler angle, the color and the situation changes from one to the other case, but in Figure 6.18C (Color Plate XXXVII), this is not the case. All the pulses travel in the same direction (straight down). If the color change is not caused by changing scan-line directions, then it must be the result of changing flow direction. Careful inspection of this figure reveals that the vessel is not perfectly straight. It is concave up (convex down). The flow is from right to left so that flow is away from the transducer on the right (negative Doppler shift or blue) and toward it on the left (positive or red, Fig. 6.18D). A view further to the left reveals a second color change caused by a downward concavity (Fig. 6.18E, Color Plate XXXVIII). Figure 6.18F (Color Plate XXXIX) shows an example of lack of color caused by a 90-degree Doppler angle. With an acceptable angle (Fig. 6.18G, Color Plate XXXIX), flow is displayed.

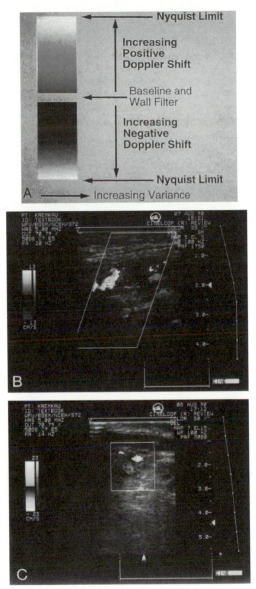

Figure 6.17. Color map information. (A) Diagram describing the information contained in a color map or color bar. The color-wheel form of map is shown in Figures 1.5 and 6.20A. It has the baseline at the bottom and the Nyquist limits joined at the top (see Color Plate XXX). (B) A luminance map. The increasing luminance of red and blue indicates increasing positive and negative, respectively, mean Doppler shifts (see Color Plate XXXI). (C) A saturation map is used to show cross-sectional flow in two vessels. The flow in the upper vessel is toward the transducer, yielding positive Doppler shifts (red). The flow in the lower vessel is away from the transducer, yielding negative Doppler shifts (blue). On this color map, red and blue progress to white (decreasing saturation and increasing luminance) with increasing positive and negative Doppler shift means, respectively (see Color Plate XXXII). (D) A hue map showing flow in the carotid artery (with reversal in the bulb) and

Illustration continued on following page

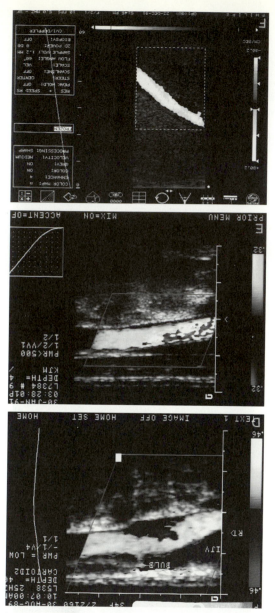

Figure 6.17. *Continued* jugular vein. Increasing positive Doppler shifts progress from dark blue to bright cyan (blue + green). Increasing negative Doppler shifts progress from dark red to bright yellow (red + green) (see Color Plate XXXIII). (E) A luminance (dark blue and red to bright blue and red) map with variance included. Increasing variance adds green to red or blue (producing yellow or cyan) from left to right across the map (see Color Plate XXXIV). (F) A saturation map on an instrument that detects echo-arrival−time shifts rather than Doppler shifts to generate a color-flow display. Red and blue progress toward white as positive and negative time shifts increase (see Color Plate XXXV). (Part A from Kremkau FW: Principles and instrumentation. In Merritt CRB (ed): Doppler Color Imaging. New York, Churchill Livingstone, 1992. Parts B to F from Kremkau FW: Principles and pitfalls of real-time color-flow imaging. In Bernstein EF (ed): Vascular Diagnosis, 4th edition. St. Louis, Mosby-Year Book, 1993. Reprinted with permission.)

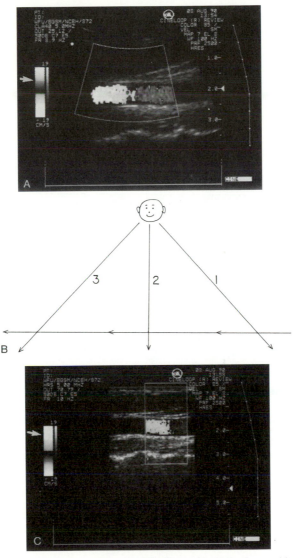

Figure 6.18. (A) In this saturation map, blue and red are assigned to positive and negative Doppler shifts, respectively, progressing to white at the extremes (see Color Plate XXXVI). (B) With the flow from right to left, an observer looking to the right (1) is looking upstream; looking to the left (3) is a downstream view. The perpendicular view (2) is neither upstream nor downstream. (C) In this map, the color assignments are reversed from those in Part A, i.e., red and blue are assigned to positive and negative Doppler shifts, respectively (see Color Plate XXXVII).

Illustration continued on following page

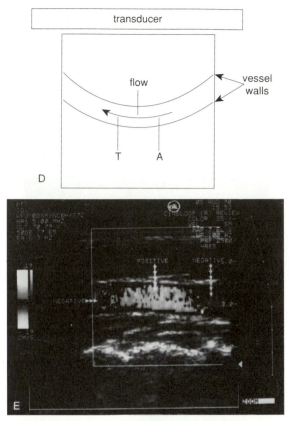

Figure 6.18. *Continued* (D) An exaggerated representation of Part C. A, flow is away from transducer; T, flow is toward the transducer. (E) Extension to the left of the color box in Part C reveals another color change caused by vessel curvature (concave down) (see Color Plate XXXVIII).

Figure 6.19A (Color Plate XL) shows various Doppler shifts as Doppler-angle changes across the display caused by the sector format: yellow, large positive shift; red, small positive; black, zero; blue, small negative; and cyan, large negative. Figures 6.19B to F show confirmations of this by the spectral displays.

In Figure 6.20 (Color Plates XLI to XLIII), some interesting questions arise. First, in Figure 6.20A (Color Plate XLI), what is the direction of blood flow? According to the color map (color wheel) in the upper left hand corner of the figure, negative Doppler shifts are coded in red and yellow, and positive Doppler shifts are blue and cyan. The color scan lines (and pulses) are steered to the left, and negative Doppler shifts (red and yellow) are received from the blood flowing within the

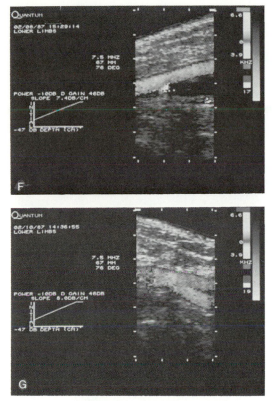

Figure 6.18. *Continued* (F) Profunda branch off the femoral artery appears to have no flow (no color within it) (see Color Plate XXXIX). (G) This view of the profunda shows color within it. The 90-degree Doppler angle in Part F causes no Doppler shift and, therefore, a lack of color (see Color Plate XXXIX). (Parts A and C from Kremkau FW: Principles of color flow imaging. J Vasc Technol *15*:104–111, 1991. Part E from Kremkau FW: Color-flow color assignments I. J Vasc Technol *15*:265–266, 1991. Reprinted with permission.)

vessel. If we are looking to the left and seeing blood flowing away from us (negative Doppler shifts), the blood must be flowing from right to left in the upper and lower horizontal portions of the vessel. What about the central portion of the vessel? The blood would have to be flowing from left to right there, but how is it, then, that negative Doppler shifts are seen there also? The answer is that this portion of the vessel is not horizontal but is angled down so that, in fact, even though the blood is flowing from left to right it is also flowing away from the transducer because of the downward direction. Thus, negative Doppler shifts are found throughout the vessel in this scan. Another way to say this is that the flow direction never crosses perpendicularly to the scan lines.

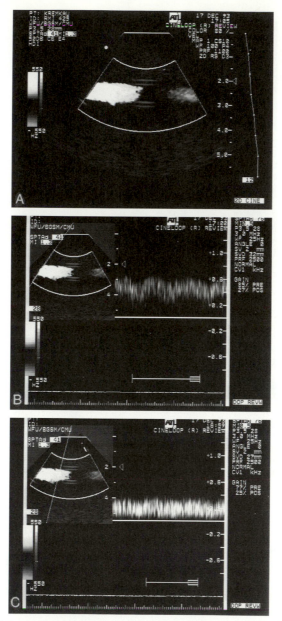

Figure 6.19. (A) Sector-format color-flow presentation of flow from left to right in a straight tube. Approximate Doppler shifts (from the color map) are yellow, 500 Hz; red, 200 Hz; black, 0 Hz; blue, −200 Hz; and cyan, −500 Hz (see Color Plate XL). The spectra in Parts B to F confirm these estimates. Doppler shifts decrease as Doppler angles increase toward the center of the color window.

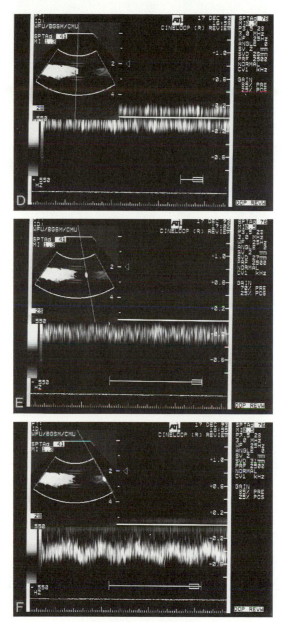

Figure 6.19. *Continued*

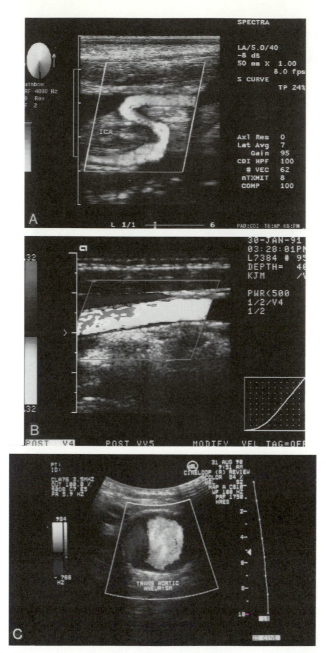

Figure 6.20. (A) A tortuous artery (see Color Plate XLI). (B) A (nearly) straight artery (see Color Plate XLII). (C) Circular flow in an aneurysm. Black between the red and blue indicates true flow reversal (see Color Plate XLIII). (Parts A and B from Kremkau FW: Color interpretation II. J Vasc Technol 16:215–216, 1992. Reprinted with permission.)

Another intriguing question regarding Figure 6.20A (Color Plate XLI) is the following: does the yellow region in the bend at the upper left indicate where the speed of the blood flow is the greatest? According to the color map, this region is where the highest negative Doppler shifts are generated, but does that mean that this is where the highest flow speeds are encountered? The answer in this case is no. The highest negative Doppler shifts are found in this region because the smallest Doppler angles are encountered there, not because high flow speeds are found there. In this region, the flow is approximately parallel to the scan lines, yielding Doppler angles around zero. There is no evidence of vessel narrowing to explain an increased flow speed. The increased Doppler shift can be explained purely on angular grounds.

In Figure 6.20B (Color Plate XLII), the region shown in cyan (aqua or blue-green) indicates positive Doppler shifts, according to the color map, whereas the blood flow in the rest of the vessel is generating negative Doppler shifts (red and yellow). Again, the scan lines are steered to the left so that negative Doppler shifts indicate that we are looking downstream, seeing flow away from the transducer. Therefore, blood flow is from right to left in this carotid artery with the head oriented to the left as usual. How can we, then, explain the positive Doppler shifts found in the upper left-hand portion of the vessel? The possibilities include turbulent flow, flow reversal, and flow speeds that exceed 32 cm/sec in this region, producing aliasing (Section 7.2). Flow reversal and turbulent flow can be eliminated because the region between the negative (red and yellow) and positive (cyan) Doppler shift regions contains no dark or black region (crossing the baseline indicates flow reversal). It is easy to distinguish between true flow reversal (which involves dark regions, as shown around the baseline of the color bar; Fig. 6.20C, Color Plate XLIII) and aliasing, which involves bright colors, as indicated at the bar extremes (Section 7.2). Thus, the aqua region is a region of flow away from the transducer that has exceeded the negative aliasing limit of 32 cm/s and has become an aliased positive Doppler shift (cyan).

Does this mean that the flow speed in the aliased aqua region exceeds 32 cm/s? In this case, the answer is no. The aliasing limit, which is one half of the PRF, has been exceeded. This aliasing limit has been converted, using the Doppler equation, to an equivalent flow speed of 32 cm/s. However, because there is no angle correction in this scan, an angle of zero was assumed in the conversion from Doppler shift to flow speed. Therefore, the aliased flow exceeds 32 cm/s only when it is parallel to the scan lines. Because the Doppler angle in this example is approximately 60 degrees, the Doppler shifts are only about one half of what they would be at zero degrees. Therefore, the flow in the aliased region exceeds approximately 64 cm/s. Care must be taken in using tagging (Figs. 6.14C and D, Color Plates XXIV and XXVII) or aliasing limits converted to flow speed units with no angle correction.

Figure 6.21 (Color Plate XLIV) shows a transverse view through the external and internal carotid arteries. The external carotid artery (ECA), according to the color map on the left, contains negative Doppler-shifted echoes (red and yellow) around its periphery and positive Doppler-shifted echoes (cyan and blue) in its central core. What is the direction of blood flow in this vessel, toward or away from the observer? Are the flow directions in the central core and periphery opposite? With the help of Figure 6.22 (Color Plate XLV), we can conclude that Figure 6.21 (Color Plate XLIV) is a downstream view in the periphery and an upstream view in the central core. However, it is not likely that the flow directions in these two regions are opposite. A better explanation needs to be found. Because the region between the dark red and the blue in the vessel corresponds to the bright yellow and cyan color bar extremes, aliasing is indicated (Section 7.2). Now, we can correctly sort out the proper interpretation of the colors in Figure 6.21 (Color Plate XLIV). The slower flows (and smaller Doppler shifts) in the periphery indicate a downstream view. That is, the negative Doppler shifts tell us that the flow is moving through the vessel away from the observer and transducer in this transverse view. Pro-

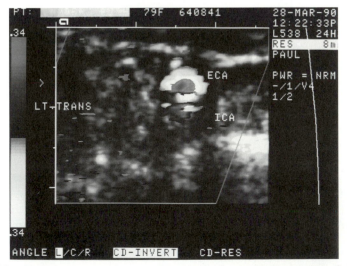

Figure 6.21. Transverse view of external and internal carotid arteries (see Color Plate XLIV). (From Kremkau FW: Color interpretation III. J Vasc Technol *16*:309–310, 1992. Reprinted with permission.)

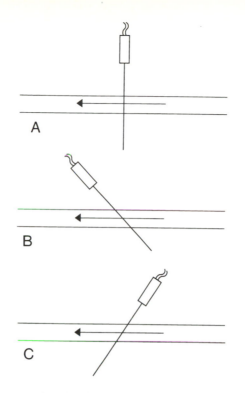

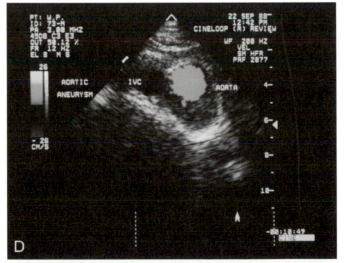

Figure 6.22. The image plane cuts in a transverse manner across the vessel. The views are (A) perpendicular, (B) upstream, and (C) downstream. Doppler shifts obtained would be (A) zero, (B) positive, and (C) negative. The image plane is being viewed edge-on in this figure. (D) Transverse view upstream (positive Doppler shift) in the aorta and downstream (negative Doppler shift) in the inferior vena cava (see Color Plate XLV). (Parts A to C from Kremkau FW: Color interpretation III. J Vasc Technol *16*:309–310, 1992. Reprinted with permission.)

gressing from the vessel's edge toward its center finds increasing Doppler shifts, which is consistent with laminar flow (dark red progresses to bright yellow). Where the yellow changes to cyan, the negative aliasing limit has been exceeded, and positive Doppler shifts result. Continuing toward the center of the vessel, the cyan changes to blue as the positive Doppler shift decreases down the bar (Fig. 7.16B, Color Plate L). The aliased Doppler shifts are the result of the fastest flow speeds away from the transducer, which exceed the aliasing limit of 0.34. Does this mean that at the point where yellow changes to cyan the flow speed is 34 cm/s? No, because the aliasing limits on the color bar are not angle corrected and, therefore, are correct only if the flow is parallel to the scan lines, i.e., parallel to the scan plane (which it obviously is not in this transverse view).

6.5
Review

Color-flow imaging acquires Doppler- or time-shifted echoes from a cross section of tissue scanned by an ultrasound beam. These echoes are then presented in color and superimposed on the gray-scale anatomic image of nonshifted echoes that were received during the scan. The flow echoes are assigned colors according to the color map chosen. Red, yellow, blue, cyan, and white indicate positive or negative Doppler shifts (approaching or receding flow). Yellow, cyan, or green is used to indicate variance (disturbed or turbulent flow). Several pulses (the number is called the ensemble length) are needed to generate a color scan line. Linear, convex, and phased arrays are used to acquire the gray-scale and color-flow information. Color controls include gain; depth gain compensation; map selection; variance on/off; persistence; ensemble length; color/gray priority; scale (PRF); baseline shift; wall filter; and the color window's angle, location, and size. Doppler color-flow instruments are pulsed-Doppler instruments and are subject to the same limitations, i.e., Doppler-angle dependence and aliasing, as are other Doppler instruments. Time-shift instruments have the same angle dependence.

The definitions of terms used in this chapter are listed next.

Autocorrelation. A rapid technique for obtaining the mean Doppler-shift frequency. This technique is used in most color-flow instruments.
Clutter. Noise in the Doppler signal generally caused by high-amplitude, Doppler-shifted echoes from the heart or vessel walls.
Color flow. The presentation of two-dimensional, real-time Doppler-

or time-shift information superimposed on a real-time, gray-scale anatomic cross-sectional image. Flow directions toward and away from the transducer (i.e., positive and negative Doppler or time shifts) are presented as different colors on the display.

Cross correlation. A rapid technique for determining time shifts in the echo's arrival. This technique is used to determine flow speed without using the Doppler effect.

Ensemble length. The number of pulses used to generate one color-flow-image scan line. Also called packet size, dwell time, or color sensitivity.

Frame rate. The number of frames displayed per second.

Hue. The color perceived as a result of the frequency of light.

Luminance. The brightness of a presented hue and saturation.

Priority. The gray-scale echo strength below which color-flow information is preferentially shown on a display.

Saturation. The amount of hue present in a mix with white.

Variance. The square of the standard deviation. One of the outputs of the autocorrelation process. A measure of spectral broadening.

Wall filter. An electric filter that passes frequencies above a set level and eliminates strong low-frequency Doppler shifts (clutter) from the pulsating heart or vessel walls.

Exercises

6.1 What colors are used on color-flow maps?

   a. red and blue
   b. yellow and cyan
   c. black and magenta
   d. green and white
   e. more than one of the above

6.2 Multiple focus is not used in color-flow imaging because

   a. it would not improve the image
   b. Doppler transducers cannot focus
   c. of the ensemble length
   d. frame rates would be too low
   e. more than one of the above

6.3 In Figure 6.20A (Color Plate XLI), red and yellow indicate negative Doppler shifts. Therefore, flow in this vessel is:

   a. from upper right to lower left
   b. from lower left to upper right

6.4 In the bend at the upper left of Figure 6.20A (Color Plate XLI), there is a yellow region in the center of the vessel. This indicates the region in the image where blood flow speed is the greatest. True or false?

6.5 In Figure 6.20B (Color Plate XLII), the region shown in cyan (aqua or blue-green) indicates:

   a. turbulent flow
   b. flow reversal
   c. flow speed exceeding 32 cm/s
   d. all of the above
   e. none of the above

6.6 Color-flow instruments present two-dimensional, color-coded images, representing _____, that are superimposed on gray-scale images, representing _____.

6.7 Which of the following on a color-flow display is (are) presented in real time?

   a. gray-scale anatomy
   b. flow direction
   c. Doppler spectrum
   d. a and b
   e. all of the above

6.8 If red represents flow toward the transducer and blue represents flow away, what color would be seen for normal flow toward the transducer? What color would be seen for aliasing flow toward the transducer? What colors would be seen for normal flow away and for aliasing flow away? What color would be seen for a positive Doppler shift or a negative shift?

6.9 Doppler color-flow instruments use an _____ technique to yield _____ flow speed in real time.

6.10 Time-shift, color-flow instruments use a _____ technique to determine flow speeds.

6.11 The angle dependencies of Doppler- and time-shift color-flow instruments are different. True or false?

6.12 The Fourier transform technique is not necessary in color-flow instruments because it is not _____ enough.

    a. slow
    b. fast
    c. bright
    d. cheap
    e. none of the above

6.13 Do the different colors appearing in Figures 6.18A (Color Plate XXXVI) and C (Color Plate XXXVII) indicate that flow is going in two different directions in the vessel?

6.14 In color-flow instruments, color is used only to represent the direction of flow. True or false?

6.15 Approximately _____ pulses are required to obtain one line of color-flow information.

    a. 1
    b. 10
    c. 100
    d. 1000
    e. 1,000,000

6.16 There are approximately _____ samples per line on a color-flow display.

    a. 2
    b. 20
    c. 200
    d. 2000
    e. 2,000,000

6.17 There are about _____ frames per second produced by a color-flow Doppler instrument.

    a. 10
    b. 20
    c. 40
    d. 80
    e. more than one of the above

6.18 Color-flow displays are not dependent on the Doppler angle. True or false?

6.19 If two colors are shown in the same vessel using a color-flow instrument, it always means flow is occurring in opposite directions in the vessel. True or false?

6.20 A region of bright color on a color-flow display always indicates the highest flow speeds. True or false?

6.21 Non-Doppler color-flow instruments detect echo arrival _____ shifts to determine flow.

6.22 The _____ technique is commonly used to detect echo Doppler shifts in color-flow instruments.

6.23 The _____ technique is used to detect echo-arrival time shifts in color-flow instruments.

6.24 The autocorrelation technique yields

    a. mean Doppler shift
    b. sign of Doppler shift
    c. spread around the mean (variance)
    d. all of the above
    e. none of the above

6.25 Which of the following reduce the frame rate of a color-flow image (more than one correct answer)?

    a. wider color window
    b. longer color window
    c. increased ensemble length
    d. higher transducer frequency
    e. higher priority setting

6.26 Lack of color in a vessel with flow may be the result of (more than one correct answer)?

    a. low color gain
    b. high wall filter setting
    c. low priority setting
    d. baseline shift
    e. high PRF

6.27 Increasing ensemble length _____ color sensitivity and accuracy and _____ frame rate.

   a. improves, increases
   b. degrades, increases
   c. degrades, decreases
   d. improves, decreases
   e. none of the above

6.28 Which controls can be used to deal with aliasing (more than one correct answer)?

   a. wall filter
   b. gain
   c. baseline shift
   d. PRF
   e. smoothing

6.29 Pink compared with red is an example of

   a. hue
   b. luminance
   c. saturation
   d. b and c
   e. none of the above

6.30 Yellow is the combination of

   a. red and green
   b. red and blue
   c. blue and green
   d. red, green, and blue

6.31 Cyan is the combination of

   a. red and green
   b. red and blue
   c. blue and green
   d. red, green, and blue

6.32 White is the combination of

   a. red and green
   b. red and blue
   c. blue and green
   d. red, green, and blue

6.33 Which control can be used to help with clutter?

- **a.** wall filter
- **b.** gain
- **c.** baseline shift
- **d.** PRF
- **e.** smoothing

6.34 Color map baselines are always represented by

- **a.** white
- **b.** black
- **c.** red
- **d.** blue
- **e.** cyan

6.35 Autocorrelation and fast Fourier transform are essentially the same. True or false?

6.36 Autocorrelation is used in both Doppler- and time-shift color-flow instruments. True or false?

6.37 If a green tag indicates that the flow speed is 50 cm/s but the Doppler angle is 60 degrees and no angle correction is used, the flow speed is actually _____ cm/s.

6.38 Doubling the width of a color window produces a(n) _____ frame rate.

- **a.** doubled
- **b.** quadrupled
- **c.** unchanged
- **d.** halved
- **e.** quartered

6.39 Steering the color window to the right or left produces a(n) _____ frame rate.

- **a.** doubled
- **b.** quadrupled
- **c.** unchanged
- **d.** halved
- **e.** quartered

6.40 Autocorrelation produces (more than one correct answer)

a. sign of Doppler shift
b. mean value of Doppler shift
c. variance
d. spectrum
e. peak Doppler shift

6.41 If the heart rate is 60 beats/min and the frame rate is 10 Hz, one edge of the color display lags the other by what fraction of the cardiac cycle?

a. one sixtieth
b. one thirtieth
c. one tenth
d. one sixth
e. one third

6.42 Steering the color window to the right or left changes

a. frame rate
b. PRF
c. Doppler angle
d. Doppler shift
e. more than one of the above

6.43 Color-flow frame rates are _____ gray-scale rates.

a. equal to
b. less than
c. more than
d. depends on color map
e. depends on priority

6.44 In a single frame, color can change in a vessel because of

a. vessel's curvature
b. sector format
c. helical flow
d. diastolic flow reversal
e. all of the above

6.45 Angle is not important in transverse color-flow views through vessels. True or false?

6.46 In Figure 6.8A, match the following:

_____ **a.** zero Doppler shift   **1.** yellow
_____ **b.** small positive   **2.** red
         shift
_____ **c.** large positive shift   **3.** black
_____ **d.** small negative   **4.** blue
         shift
_____ **e.** large negative   **5.** cyan
         shift

6.47 In Figure 6.9C (Color Plate XII), the mean Doppler shifts in the vessel are less than _____ Hz.

a. 10
b. 25
c. 50
d. 100
e. 200

6.48 What is the direction of flow indicated by red in the vessel in Figure 6.14B (Color Plate XXV)?

6.49 The flow in the aneurysm of Figure 6.20C (Color Plate XLIII) is _____.

a. clockwise
b. counterclockwise
c. left to right
d. top to bottom
e. right to left.

6.50 The dark red and blue colors in Figure 6.22D (Color Plate XLV) show that flow in the vessels is at speeds less than 26 cm/s. True or false?

7

Artifacts, Performance, and Safety

Several artifacts are encountered in Doppler ultrasound.[43] These are incorrect presentations of flow information. The most common of these is aliasing. However, others occur, including shadowing, range ambiguity, spectrum mirror image, location mirror image, and electromagnetic interference. Artifacts encountered in sonography are discussed in Section 2.4 and in Chapter 6 of reference 1.

Several devices (Fig. 7.1) are available to determine if sonographic and Doppler ultrasound instruments are operating correctly and consistently. Those that test the operation of the Doppler instrument as a whole are discussed in Section 7.3. Those that measure the beams produced by transducers and those that measure the acoustic output of instruments are discussed in Chapter 7 of reference 1. The system's performance is important for evaluating the instrument as a diagnostic tool. Beam profiles are important when evaluating and choosing transducers. The acoustic output of an instrument is important when considering bioeffects and safety.

Risk and safety considerations are always relevant in medical diagnostic techniques. It is desirable to gain information that is useful in guiding patient management while, at the same time, minimizing any risk resulting from the diagnostic procedure. The biologic effects of ultrasound exposure have been studied in cells, plants, and experi-

219

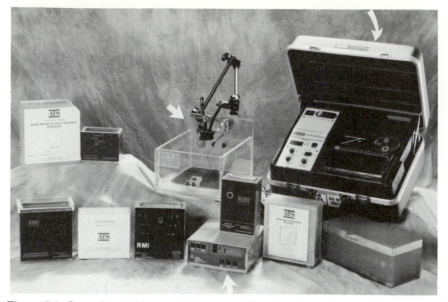

Figure 7.1. Several test objects and phantoms. The string test object and flow phantom discussed in Section 7.1 are indicated by the arrows and curved arrow, respectively. The remaining eight devices are used to evaluate sonographic instruments, as discussed in Chapter 7 of reference 1.

mental animals, and several epidemiologic studies have been performed. From this information, an approach is developed to the appropriate and prudent use of Doppler ultrasound as a medical diagnostic tool.

In this chapter, we consider the following questions. What causes spectral and color-flow presentations to appear incorrectly? How can specific artifacts be recognized and handled properly to avoid the pitfalls and misdiagnoses they can cause? How do we determine whether or not a Doppler instrument is working properly? What devices are available for testing the performance characteristics of Doppler instruments? Are there any known risks in the use of Doppler ultrasound? How can an operator of a Doppler ultrasound instrument minimize exposure of the patient to ultrasound? The following terms are discussed in this chapter:

aliasing	phantom
cavitation	range ambiguity
mechanical index	shadowing
mirror image	test object
Nyquist limit	thermal index

7.1
Spectral Artifacts

Aliasing is the most common artifact encountered in Doppler ultrasound. The word alias comes from Middle English elles, Latin alius, and Greek allos, all of which mean "other" or "otherwise." Contemporary meanings for the word include (as an adverb) "otherwise called" or "otherwise known as" and (as a noun) "an assumed or additional name." In its technical use, aliasing indicates the improper representation of information that has been insufficiently sampled. The sampling can be of a spatial or a temporal nature. Inadequate spatial sampling can result in improper conclusions about the object or population sampled. For example, we could assemble 10 families, each consisting of a father, a mother, and a child, and line them up in the order: father, mother, child, father, mother, child, etc. If we wanted to sample the contents of these families by taking 10 photographs, we could choose to photograph one of every three persons (i.e., the first, fourth, seventh, etc., persons in the line). However, if we did this, we would conclude that all families are made up of three adult men, no women, and no children. Spatial undersampling of one third of the population in this example resulted in an incorrect conclusion regarding the total population.

Another example of inadequate spatial sampling is shown in Figure 7.2. In Figure 7.2A, we see what we might call a "Doppler flower," containing 12 double-pointed petals. Each petal is made up of four lines. If we sample at the intersections of these lines, we get a 48-point dot-to-dot child's puzzle, as shown in Figure 7.2B. Connecting the dots properly yields the flower shown in Figure 7.2A. In Figure 7.2C, the even-numbered dots from Figure 7.2B have been eliminated; there are now 24 dots (samples). When these dots are connected, a reasonable representation of the original flower results, but it is not as good as the representation in Figure 7.2B. The higher frequency information that describes the double pointing of the petals has been lost. In Figure 7.2D, the even-numbered dots from Figure 7.2C have been eliminated. This representation of the flower, which contains 12 samples, yields a 12-sided polygon, approximating a circle and poorly representing the original flower. The lower frequency information about the 12 petals has been lost. Figures 7.2E and F each eliminate one half of the previous samples, yielding a hexagon and a triangle, respectively. Figure 7.2F gives virtually no information regarding the round, double-pointed, 12-petaled flower.

In these examples, we see that inadequate spatial sampling yields an incorrect representation of the object sampled. This is similar to a

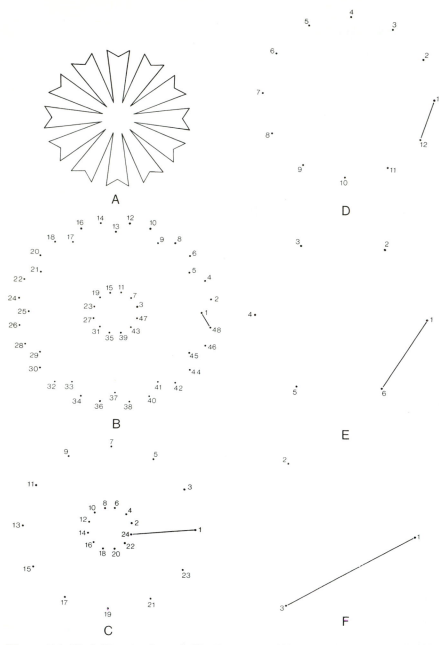

A

B

C

D

E

F

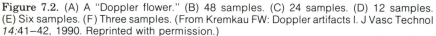

Figure 7.2. (A) A "Doppler flower." (B) 48 samples. (C) 24 samples. (D) 12 samples. (E) Six samples. (F) Three samples. (From Kremkau FW: Doppler artifacts I. J Vasc Technol *14*:41–42, 1990. Reprinted with permission.)

disguise (false appearance or assumed identity) or alias. As the sampling was reduced, we first lost the double-pointed character of each petal, then the presence of the 12 petals, and finally, the circular nature of the flower. In each case, we were experiencing spatial aliasing. Another example of spatial aliasing is given in Figure 7.3.

An optical form of temporal aliasing occurs in motion pictures when wagon wheels appear to rotate at various speeds and in a reverse direction. Similar behavior is observed when a fan is lighted with a strobe light (Figs. 7.4 to 7.6).

There is an upper limit to Doppler shift that can be detected by pulsed instruments. If the Doppler-shift frequency exceeds one half the pulse repetition frequency (normally in the 5- to 30-kHz range), temporal aliasing occurs. Improper Doppler-shift information (improper direction and improper value) results. Higher pulse repetition frequencies (Table 7.1) permit higher Doppler shifts to be detected but also increase the chance of a range ambiguity artifact (discussed later in this section). Continuous-wave Doppler instruments do not have this limitation (but neither do they provide depth localization).

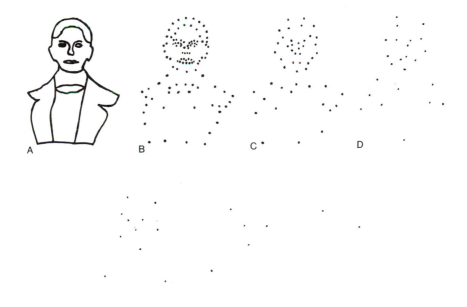

Figure 7.3. (A) A freehand drawing of Christian Doppler. (B) 96 samples from (A), (C) 48 samples, (D) 24 samples, (E) 12 samples, (F) six samples, and (G) three samples. In the last three cases, connecting the dots would yield an image that would bear no resemblance to Part A. Indeed, in Part G, a triangle would result. These cases are undersampled, yielding an "aliased" result.

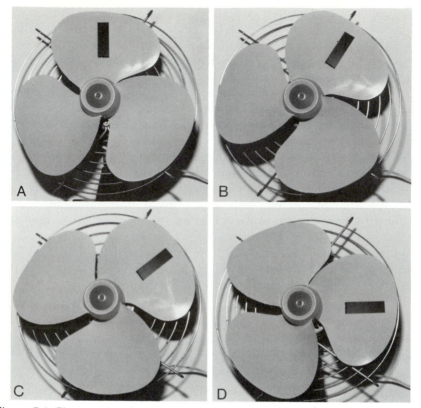

Figure 7.4. Photographs of 1000-rpm clockwise rotating fan at times (A) t = 0, (B) 5, (C) 10, and (D) 15 ms. The pictures are taken with a strobe light at a rate of 200 per second (12 per rotation) so that the clockwise rotation is observed. (From Kremkau FW: Doppler artifacts II. J Vasc Technol *14*:123–124, 1990. Reprinted with permission.)

Figure 7.7 illustrates aliasing in the popliteal artery and in the heart of a normal subject. This figure also illustrates how aliasing can be reduced or eliminated (Table 7.2) by increasing the pulse repetition frequency, increasing the Doppler angle (which decreases the Doppler shift for a given flow), or by baseline shifting. The latter is an electronic "cut-and-paste" technique that moves the misplaced aliasing peaks over to their proper location. It is a successful technique as long as there are no legitimate Doppler shifts in the region of the aliasing. If there are, they will be moved over to an inappropriate location along with the aliasing peaks. (This would happen if the baseline were shifted farther down in Fig. 7.7E.) Other approaches to eliminating aliasing include changing to a lower frequency Doppler transducer or changing to a continuous-wave mode of operation.

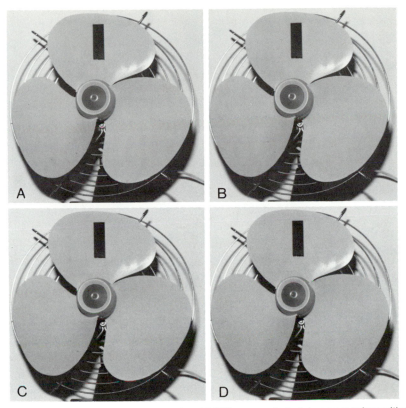

Figure 7.5. The fan speed is increased to 12,000 rpm so that pictures are taken with the blades in the same position each time. The fan appears to be stationary. (From Kremkau FW: Doppler artifacts II. J Vasc Technol *14*:123–124, 1990. Reprinted with permission.)

In Figure 7.7A, we can see that aliasing occurs at Doppler shifts greater than 1.75 kHz. The aliased peaks add another 1.25 kHz of Doppler shift; therefore, the correct peak shift is 3.0 kHz. With the higher pulse repetition frequency in Figure 7.7C, this result is confirmed. Thus, at the lower pulse repetition frequency, the peak shift could be determined, and baseline shifting is not necessary (but is convenient). However, if the peaks were buried in other portions of the Doppler signal (Fig. 7.7F), baseline shifting would not help. A higher pulse repetition frequency or a lower operating frequency might.

Aliasing occurs with the pulsed system because it is a sampling system. That is, a pulsed system acquires samples of the desired Doppler-shift frequency from which it must be synthesized (see Fig. 5.11). If samples are taken often enough, the correct result is achieved.

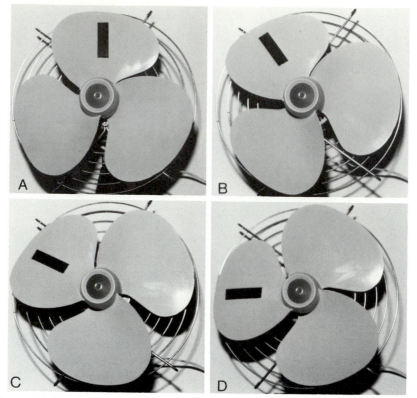

Figure 7.6. The fan speed is 11,000 rpm. (A to D) Thus the blades rotate 330 degrees between photographs. The fan appears (incorrectly) to be rotating counterclockwise at 1000 rpm. (From Kremkau FW: Doppler artifacts II. J Vasc Technol *14*:123–124, 1990. Reprinted with permission.)

Table 7–1

Aliasing and Range-Ambiguity Artifact Values

Pulse Repetition Frequency (kHz)	Doppler Shift Above Which Aliasing Occurs (kHz)	Range Beyond Which Ambiguity Occurs (cm)
5.0	2.5	15
7.5	3.7	10
10.0	5.0	7
12.5	6.2	6
15.0	7.5	5
17.5	8.7	4
20.0	10.0	3
25.0	12.5	3
30.0	15.0	2

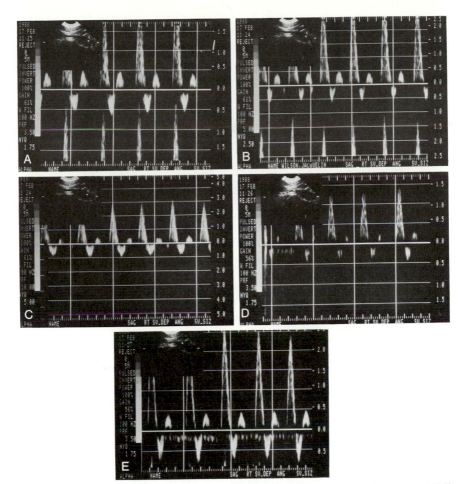

Figure 7.7. (A) Aliasing in the popliteal artery. (B) The pulse repetition frequency (PRF) is increased. (C) PRF is increased again. (D) Doppler angle is increased. (E) Baseline is shifted down. (F) An example of aliasing in Doppler echocardiography. (Parts A to E from Taylor KJW, Holland S: Doppler ultrasound I. Basic principles, instrumentation and pitfalls. Radiology *174*:297–307, 1990. Reprinted with permission.)

Illustration continued on following page

Table 7–2

Methods of Reducing or Eliminating Aliasing

Increase the pulse repetition frequency
Increase the Doppler angle
Shift the baseline
Use a lower operating frequency
Use a continuous-wave device

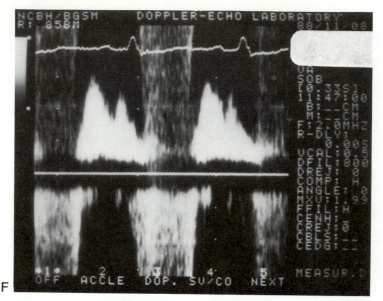

Figure 7.7. *Continued*

Figure 7.8 shows temporal sampling of a signal. Sufficient sampling yields the correct result. Insufficient sampling yields an incorrect result.

The Nyquist limit or frequency describes the minimum number of samples required to avoid aliasing. There must be at least two samples per cycle of the desired wave for it to be obtained correctly. For a complicated signal, such as a Doppler signal containing many frequencies (see Fig. 5.15), the sampling rate must be such that at least two samples occur for each cycle of the highest frequency present. To restate this rule, if the highest Doppler-shift frequency present in a signal exceeds one half the pulse repetition frequency, aliasing will occur (Fig. 7.9).

In an attempt to solve the aliasing problem by increasing the pulse repetition frequency, the range ambiguity[44] problem may be encountered. This occurs when a pulse is emitted before all the echoes from the previous pulse have been received. When this happens, early echoes from the last pulse are simultaneously received with late echoes from the previous pulse. This causes difficulty with the ranging process described in Chapter 2 and Section 5.2. The instrument is unable to determine whether an echo is an early one (superficial) from the last pulse or a late one (deep) from the previous pulse (Fig. 7.10). To avoid

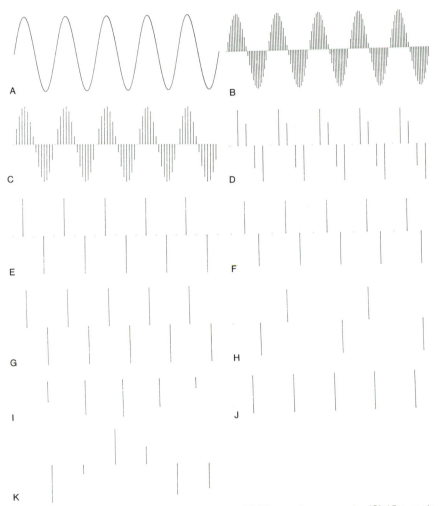

Figure 7.8. Sample of (A) a five-cycle voltage; (B) 25 samples per cycle; (C) 15 samples per cycle; (D) five samples per cycle; (E) four samples per cycle; (F) three samples per cycle; (G) two samples per cycle; (H) one sample per cycle; (I) one sample per cycle; (J) one sample per cycle; and (K) one sample per cycle. In the last four cases, aliasing occurs.

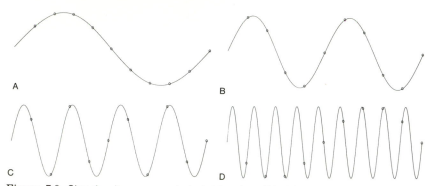

Figure 7.9. Signal voltages sampled at 10 points (O). (A) One cycle, (B) two cycles, (C) four cycles, and (D) nine cycles. As the signal's frequency is increased, aliasing occurs when the Nyquist limit is exceeded (in this case beyond five cycles). Thus, Part D is aliasing. Connecting the o's with a smooth curve would yield a one-cycle representation of what is actually a nine-cycle signal voltage.

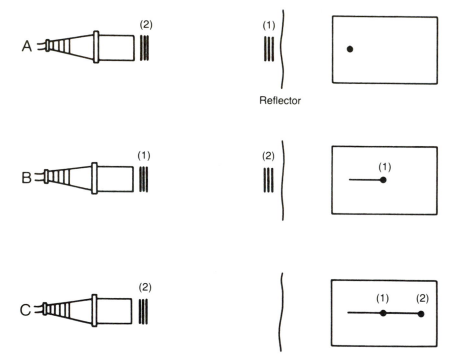

Figure 7.10. Ambiguity caused by sending out a pulse before an echo from the previous pulse is received. (A) A pulse (2) is sent out just as a previous pulse (1) is reflected. (B) The spot begins to move across the display. The first echo arrives at the transducer when the second pulse reflects. (C) The second echo arrives at the transducer, putting a bright spot (2) on the display at the position corresponding to the reflector. The spot (1) in the center of the display that results from the arrival of the earlier echo indicates a reflector at a location where there is none. (D) Transvaginal image shows the pulsed Doppler range gate (arrow) set at 33 mm within an ovary. (E) The resulting Doppler spectrum shows a waveform typical of the external iliac artery. (F) An identical signal was obtained

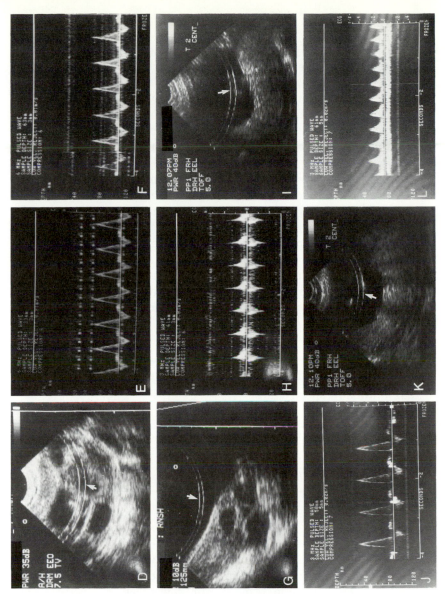

Figure 7.10. *Continued* when the range was increased to 63 mm, proving that the signal actually originated from the external iliac artery at this depth. (G) A strong arterial Doppler signal was obtained in this examination when the range gate (arrow) was placed within the urinary bladder at a depth of 31 mm. (H) An identical signal was detected when the range gate depth was increased to 61 mm, indicating that the signal actually arose from an artery at this depth. (I) With the range gate (arrow) placed at a depth of 50 mm in the uterus of a pregnant woman, at 16 weeks' gestation, signals (J) typical of the external iliac artery were detected. (K) Slight adjustment of the range gate (arrow) produced the desired umbilical artery signal (L), eliminating the artifactual iliac artery signal caused by range ambiguity. (Parts D to L from Gill RW, Kossoff MB, Kossoff G, et al: New class of pulsed Doppler US ambiguity at short ranges. Radiology *173*:272, 1989. Reprinted with permission.)

231

this difficulty, it simply assumes that all echoes are derived from the last pulse and that these echoes have originated from some depth, as determined by the 13-μs/cm rule (Section 2.1). As long as all echoes are received before the next pulse is sent out, this is true. However, with high pulse repetition frequencies, this may not be the case. Doppler-flow information may, therefore, come from locations other than the assumed one (the gate location). In effect, multiple gates or sample volumes are operating at different depths. Table 7.1 lists, for various pulse repetition frequencies, the ranges beyond which ambiguity occurs. Table 7.3 lists, for various depths, the maximum Doppler shift frequency (Nyquist limit) that avoids aliasing *and* the range ambiguity problem. The maximum flow speeds that avoid aliasing for given angles are also listed. Instruments sometimes increase the pulse repetition frequency (to avoid aliasing) into the range at which range ambiguity occurs. Multiple sample gates are shown on the display to indicate this condition. An approximate relationship between maximum flow speed and maximum depth to avoid both aliasing and range ambiguity is as follows (θ is Doppler angle).

$$\text{maximum flow speed (cm/s)}$$
$$= \frac{3000}{\text{maximum depth (cm)} \times \text{frequency (MHz)} \times \text{cosine } \theta}$$
$$v_m = \frac{3000}{d_m \, f \cos \theta}$$

maximum depth ↑ maximum flow speed ↓
frequency ↑ maximum flow speed ↓
Doppler angle ↑ maximum flow speed ↑

The mirror-image artifact described in Section 2.4 can also occur with Doppler systems. This means that an image of a vessel and a source of Doppler-shifted echoes can be duplicated on the opposite side

Table 7–3

Aliasing and Range-Ambiguity Limits

Depth (cm)	Pulse Repetition Frequency (kHz)	Nyquist Limit (kHz)	Maximum Flow Speed (cm/s)		
			0	30	60
1	77.0	38.0	585	673	1170
2	38.0	19.0	293	336	585
4	19.0	10.0	146	168	293
8	10.0	4.8	73	84	146
16	4.8	2.4	37	42	73

For various depths, the maximum pulse repetition frequency that avoids range ambiguity and the corresponding maximum Doppler shift frequency (Nyquist limit) that avoids aliasing are listed. Maximum flow speeds corresponding to the maximum Doppler shift are also listed for three Doppler angles (degrees), assuming a 5-MHz operating frequency.

of a strong reflector. The duplicated vessel that contains flow could be misinterpreted as an additional vessel. It has a spectrum similar to that for the real vessel. Figure 7.11 shows an example of image and spectrum duplication of the subclavian artery. The strong reflector in this case is the air at the pleura boundary.

A mirror image of a Doppler spectrum can appear on the opposite side of the baseline when flow is unidirectional, and it should appear only on one side of the baseline. This is an electronic duplication of the spectral information. It can occur when the receiver gain is set too high (causing overloading in the receiver and cross talk between the two flow channels, Fig. 7.12). It can also occur when Doppler angle is near 90 degrees (Fig. 7.13). Here, the duplication is usually legitimate. This is because the beams are focused and not cylindric in shape. Thus, although the axis of the beam is perpendicular to the direction of flow, one edge of the beam can be looking upstream and the other edge, downstream.

Occasionally, a spectral trace can show a straight line adjacent to and parallel to the baseline, often on both sides, as in Figure 7.14A. Apparently, this is the result of 60-Hz interference from power lines or the power supply. It can make a determination of low or absent diastolic flow difficult. Electromagnetic interference from power lines and nearby equipment can also cloud the spectral display with lines or "snow" (see Fig. 7.14B).

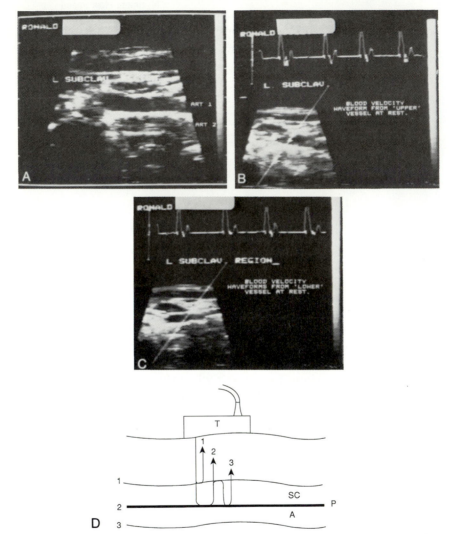

Figure 7.11. (A) Subclavian artery (ART 1) and mirror image (ART 2). (B) Flow signal from artery. (C) Flow signal from mirror image. (D) Multiple reflections produce mirror image. Paths 1 and 2 are legitimate, but Path 3 arrives late and produces the artifactual deep arterial wall. T, transducer, SC, subclavian artery, A, mirror-image artifact, P, pleura. (Part D from Kremkau FW: Principles and pitfalls of real-time color-flow imaging. In Bernstein EF (ed): Vascular Diagnosis, 4th edition. St. Louis, Mosby-Year Book, 1993. Reprinted with permission.)

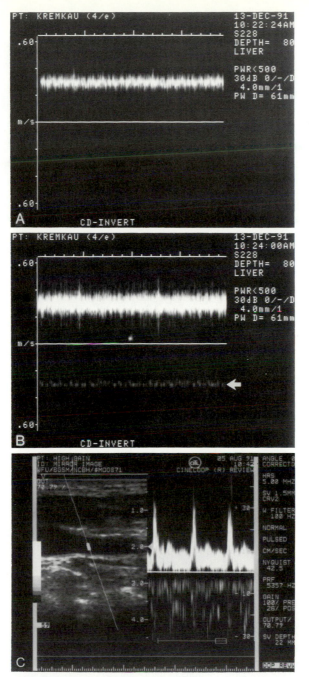

Figure 7.12. (A) Spectrum of a string moving at 30 cm/s. (B) Increased gain produces spectral broadening (Section 5.4) and mirror image (arrow). (C) High gain produces mirror image of carotid artery spectrum below the baseline. (Part C from Kremkau FW: Doppler principles. Semin Roentgenol 27:6–16, 1992. Reprinted with permission.)

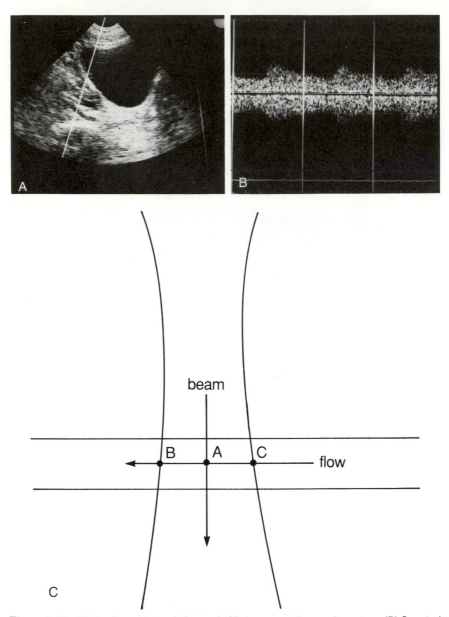

Figure 7.13. (A) The Doppler angle is nearly 90 degrees at the ovarian artery. (B) Spectral mirror image with low-resistance flow on both sides of the baseline. (C) Because beams are focused and not cylindric, portions of the beam (C) can experience flow toward while other portions (B) can experience flow away when the beam axis intersects (A) the flow at 90 degrees. (Parts A and B from Taylor KJW, Holland S: Doppler ultrasound I. Basic principles, instrumentation and pitfalls. Radiology *174*:297–307, 1990. Reprinted with permission.)

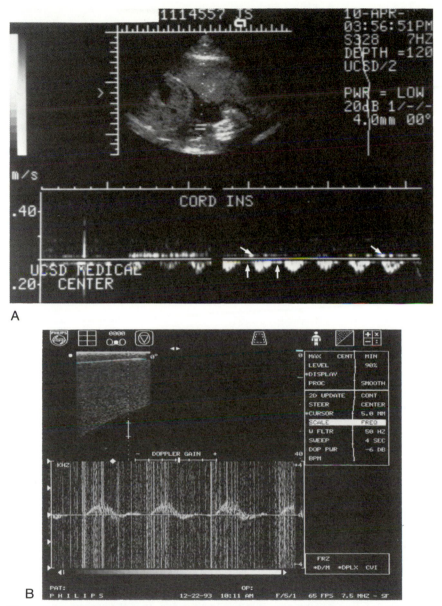

Figure 7.14. (A) Sixty-hertz interference (arrows) above and below the baseline. (B) Interference from nearby electric equipment clouds the spectral display with "snow."

7.2
Color-Flow Artifacts

Artifacts that occur with color-flow imaging[38,39,43] are color presentations of artifacts that are seen in gray-scale imaging (Section 2.4) and Doppler spectral displays (Section 7.1). Several artifacts are encountered in color-flow ultrasound. These are incorrect presentations of two-dimensional flow information. The most common of these is aliasing (Section 7.1). However, others occur, including an anatomic mirror image, Doppler-angle effects, shadowing, clutter, and others. Aliasing occurs when the Doppler shift exceeds the Nyquist limit (see Figs. 6.9E, 6.17B and E, 6.20B, 6.21, and 7.15; Color Plates XIV, XXXI, XXXIV, XLII, XLIV, and XLVI to XLVIII). The result is incorrect flow direction on the color-flow image (Fig. 7.16; Color Plates XLIX to LI). Increasing the flow speed range (which is actually an increase in the pulse repetition frequency) can solve the problem (Fig. 7.17; as above, Color Plates LII to LVI). However, too high a range can cause a loss of flow information, particularly if the wall filter is set high (see Figs. 6.9C and 7.17D and E; Color Plates XII, LV, and LVI). It can also cause

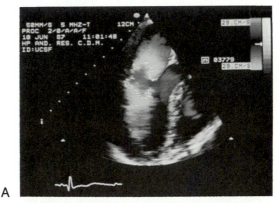

A

Figure 7.15. (A) Transesophageal cardiac color-flow image of the long axis in diastole. The blue colors between the left atrium (upper) and left ventricle (lower) represent blood traveling away from the transducer. However, when the flow speeds exceed the Nyquist limit (29 cm/s), aliasing (Section 7.1) occurs, and the yellow and orange colors replace the blue colors (see Color Plate XLVI). (B) Color-flow presentation of common carotid artery flow, including flow reversal and aliasing. The two can be distinguished because the boundary between the different directions with flow reversal passes through the baseline (black), whereas the aliasing boundary passes through the upper and lower extremes of the color bar (white). In this particular color bar assignment, the maximum positive Doppler shifts are assigned the color green so that there is a thin green region that shows the exact boundary where aliasing occurs. The aliasing occurs in the distal portion of the vessel

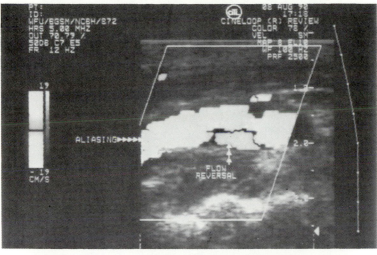

B

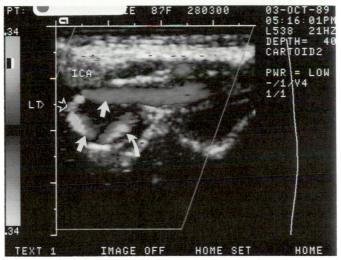

C

Figure 7.15. *Continued* because it is curving down, reducing the Doppler angle between the flow and the scan lines (see Color Plate XLVI). (Part B from Kremkau FW: Doppler principles. Semin Roentgenol 27:6–16, 1992. Reprinted with permission.) (C) In a tortuous internal carotid artery, negative Doppler shifts are indicated in the red regions (solid straight arrows). Two regions of positive Doppler shifts (blue) are seen (open arrow and curved arrow). In the latter, legitimate flow toward the transducer is indicated. In the former, the flow away from the transducer has yielded high Doppler shifts (because of a small Doppler angle, i.e., flow is approximately parallel to scan lines), which produces a color shift to the opposite side of the map that is caused by aliasing. The boundaries from and to normal negative Doppler shifts into and out of the aliased region are bright yellow and cyan from the ends of the color bars. The transition from unaliased negative Doppler shift into unaliased positive Doppler shift (near the bottom) is black, representing the baseline of the color bar (see Color Plate XLVIII). (Part C from Kremkau FW: Principles of color flow imaging. J Vasc Technol 15:104–111, 1991. Reprinted with permission.)

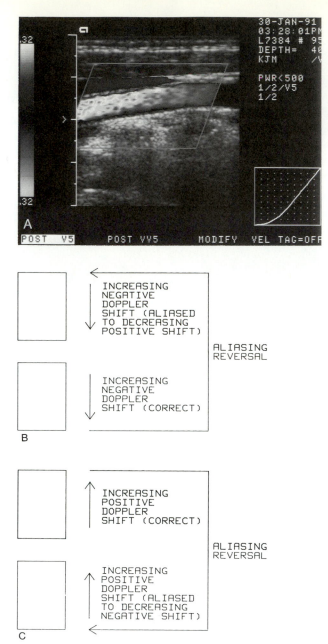

Figure 7.16. (A) Positive (blue) Doppler shifts are shown in the arterial flow in this image (see Color Plate XLIX). These are actually negative Doppler shifts that have exceeded the lower Nyquist limit (converted here to the equivalent flow speed, −0.32 m/s) and wrapped around to the positive portion of the color bar (B) (see Color Plate L). Positive shifts that exceed the +0.32-m/s limit would alias to the negative side (C) (see Color Plate LI). (From Kremkau FW: Principles and pitfalls of real-time color-flow imaging. In Bernstein EF (ed): Vascular Diagnosis, 4th edition. St. Louis, Mosby-Year Book, 1993. Reprinted with permission.)

240

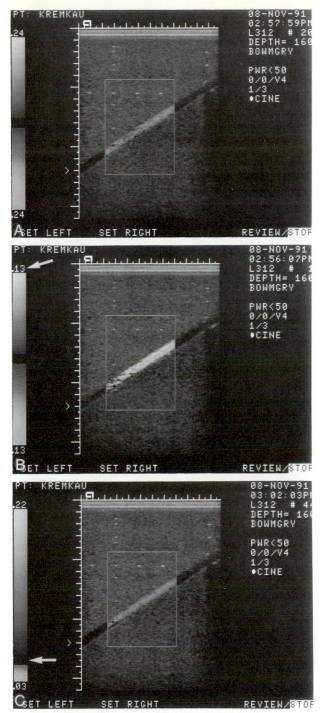

Figure 7.17. (A) Flow is toward the upper right, producing positive Doppler shifts (see Color Plate LI). (B) The pulse repetition frequency (PRF) and Nyquist limit (0.13) are too low, resulting in aliasing (negative Doppler shifts) at the center of the flow in the vessel

Illustration continued on following page

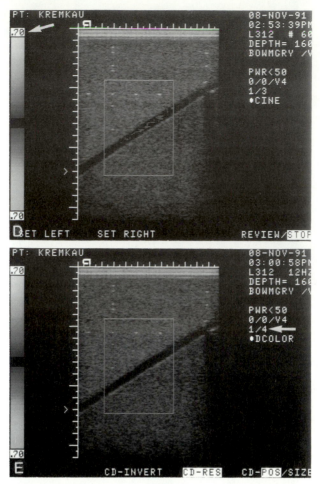

Figure 7.17. *Continued* (Fig. 7.16C) (see Color Plate LI). (C) With the same PRF setting as in (B), the aliasing has been eliminated by shifting the baseline (arrow) down 10 cm/s below the center of the color bar (see Color Plate LIV). (D) Here the Nyquist limit setting (0.70) is too high, causing the detected Doppler shifts to be well down the positive scale and producing a dark red appearance (see Color Plate LV). (E) With the Nyquist limit set as in (D), an increase in the wall-filter setting (arrow) eliminates what little color-flow information there was in part D (see Color Plate LV). From Kremkau FW: Principles and pitfalls of real-time color-flow imaging. In Bernstein EF (ed): Vascular Diagnosis, 4th edition. St. Louis, Mosby-Year Book, 1993. Reprinted with permission.)

range ambiguity, which places echoes and Doppler gates at incorrect depth locations. Baseline shifting can decrease or eliminate the effect of aliasing (see Fig. 7.17C, Color Plate LIV), as in spectral displays.

In the mirror (or ghost) artifact (Fig. 7.18, Color Plates LVII and LVIII), an image of a vessel and source of Doppler-shifted echoes can be duplicated on the opposite side of a strong reflector (e.g., pleura or

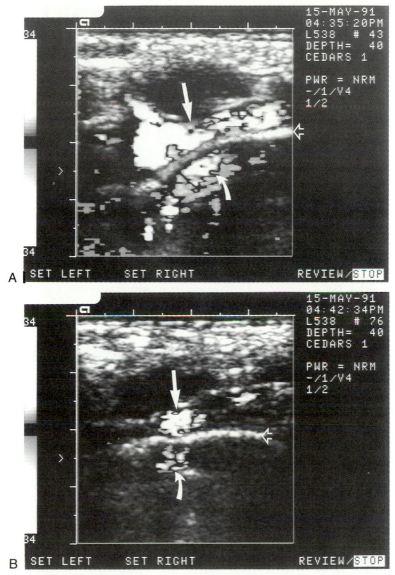

Figure 7.18. Color-flow imaging of the subclavian artery (straight arrow) in longitudinal (A) and transverse (B) views. The pleura (open arrow) causes the mirror image (curved arrow) (see Color Plates LVII and LVIII). Figure 7.11D shows a diagram of how this artifact occurs.

diaphragm). This is a color-flow extension of Figure 7.11. Shadowing can weaken or eliminate Doppler-shifted echoes beyond the shadowing object (Fig. 7.19, Color Plate LIX). This is the color-flow extension of Figure 2.47. Clutter results from tissue, heart, or vessel wall motion

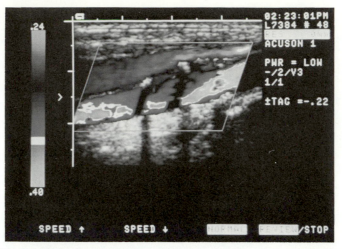

Figure 7.19. Shadowing from a calcified plaque follows the gray-scale scan lines straight down while following the angled color scan lines parallel to the sides of the parallelogram. This image also shows an example of (white) tagging at −0.22 cm/s (see Color Plate LIX). (From Kremkau FW: Principles and instrumentation. In Merritt CRB (ed): Doppler Color Imaging. New York, Churchill Livingstone, 1992. Reprinted with permission.)

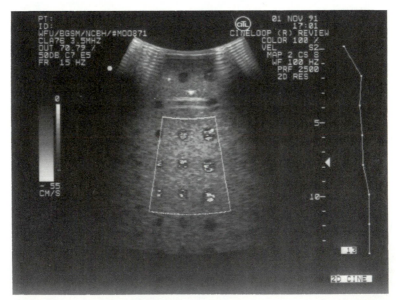

Figure 7.20. Color appears in echo-free (cystic) regions of a tissue-equivalent phantom. The color gain has been increased sufficiently to produce this effect. The instrument tends to write color information preferentially in areas in which non-Doppler shifted echoes are weak or absent (see Color Plate LX). (From Kremkau FW: Principles and pitfalls of real-time color-flow imaging. In Bernstein EF (ed): Vascular Diagnosis, 4th edition. St. Louis, Mosby-Year Book, 1993. Reprinted with permission.)

(see Fig. 6.9A, Color Plate X). It is eliminated by wall filters. Doppler-angle effects include zero Doppler shift when the Doppler angle is 90 degrees (see Fig. 6.18F, Color Plate XXXIX) and the change of color in a straight vessel viewed with a sector transducer (see Fig. 6.18A, Color Plate XXXVI). Noise in the color-flow electronics can mimic flow, particularly in hypoechoic or anechoic regions (Fig. 7.20, Color Plate LX).[45] All these artifacts can hinder a proper interpretation and diagnosis. They must be avoided or properly handled when encountered.

7.3
Performance

Test objects and tissue- and blood-mimicking phantoms are commercially available for the evaluation of Doppler instruments (Figs. 7.21 and 7.22; Color Plate LXI). These are useful for testing the effective penetration of the Doppler beam, the ability to discriminate between different flow directions, the accuracy of sample volume location, and the accuracy of the measured flow speed.[46-48] Doppler-flow phantoms use a flowing blood-mimicking liquid (e.g., Sephadex in water, polystyrene microspheres suspended in a water and glycerol mixture, a mixture of water and machine cutting oil, and aqueous starch suspensions). Doppler test objects use a moving solid object (usually a string) for scattering the ultrasound. The latter can be calibrated more easily and can produce pulsatile and reverse motions (see Fig. 7.21). The former have some difficulties, such as the presence of bubbles and nonuniform flow, but can be arranged to simulate clinical conditions more easily, such as tissue attenuation (see Fig. 7.22). They can be calibrated with an electromagnetic flowmeter or by volume collection over time. Figures 5.9B and C illustrate the use of a string test object in the evaluation of a Doppler-angle correction. Figures 7.12A and B show the use of a string test object in evaluating spectral mirror image. Figure 5.12 illustrates the use of a flow phantom in determining accuracy of the gate location indicator on the anatomic display. Figure 6.19 (Color Plate XL) shows the use of a flow phantom to illustrate the effect of Doppler angle on Doppler shift. Figure 7.17 (Color Plates LII to LVI) illustrates the evaluation of aliasing, Nyquist limit, baseline shifting, and wall filter operation with a flow phantom.

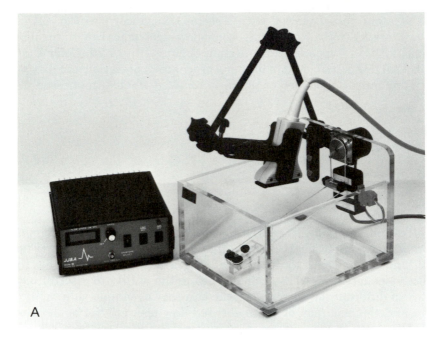

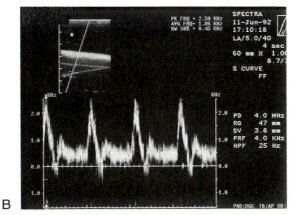

Figure 7.21. (A) Moving string test object and controller (JJ&A Mark 4). (B) Spectral display of moving string operating in pulsatile mode.

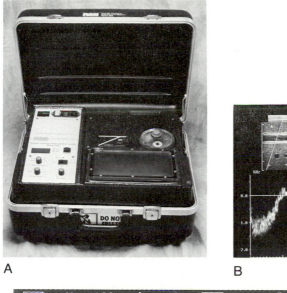

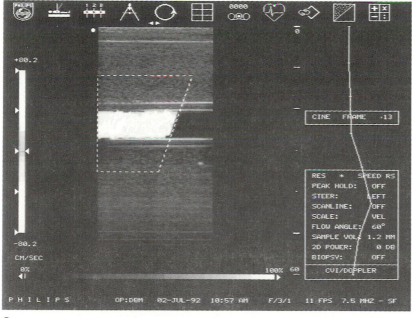

Figure 7.22. (A) Doppler flow phantom (RMI model 425). (B) Spectral display from flow phantom. (C) Color-flow image from flow phantom (see Color Plate LXI.)

7.4
Safety

The biologic effects and safety of diagnostic ultrasound have received considerable attention during the past few years. Several review articles, textbooks, and institutional documents have been published.[49-60] In this section, we review the knowledge obtained in regard to the bioeffects in cells, plants, and experimental animals; the mechanisms of interaction between ultrasound and biologic cells and tissues; regulatory activities; epidemiology; risk and safety considerations; and elements of prudent practice.

As with any diagnostic test, there may be some risk (some probability of damage or injury) with the use of diagnostic ultrasound. This risk, if known, must be weighed against the perceived benefit to determine the appropriateness of the diagnostic procedure. A knowledge of how to minimize the risk (even if it is unidentified) is useful to everyone involved in diagnostic ultrasound. The sources of information used in developing a policy regarding the use of diagnostic ultrasound (whether it be an individual, departmental, institutional, national, or world policy) are diagrammed in Figure 7.23. They include bioeffects data from experimental systems, output data from diagnostic instruments, and knowledge and experience regarding how the diagnostic information obtained is of benefit in the management of patients. A comparison of the first two components allows an assessment of the risk; the combination of the latter two components yields an awareness of benefit. It seems reasonable to assume that there is some risk (however small) in the use of diagnostic ultrasound because ultrasound is a form of energy and has, at least, the potential to produce a biologic effect that could constitute a risk. Even if this risk is so minimal that it is difficult

Figure 7.23. Ultrasound risk and benefit information. Risk information comes from experimental bioeffects, epidemiology, and instrument output data. Benefit information comes from knowledge and experience in diagnostic ultrasound use and efficacy. Together they lead to a policy on the prudent use of diagnostic ultrasound in medicine.

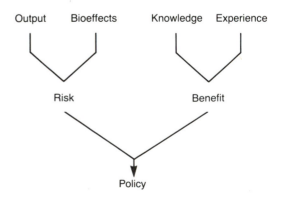

to identify, prudent practice dictates that routine measures be implemented to minimize the risk while obtaining the necessary information to achieve the benefit.

Our knowledge of the bioeffects resulting from ultrasound exposure comes from several sources (Fig. 7.24). They include experimental observations in cell suspensions and cultures, plants, and experimental animals; epidemiologic studies with humans; and an understanding of mechanisms of interaction, such as heating and cavitation. These categories are discussed separately in the following sections.

Cells

Several end points have been used in studies of the effects of ultrasound on cells in suspension or in culture. Ultrastructural changes and altered motility patterns in fibroblasts have been reported. These results have not been independently confirmed. Single-strand breaks in the DNA of human leukocytes after exposure to ultrasound have been observed. Various continuous and pulsed exposure frequencies and intensities were used, some involving cavitation and some not. Only one (94 W/cm^2 spatial peak temporal average at 8 MHz continuous wave) yielded a significantly increased frequency of breaks, which may have resulted from the chemical activity associated with transient cavitation. For virtually all bioeffects found in cell suspensions, cavitation appears to be involved.

The most extensively studied end point with ultrasound exposure of cells is sister chromatid exchange (Fig. 7.25). During a 10-year period, about two dozen reports have been published on this subject. Most studies yielded negative results; a few were positive. Of importance is the fact that there is no independent confirmation of a published positive effect. Attempts to do so led to the conclusion that the cause

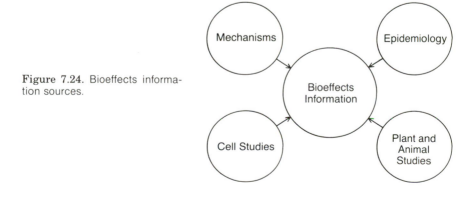

Figure 7.24. Bioeffects information sources.

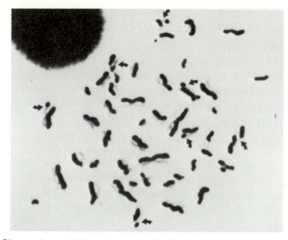

Figure 7.25. Sister chromatid exchange is indicated by arrows. Bromodeoxyuridine-substituted Giemsa-stained human lymphocyte metaphase. (From Kremkau FW: Biologic effects and safety. In Rumack CM, Wilson SR, Charboneau JW (eds): Diagnostic Ultrasound. St. Louis, Mosby-Year Book, 1991, pp. 19–29. Reprinted with permission. Courtesy of Morton W. Miller.)

for the small but statistically significant effects is unknown, but ultrasound exposure either does not produce increased exchanges or the effect is not reproducible and is too small to be consistently produced.[50] Even if ultrasound were shown to produce increased exchanges consistently with all this activity, sister chromatid exchanges usually have no genetic effect and, therefore, do not constitute a risk.

Because cells in suspension or in culture are so different from the case in an intact patient in a clinical environment, restraint must be exercised in extrapolating in vitro results to clinical situations. Cellular studies are useful in determining mechanisms of interaction and guiding the design of experimental animal studies and epidemiologic studies. The American Institute of Ultrasound in Medicine (AIUM) Official Statement on In Vitro Biological Effects[51] follows:

> It is difficult to evaluate reports of ultrasonically induced in vitro biological effects with respect to their clinical significance. The predominant physical and biological interactions and mechanisms involved in an in vitro effect may not pertain to the in vivo situation. Nevertheless, an in vitro effect must be regarded as a real biological effect. Results from in vitro experiments suggest new endpoints and serve as a basis for design of in vivo experiments. In vitro studies provide the capability to control experimental variables and thus offer a means to explore and evaluate specific mechanisms. Although they may have limited applicability to in vivo biological effects, such studies can disclose fundamental intercellular or intracellular interactions. While it is valid for authors to place their results in context and to suggest further relevant investigations, reports

of in vitro studies which claim direct clinical significance should be viewed with caution.

Plants

The primary components of plant tissues—stems, leaves, and roots—contain gas-filled channels between the cell walls. Plants have thus served as useful biologic models for studying the effects of cavitation. Through this mechanism, normal cellular organization and function can be disturbed. Irreversible effects appear to be limited to cell death. Reversible effects include chromosomal abnormalities, mitotic index reductions, and growth-rate reduction. Membrane damage induced by microstreaming shear stress appears to be the cause of the cell death in leaves. Intensity thresholds for the lysis of leaf cells are much higher with pulsed ultrasound than they are with continuous-wave devices. Apparently, the response of bubbles within the tissues to continuous and pulsed fields is different.

Animals

With experimental animals, mostly mice and rats, the reported in vivo effects include fetal weight reduction, postpartum fetal deaths, fetal abnormalities, tissue lesions, hind limb paralysis, blood flow stasis, wound repair enhancement, and tumor regression. Recent negative studies include B cell development, ovulatory response, and teratogenicity, all in mice.[50]

Many studies on fetal weight reduction in mice and rats have been performed. All rat and several mouse studies yielded negative results. A linear dose-effect dependence on the exposure condition versus average fetal weight was reported in which the dose parameter was defined as I^2t, where I is the spatial average exposure intensity and t is the exposure time. This exposure dependence was not independently confirmed. In one attempt, no effect on fetal weight was found at values of the dose parameter large enough to produce measurable heating in the fetal and maternal tissues.

Focal lesion production is a well-documented bioeffect from at least three laboratories. It was observed over a wide range of intensity and exposure duration conditions (Fig. 7.26).

In 1992, the AIUM issued the following statement (American Institute of Ultrasound in Medicine Statement on Non-Human Mammalian In Vivo Biological Effects, approved October 1992).

> Information from experiments using laboratory mammals has contributed significantly to our understanding of ultrasonically induced biologic effects and the mechanisms that are most likely responsible. The following

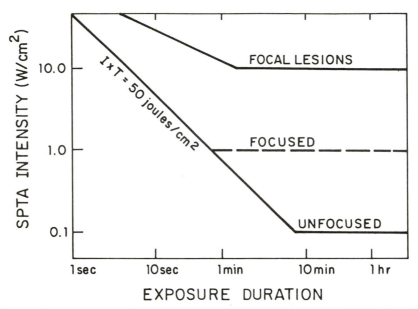

Figure 7.26. Comparison of the minimum spatial peak temporal average (SPTA) intensities required for ultrasonic bioeffects specified in American Institute of Ultrasound in Medicine Statement on Mammalian Bioeffects. The minimum levels required for focal lesions are also shown on the figure for comparison. Note that logarithmic scaling was used for the axes of this figure so that the horizontal lines are separated by factors of 10 in intensity. (From Bioeffects Conference Subcommittee: Bioeffects and Safety of Diagnostic Ultrasound. Laurel, MD, American Institute of Ultrasound in Medicine, 1993. Reprinted with permission.)

statement summarizes observations relative to specific ultrasound parameters and indices. The history and rationale for this statement are provided in *Bioeffects and Safety of Diagnostic Ultrasound*.[52,53]

In the low megahertz frequency range there have been no independently confirmed adverse biologic effects in mammalian tissues exposed in vivo under experimental ultrasound conditions, as follows.

1. When a thermal mechanism is involved, these conditions are unfocused-beam intensities* below 100 mW/cm^2, focused-beam intensities† below 1 W/cm^2, or thermal index values less than 2. Furthermore, such effects have not been reported for higher values of thermal index when it is less than

$$6 - \frac{\log_{10}t}{0.6}$$

---

*Free-field spatial peak temporal average for continuous-wave and pulsed exposure.
†Quarter-power (-6 dB) beam width smaller than four wavelengths or 4 mm, whichever is less at the exposure frequency.

where t is exposure time ranging from 1 to 250 minutes, including off-time for pulsed exposure.

2. When a nonthermal mechanism is involved (for diagnostically relevant ultrasound exposures), in tissues that contain well-defined gas bodies, these conditions are in situ peak rarefactional pressures below approximately 0.3 MPa or mechanical index values less than approximately 0.3. Furthermore, for other tissues no such effects have been reported.

Figure 7.26 illustrates the intensity and time relations given in part 1 of the statement. Figure 7.27 shows the thermal index versus exposure time, as given in part 1 of the statement. Figure 7.28 presents the pressure versus frequency for a mechanical index value of 0.3, as given in part 2 of the statement. These indexes are described in the next section on mechanisms.

Mechanisms

The mechanisms of action by which ultrasound could produce biologic effects can be characterized into two groups: heating and mechanical. Attenuation of the beam in tissue is primarily caused by absorption, that is, conversion of ultrasound to heat. Thus, ultrasound produces a temperature rise as it propagates through tissues. The heating produced depends on the applied intensity and frequency of the sound (because the absorption coefficient is approximately proportional to

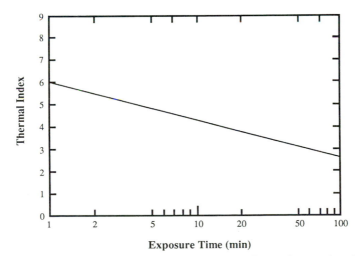

Exposure Time (min)

Figure 7.27. Thermal index versus exposure time on a log-linear plot, as given in Part 1 of the American Institute of Ultrasound in Medicine statement. (From Bioeffects Conference Subcommittee: Bioeffects and Safety of Diagnostic Ultrasound. Laurel, MD, American Institute of Ultrasound in Medicine, 1993. Reprinted with permission.)

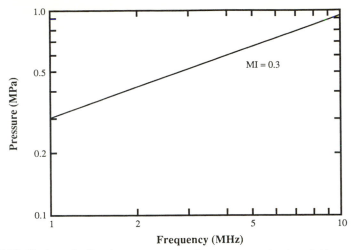

Figure 7.28. Peak rarefactional pressure versus frequency on a log-log plot for a mechanical index (MI) of 0.3. (From Bioeffects Conference Subcommittee: Bioeffects and Safety of Diagnostic Ultrasound. Laurel, MD, American Institute of Ultrasound in Medicine, 1993. Reprinted with permission.)

frequency) and on the beam focusing and tissue perfusion. Heating increases as the intensity or frequency is increased. For a given transducer output intensity, at greater tissue depths, heating is decreased at higher frequencies because of the increased attenuation, which reduces the intensity arriving at depth. Temperature rises are considered significant if they are greater than 2°C. Intensities greater than a few hundred milliwatts per square centimeter can produce such temperature rises. Absorption coefficients are higher in bone than they are in soft tissues. Bone heating, particularly in the fetus, therefore, should receive special consideration.

Heating has been shown to be an important consideration in some bioeffects reports. Mathematic models have been developed for calculating temperature rises in tissues.[52,54,55] These have been used, for example, to calculate the estimated intensities required for a given temperature rise (e.g., 2°C). In 1992, the AIUM developed conclusions regarding heat,[52,53] as follows:

I. Excessive temperature increase can result in toxic effects in mammalian systems. The biologic effects observed depend on many factors, such as the exposure duration, the type of tissue exposed, its cellular proliferation rate, and its potential for regeneration. Age and stage of development are important factors when considering fetal and neonatal safety. Temperature increases of several degrees Celsius above the normal core range can occur naturally;

there have been no significant biologic effects observed resulting from such temperature increases except when they are sustained for extended time periods.

A. For exposure durations up to 50 hours, there have been no significant biologic effects observed due to temperature increases less than or equal to 2°C above normal.

B. For temperature increases greater than 2°C above normal, there have been no significant biologic effects observed due to temperature increase less than or equal to

$$6 - \frac{\log_{10}t}{0.6}$$

where t is the exposure duration ranging from 1 to 250 minutes. For example, for temperature increases of 4°C and 6°C, the corresponding limits for the exposure duration t are 16 min and 1 min, respectively.

C. In general, adult tissues are more tolerant of temperature increases than fetal and neonatal tissues. Therefore, higher temperatures and/or longer exposure durations would be required for thermal damage.

II. The temperature increase during exposure of tissues to diagnostic ultrasound fields is dependent upon (a) output characteristics of the acoustic source such as frequency, source dimensions, scan rate, power, pulse repetition frequency, pulse duration, transducer self heating, exposure time and wave shape and (b) tissue properties such as attenuation, absorption, speed of sound, acoustic impedance, perfusion, thermal conductivity, thermal diffusivity, anatomical structure and nonlinearity parameter.

III. For similar exposure conditions, the expected temperature increase in bone is significantly greater than in soft tissues. For this reason, conditions where an acoustic beam impinges on ossifying fetal bone deserve special attention due to its close proximity to other developing tissues.

IV. Calculations of the maximum temperature increase resulting from ultrasound exposure in vivo should not be assumed to be exact because of the uncertainties and approximations associated with the thermal, acoustic and structural characteristics of the tissues involved. However, experimental evidence shows that calculations are capable of predicting measured values within a factor of two. Thus, it appears reasonable to use calculations to obtain safety guidelines for clinical exposures where temperature measurements are not feasible. To provide a display of real-time estimates of tissue temperature increases as part of a diagnostic system, simplifying approximations are used to yield values called Thermal Indices*. Under most clinically relevant conditions, the soft-tissue thermal index, TIS, and the bone thermal index, TIB, either overestimate or closely approximate the best available estimate of the maximum temperature increase (ΔT_{max}). For example, if TIS = 2, then $\Delta T_{max} \leq 2°C$.

V. The current FDA regulatory limit for $I_{SPTA.3}$ is 720 mW/cm^2. For this, and lesser intensities, the best available estimate of the maximum temperature increase in the conceptus can exceed 2°C.

VI. The soft-tissue thermal index, TIS, and the bone thermal index, TIB, are useful for estimating the temperature increase in vivo. For this purpose, these thermal indices are superior to any single ultrasonic field quantity such as the derated spatial-peak, temporal-average intensity, $I_{SPTA.3}$. That is, TIS and TIB track changes in the maximum temperature increases, ΔT_{max}, thus allowing for implementation of the ALARA principle, where $I_{SPTA.3}$ does not. For example,

A. At a constant value of $I_{SPTA.3}$, TIS increases with increasing frequency and with increasing source diameter.

B. At a constant value of $I_{SPTA.3}$, TIB increases with increasing focal beam diameter.

Experimental measurements have been performed that show reasonable confirmation of the mathematic calculations. Bone heating was not found experimentally to be significantly greater than that calculated for soft tissues. The biologic consequences of hyperthermia include fetal absorption or abortion, growth retardation, microphthalmia, cataract production, abdominal wall defects, renal agenesis, palate defects, reduction in brain wave, microencephaly, anencephaly, spinal cord defects, amyoplasia, forefoot hypoplasia, tibial and fibular deformations, and abnormal tooth genesis. There are about 80 known biologic effects caused by hyperthermia. None have occurred at temperatures less than 39°C. Above this level, the occurrence of a biologic effect depends on the temperature and exposure time, as shown in Figure 7.29.

---

*The Thermal Indices are the nondimensional ratios of the estimated temperature increases to 1°C for specific tissue models (see the Standard for Real-Time Display of Thermal and Mechanical Acoustic Output Indices on Diagnostic Ultrasound Equipment, AIUM/NEMA, 1992).[59]

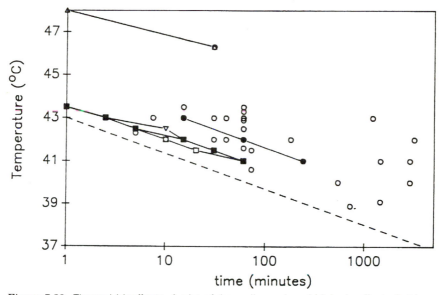

Figure 7.29. Thermal bioeffects. A plot of thermally produced biologic effects that have been reported in the literature in which the temperature elevation and exposure durations are provided. Each data point represents either the lowest temperature reported for any duration or the shortest duration for any temperature reported for a given effect. The solid lines represent multiple data points that are related to a single effect. The dashed line represents a lower boundary ($t_{43} = 1$) for observed thermally induced biologic effects. (From Miller MW, Ziskin MC: Biological consequences of hyperthermia. Ultrasound Med Biol 15:707–722, 1989. Reprinted with permission.)

Cavitation is the production and dynamics of bubbles in a liquid medium.[54,56,58] A propagating sound wave is one means by which cavitation can occur. Two types of cavitation are recognized. Stable cavitation is the term used to describe bubbles that oscillate in diameter with the passing pressure variations of the sound wave. Streaming of surrounding liquid can occur in this situation and result in shear stresses on suspended cells or intracellular organelles. The detection of cavitation in tissues under continuous-wave, high-intensity conditions was reported. Transient (collapse) cavitation occurs when bubble oscillations are so large that the bubble collapses (Fig. 7.30A), producing pressure discontinuities (shock waves), localized extremely high temperatures, and light emission in clear liquids (see Fig. 7.30B). Transient cavitation has the potential to produce significant destructive effects. It is the means by which laboratory cell disruptors operate.

Theory has been developed that predicts that ultrasound could produce transient cavitation under diagnostically relevant conditions in water. This theory also incorporates a range of bubble sizes, which

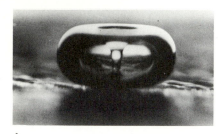

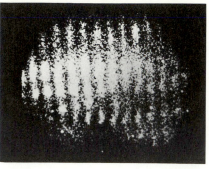

A   B

Figure 7.30. (A) Photograph of liquid jet produced by collapsing cavitation bubble. Width of bubble is approximately 1 mm. (B) Photograph taken from television monitor of image intensifier system, showing light emission from an acoustic standing wave produced in amniotic fluid at 37°C. The vertical bands are separated by approximately 0.75 mm or one half of the wavelength for the applied acoustic frequency of 1.0 MHz. The light emission is caused by transient cavitation in the standing wave. (From Kremkau FW: Biologic effects and safety. In Rumack CM, Wilson SR, Charboneau JW (eds): Diagnostic Ultrasound. St. Louis, Mosby-Year Book, 1991, pp. 19–29. Reprinted with permission. Courtesy of Lawrence A. Crum.)

yields a predicted dependence of the cavitation threshold on pressure and frequency. Experimental verification of this dependence was carried out with stabilized microbubbles in water. The thresholds for cavitation in soft tissue and body liquids were recently determined. The AIUM summarized information on the cavitation mechanism in its conclusions regarding gas bodies[52,53] as follows:

1. The temporal peak outputs of some currently available diagnostic ultrasound devices can exceed the threshold for cavitation in vitro and can generate levels that produce extravasation of blood cells in the lungs of laboratory animals.
2. A mechanical index (MI)* has been formulated to assist users in evaluating the likelihood of cavitation-related adverse biological effects for diagnostically relevant exposures. The MI is a better indicator than derated spatial peak, pulse average intensity ($I_{\text{SPTA.3}}$) or derated peak rarefactional pressure ($P_{r.3}$) for known adverse nonthermal biological effects of ultrasound.
3. Thresholds for adverse nonthermal effects depend upon tissue characteristics and ultrasound parameters such as pressure amplitude, pulse duration and frequency. Thus far, biologically significant, adverse, nonthermal effects have only been identified with certainty

---

*The MI is equal to the derated peak rarefactional pressure (in MPa) at the point of the maximum pulse intensity integral divided by the square root of the ultrasonic center frequency (in MHz).[59]

for diagnostically relevant exposures in tissues that have well-defined populations of stabilized gas bodies. For extravasation of blood cells in postnatal mouse lung, the threshold values of MI increase with decreasing pulse duration in the 1–100 μs range, increase with decreasing exposure time and are weakly dependent upon pulse repetition frequency. The threshold value of MI for extravasation of blood cells in mouse lung is approximately 0.3. The implications of these observations for human exposure are yet to be determined.

4. No extravasation of blood cells was found in mouse kidneys exposed to peak pressures in situ corresponding to an MI of 4. Furthermore, for diagnostically relevant exposures, no independently confirmed, biologically significant adverse effects have been reported in mammalian tissues that do not contain well-defined gas bodies.

Experimental measurements have been performed that show reasonable confirmation of the theoretic calculations (Fig. 7.31). The only well-documented mammalian biologic consequence of gas bodies in an

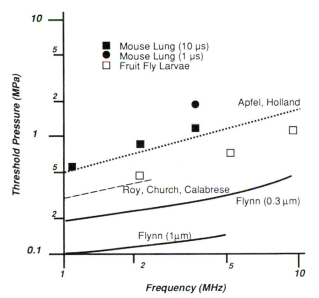

Figure 7.31. Threshold, in situ, rarefactional pressures for biologic effects in vivo of low-temporal-average–intensity pulsed ultrasound. Pulse durations are shown in parenthesis in the legend. Also shown for reference purposes are values for the mechanical index and the local spatial peak, pulse average intensity. In all cases, the tissues contain identifiable small stabilized gas bodies. As in diagnostic ultrasound, all exposures consisted of repetitive pulses ($\leq$10 μs). Total exposure times were less than 5 minutes. (From Bioeffects Conference Subcommittee: Bioeffects and Safety of Diagnostic Ultrasound. Laurel, MD, American Institute of Ultrasound in Medicine, 1993. Reprinted with permission.)

ultrasound beam is blood cell extravasation in an inflated lung. This has not occurred at acoustic pressure amplitudes less than 0.3 MPa. Above this level, its occurrence depends on frequency, exposure time, and pulsing conditions.

Instrument Outputs

Several reports and compilations of output data have been published. The instrument output may be expressed in many ways. Intensity is the most popular quantity presented to describe instrument output. There are several intensities that may be used. The spatial peak temporal average (SPTA) intensity[1] is used in the AIUM Statement on Mammalian Bioeffects and relates reasonably well to a thermal mechanism of interaction. It is the output intensity most commonly presented. Table 7.4 gives a compilation of the ranges of SPTA intensities from several sources. Output intensities have a large range, with the highest being 250,000 times the lowest. Imaging instruments dominate the lower portion of the range; Doppler instruments dominate the higher portion. Within specific classes of instruments, intensity ranges vary by factors as small as 24 (phased arrays, stopped) and as large as 4800 (linear arrays, scanning). In general, spectral Doppler outputs are highest, gray-scale imaging scans are lowest, with color-flow imaging in between. Pulsed-Doppler output data are shown in Figure 7.32.

These output intensity measurements are usually made with the use of hydrophones and radiation-force balances[1] located in the beam in a water bath. The attenuation of the beam in water is low compared

Table 7–4	
Spatial Peak Temporal Average Output Intensities (in milliwatts per square centimeter)	
All instruments	0.01–2500
Imaging instruments	0.01– 680
scanning	0.01– 440
linear array	0.01– 48
phased array	0.1 – 85
mechanical	0.1 – 440
stopped	0.5 – 680
linear array	3.8 – 332
phased array	10.1 – 240
mechanical	1.6 – 680
static	0.5 – 200
Doppler instruments	0.6 –2500
Continuous-wave obstetrics	0.6 – 80
Continuous-wave cardiac/ peripheral vascular	20 –2500
pulsed	40 –1945

with that in tissues so that an intensity at a comparable location within the tissue would be less than that in water. Models for accounting for the tissue attenuation have been applied.[52,54,59]

To compare instrument output intensities with bioeffects knowledge (AIUM Statement on Non-Human Mammalian In Vivo Biological Effects), let us assume a 7-dB average tissue attenuation. This corresponds to an intensity reduction of 80 percent. Reducing the values in Table 7.4 by 80 percent yields upper limits, as given in Table 7.5. Because most of the bioeffects studies were done in small animals, such as mice and rats, the attenuation would be negligible, and the values in Table 7.5 can be compared with the AIUM statement value of 1 W/cm^2 for focused beams because virtually all diagnostic ultrasound uses focused beams. It can be seen from this comparison that, on the basis of experimental animal studies, clinical bioeffects would not be expected to occur from the output intensities used in current and past diagnostic instrumentation.

Regulatory Activities

Manufacturers are required to submit premarket notifications to the Food and Drug Administration (FDA) prior to marketing a device for a specific application. The FDA then reviews this notification to

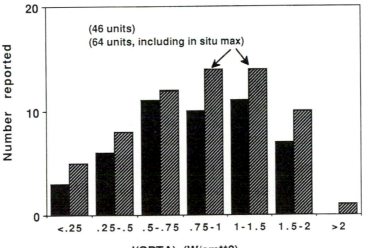

Figure 7.32. Histogram showing the spatial peak temporal average intensities [I(SPTA)] for pulsed Doppler, as reported by manufacturers participating in the American Institute of Ultrasound in Medicine commendation process. (From Ide M, Zagzebski JA, Duck FA: Acoustic output of diagnostic equipment. Ultrasound Med Biol 15[suppl. 1]: 47–65, 1989. Reprinted with permission.)

Table 7–5

Upper Limits of Attenuated* Spatial Peak Temporal Average Output Intensities (in milliwatts per square centimeter) from Table 7–4

All instruments	500
Imaging instruments	136
Scanning	88
Stopped	136
Doppler instruments	500
Continuous wave	500
Pulsed	389

*7 dB to account for human tissue path.

determine if the device is substantially equivalent, with regard to safety and effectiveness, to instruments on the market prior to the enactment of the regulatory act (1976). If the device is determined to be substantially equivalent, the manufacturer may then market it for that application. Part of the FDA evaluation involves output data for the instrument, which are then compared with maximum values found for pre-1976 devices. These values are given in the 510(k) Guide for Measuring and Reporting Acoustic Output of Diagnostic Ultrasound Medical Devices and are presented here in Table 7.6. Some of the values have been updated since the 1985 publication of this guide. The current values are shown in the table. Until recently, fetal Doppler was not approved by the FDA, primarily because of efficacy considerations. However, some devices are now approved for this application. Part of the requirements for this approval is the real-time display of output information on the instrument. Recently, the development of a voluntary output display standard was undertaken by a joint committee involving the AIUM, FDA, National Electrical Manufacturers Association (NEMA), and several other ultrasound-related professional societies. The goal of this activity was to develop a voluntary standard that would provide a parallel pathway to the current regulatory 510(k) process. It would allow an exemption from the upper limits given in

Table 7–6

510(k) Guide SPTA In Situ Intensity Upper Limits (mW/cm^2)

Cardiac	430
Peripheral vessel	720
Ophthalmic	17
Fetal imaging and other*	94

*Abdominal, intra-operative, pediatric, small organ (breast, thyroid, testes), neonatal cephalic, adult cephalic.

the 510(k) guide (except an overall limit of 720 mW/cm^2 SPTA would still apply) in exchange for presenting output information on the display. The standard[59] includes two indexes that would be displayed: thermal and mechanical. The thermal index is defined as the transducer acoustic output power divided by the estimated power required to raise the tissue temperature by 1°C. The mechanical index is equal to the peak rarefactional pressure divided by the square root of the center

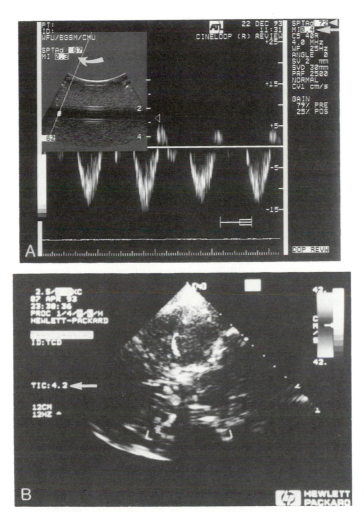

Figure 7.33. (A) A spectral display indicating attenuation-compensated spatial peak temporal average intensity (arrowhead upper right) and mechanical index (arrow). The values for the gray-scale image are shown on the inset at upper left (curved arrow). (B) The thermal index (arrow) value is indicated on this image of transcranial flow.

frequency of the pulse bandwidth. In the case of both indices, display would not be required if the instrument were incapable of exceeding index values of 1. The standard was adopted by the AIUM and NEMA in 1992. Displays including mechanical index and SPTA intensity (incorporating tissue attenuation) appeared in 1991 (Fig. 7.33A). Displays including thermal index appeared in 1993 (see Fig. 7.33B).

Epidemiology

A dozen or so studies of an epidemiologic nature have been conducted and published.[51] These indicate that epidemiologic studies and surveys in widespread clinical usage over 25 years yield no evidence of any adverse effect from diagnostic ultrasound. One recent study included 806 children, approximately one half of whom had been exposed to diagnostic ultrasound in utero. The study measured Apgar scores, gestational age, head circumference, birth weight and length, congenital abnormalities, neonatal infection, congenital infection at birth, conductive and nerve measurements of hearing, visual acuity and color vision, cognitive function, behavior, and complete and detailed neurologic examinations from ages 7 to 12 years. No biologically significant differences between exposed and unexposed children were found. Another study included head circumference, height, and weight of 149 sibling pairs of the same sex, one of whom had been exposed to diagnostic ultrasound in utero. No statistically significant differences of head circumference at birth or of height and weight between birth and 6 years of age were found between ultrasound-exposed and unexposed siblings.

Although these studies have limitations and some flaws, they have not revealed a risk in clinical use of diagnostic ultrasound. The AIUM developed and approved in 1987 the following statements[51] regarding epidemiology:

1. Widespread clinical use over 25 years has not established any adverse effect arising from exposure to diagnostic ultrasound.
2. Randomized clinical studies are the most rigorous method for assessing potential adverse effects of diagnostic ultrasound. Studies using this methodology show no evidence of an effect on birthweight in humans.*
3. Other epidemiologic studies have shown no causal association of diagnostic ultrasound with any of the adverse fetal outcomes studied.*

---

*The acoustic exposure levels in these studies may not be representative of the full range of current fetal exposures.

Prudent Use

Epidemiologic studies have shown no known risk in the use of diagnostic ultrasound. Experimental animal studies show that bioeffects occur at intensities higher than those expected at relevant tissue locations during ultrasound imaging and flow measurements. Thus, a comparison of instrument output data adjusted for tissue attenuation with experimental bioeffects data does not indicate any risk. We must be open to the possibility that an unrecognized, but nonzero, risk may exist, however. Such risk, if it does exist, may have eluded detection up to this point because it is either subtle or delayed or has incidence rates close to normal values. As more sensitive end points are studied over longer periods of time or with larger populations, such a risk may be identified. On the other hand, future studies may not yield any positive effects, thus strengthening the possibility that medical ultrasound imaging is without detectable risk.

In the meantime, with no known risk and with a known benefit to the procedure, a conservative approach to imaging (Fig. 7.34) should be used.[51] That is, ultrasound imaging should be used when medically indicated with minimum exposure of the patient and fetus. Exposure is minimized by minimizing instrument output and exposure time during a study. Doppler instrument outputs can be significantly higher than those for imaging (see Table 7.4). Thus, it seems most likely that the greatest potential for risk in ultrasound diagnosis (although no specific risk has been identified even in this case) occurs in fetal spectral Doppler studies. These combine potentially high-output intensities with stationary geometry and the (presumably more sensitive) fetus.

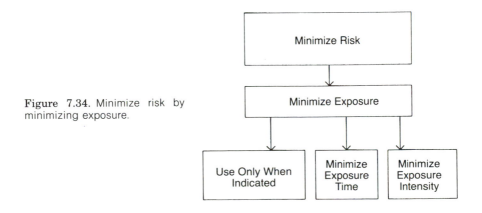

Figure 7.34. Minimize risk by minimizing exposure.

The World Health Organization has stated that "the benefits of this imaging modality far outweigh any presumed risks."[60] The AIUM[51,52] issued the following statement on clinical safety (October 1982, revised October 1983 and March 1988, reaffirmed March 1993):

> Diagnostic ultrasound has been in use since the late 1950's. Given its known benefits and recognized efficacy for medical diagnosis, including use during human pregnancy, the American Institute of Ultrasound in Medicine herein addresses the clinical safety of such use:
>
>> No confirmed biological effects on patients or instrument operators caused by exposure at intensities typical of present diagnostic ultrasound instruments have ever been reported. Although the possibility exists that such biological effects may be identified in the future, current data indicate that the benefits to patients of the prudent use of diagnostic ultrasound outweigh the risks, if any, that may be present.

In conclusion, extensive mechanistic, in vitro, in vivo, and epidemiologic studies have revealed no known risk with the current ultrasound instrumentation used in medical diagnosis. However, a prudent and conservative approach to ultrasound safety is to assume that there may be unidentified risk that should be minimized in medically indicated ultrasound studies by minimizing exposure time and output.

It is difficult to make firm statements about the clinical safety of diagnostic ultrasound. The experimental and epidemiologic bases for risk assessment are incomplete. However, much work has been done, with no evidence of clinical harm revealed. Patients should be informed that there currently is no basis for judging that diagnostic ultrasound produces any harmful effects in patients. However, unobserved effects could be occurring. Thus, ultrasound should not be used indiscriminantly. The AIUM Clinical Safety Statement forms an excellent basis for formulating a response to a patient's questions and concerns. Prudence in practice is exercised by minimizing the exposure time and output. A display of instrument outputs in the form of amplitudes or intensities or the display of thermal and mechanical indexes greatly facilitates this approach to prudent use.

7.5

Review

Artifacts with Doppler ultrasound include aliasing, range ambiguity, image and Doppler signal mirroring, spectral trace mirroring, and electrical interference. Aliasing is the most common artifact. It occurs when the Doppler-shift frequency exceeds one half of the pulse repetition frequency. It can be reduced or eliminated by increasing the pulse repetition frequency or Doppler angle, using baseline shift, reducing operating frequency, or using a continuous-wave instrument.

Doppler performance evaluation devices of two types are available: those that use a blood-mimicking fluid and those that use a moving string. They are useful for evaluating the performance (e.g., spectral scale accuracy) of Doppler instruments.

Extensive mechanistic, in vitro, in vivo, and epidemiologic studies have revealed no known risk with the current ultrasound instrumentation used in medical diagnosis. A prudent and conservative approach, however, to ultrasound safety is to assume that there may be unidentified risk, which should be minimized in medically indicated ultrasound studies by minimizing exposure. The output display indexes facilitate this conservative approach to patient safety.

The definitions of terms used in this chapter are listed next.

Aliasing. Improper Doppler-shift information from a pulsed-Doppler or color-flow instrument when the true Doppler shift exceeds one half of the pulse repetition frequency.

Cavitation. Production and behavior of bubbles in sound.

Mechanical index. An indicator of nonthermal mechanism activity. Equal to peak rarefactional pressure divided by the square root of the center frequency of the pulse bandwidth.

Mirror image. In sonography, duplication of an object on the opposite side of a strong reflector. In Doppler, duplication of the spectrum on the other side of the baseline.

Nyquist limit. The Doppler-shift frequency above which aliasing occurs. One half of the pulse repetition frequency.

Phantom. Tissue-equivalent materials that have some characteristics representative of tissues (e.g., scattering or attenuation properties).

Range ambiguity. Improper placement of late echoes (from a previous pulse) received after the next pulse is emitted.

Shadowing. Reduction in echo amplitude from reflectors that lie behind a strongly reflecting or attenuating structure.

Test object. A device designed to measure some characteristic of an ultrasound system without having tissuelike properties.

Thermal index. An indicator of thermal mechanism activity (estimated temperature rise). Equal to transducer acoustic output power divided by the estimated power required to raise the tissue temperature by 1°C.

Exercises

7.1 The most common artifact encountered in Doppler ultrasound is

a. aliasing
b. range ambiguity
c. spectrum mirror image
d. location mirror image
e. electromagnetic interference

7.2 Which of the following can reduce or eliminate aliasing?

a. increase pulse repetition frequency
b. increase Doppler angle
c. increase operating frequency
d. use continuous wave
e. more than one of the above

7.3 Which of the following can decrease or eliminate aliasing?

a. decrease pulse repetition frequency
b. decrease Doppler angle
c. increase operating frequency
d. baseline shifting
e. more than one of the above

7.4 To avoid aliasing, a signal voltage must be sampled at least _____ times per cycle.

a. 1
b. 2
c. 3
d. 4
e. 5

7.5 If the highest Doppler shift frequency present in a signal exceeds _____ the pulse repetition frequency, aliasing will occur.

a. one tenth
b. one half
c. 2 times
d. 5 times
e. 10 times

7.6 When a pulse is emitted before all the echoes from the previous pulse have been received, which artifact occurs?

a. aliasing
b. range ambiguity
c. spectrum mirror image
d. location mirror image
e. speckle

7.7 When the receiver gain is set too high, which artifact is likely to occur?

a. aliasing
b. range ambiguity
c. spectrum mirror image
d. location mirror image
e. speckle

7.8 When a strong reflector is located in the scan plane, which of the following artifacts is likely to occur?

a. aliasing
b. range ambiguity
c. spectrum mirror image
d. location mirror image
e. speckle

7.9 Increasing the pulse repetition frequency to avoid aliasing can cause:

a. baseline shift
b. range ambiguity
c. spectrum mirror image
d. location mirror image
e. speckle

7.10 Which of the following decreases the likelihood of a range ambiguity artifact?

a. decreasing operating frequency
b. decreasing pulse repetition frequency
c. decreasing Doppler angle
d. baseline shift
e. increasing pulser output

7.11 Range ambiguity can occur in which of the following?

    a. imaging instruments
    b. duplex instruments
    c. pulsed-Doppler instruments
    d. color-flow instruments
    e. all of the above

7.12 Range ambiguity produces which error in echo presentation?

    a. range too long
    b. range too short
    c. intensity too high
    d. Doppler shift too high
    e. Doppler shift too low

7.13 If a pulse is emitted 65 μs after the previous one, echoes returning from beyond _____ cm will produce range ambiguity.

    a. 1
    b. 2
    c. 3
    d. 4
    e. 5

7.14 To avoid aliasing and range ambiguity, if the maximum depth is 5 cm, the frequency is 2 MHz, and the Doppler angle is zero, what is the maximum flow speed?

    a. 100 cm/s
    b. 200 cm/s
    c. 300 cm/s
    d. 400 cm/s
    e. 500 cm/s

7.15 Does solving aliasing by decreasing the operating frequency increase the possibility of a range ambiguity artifact?

7.16 If the operating frequency is increased to decrease the possibility of range ambiguity (by increasing attenuation), does the possibility of aliasing increase?

7.17 If a pulsed-Doppler sample volume is located at a depth of 8 cm, the sampled echoes arrive at what time following the emission of the pulse?

    a. 25 μs
    b. 50 μs
    c. 75 μs
    d. 104 μs
    e. 117 μs

7.18 In Exercise 7.17, if the pulse repetition frequency is set at 11 kHz, a second gate would be located at which depth?

    a. 1 cm
    b. 2 cm
    c. 3 cm
    d. 4 cm
    e. 5 cm

7.19 If the pulse repetition frequency is 4 kHz, which of the following Doppler shifts will alias?

    a. 1 kHz
    b. 2 kHz
    c. 3 kHz
    d. 4 kHz
    e. more than one of the above

7.20 If the pulse repetition frequency is 10 kHz, which of the following Doppler shifts will alias?

    a. 1 kHz
    b. 2 kHz
    c. 3 kHz
    d. 4 kHz
    e. none of the above

7.21 Connect the dots (samples) in Figure 7.35 to get the Doppler-shift frequency. How many cycles are in each example?

    a. _____
    b. _____
    c. _____
    d. _____
    e. _____

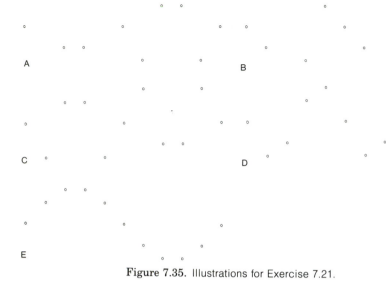

A   B

C   D

E

Figure 7.35. Illustrations for Exercise 7.21.

7.22 The frequencies that were sampled in Exercise 7.21 are shown in Figure 7.36. In which example(s) has aliasing occurred?

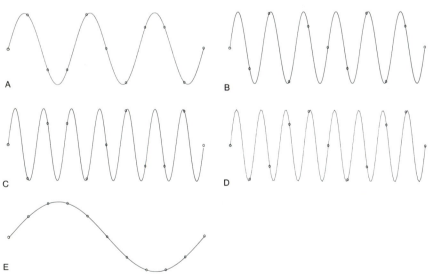

A   B

C   D

E

Figure 7.36. Illustrations for Exercise 7.22.

7.23 Which of the following instruments can produce aliasing?

    a. continuous-wave Doppler
    b. pulsed Doppler
    c. duplex
    d. color flow
    e. more than one of the above

7.24 Doppler performance evaluation devices fall into two groups: those that use a blood-mimicking _____ and those that use a moving _____ for scattering the ultrasound.

7.25 Heating depends most directly on

    a. thermal index
    b. SATP intensity
    c. SPTP intensity
    d. mechanical index

7.26 The available epidemiologic data are sufficient to make a final judgment on the safety of diagnostic ultrasound. True or false?

7.27 Exposure is minimized by using diagnostic ultrasound

    a. only when indicated
    b. with minimum output
    c. with minimum time
    d. all of the above
    e. none of the above

7.28 There is no possible hazard involved in the diagnostic use of ultrasound. True or false?

7.29 Ultrasound should not be used as a diagnostic tool because of the bioeffects it can produce. True or false?

7.30 No independently confirmed significant bioeffects in mammalian tissues have been reported at intensities below

    a. 10 W/cm^2 SPTP
    b. 100 mW/cm^2 SPTA
    c. 10 mW/cm^2 SPTA
    d. 10 mW/cm^2 SATA
    e. 1 mW/cm^2 SATP

7.31 Is there any knowledge of what types of injuries or risks occur with diagnostic ultrasound in patients and under what conditions? Yes or no?

7.32 Is there any knowledge of any bioeffects that ultrasound produces in small animals under experimental conditions? Yes or no?

7.33 Which of the following are mechanisms by which ultrasound can produce bioeffects? (More than one correct answer.)

    a. direction ionization
    b. absorption
    c. photoelectric effect
    d. cavitation
    e. Compton effect

7.34 Which of the following relates to heating?

    a. impedance
    b. sound speed
    c. absorption
    d. refraction
    e. diffraction

7.35 The SPTA intensity below which bioeffects in experimental animals have not been confirmed in the 0.5 to 10-MHz frequency range for focused beams is

    a. 100 μW/cm^2
    b. 1 mW/cm^2
    c. 1 W/cm^2
    d. 100 W/cm^2
    e. 100 kW/cm^2

7.36 The following end point is documented in the scientific literature well enough that a risk assessment for diagnostic ultrasound can be based on it:

    a. fetal weight
    b. sister chromatid exchange
    c. fetal abnormalities
    d. carcinogenesis
    e. none

7.37 More than one epidemiologic study has shown a statistically significant effect of ultrasound exposure on which of the following end points?

a. fetal activity
b. birth weight
c. fetal abnormalities
d. dyslexia
e. none

7.38 Which of the following acoustic parameters have been documented in ultrasound epidemiologic studies published thus far?

a. frequency
b. exposure time
c. intensity and pulsing conditions
d. scanning patterns
e. none

7.39 A typical output intensity (SPTA) for an ultrasound imaging instrument is

a. 1540 W
b. 13 kW/mm^2
c. 3.5 MHz
d. 1 mW/cm^2
e. 2 dB/cm

7.40 Which of the following typically have the highest output intensity?

a. fetal monitor Doppler
b. duplex pulsed Doppler
c. color-flow imager
d. mechanical gray-scale imager
e. phased-array, gray-scale imager

7.41 The attenuation of 3.5-MHz ultrasound in soft tissue is such that the intensity at a depth of 8 cm is approximately which fraction of that at the transducer face (skin surface)?

a. 90 percent
b. 50 percent
c. 20 percent
d. 4 percent
e. 0.01 percent

7.42 To minimize whatever (unidentified) risk there may be with Doppler ultrasound, the following should be done. (More than one correct answer.)

a. scan for family album pictures
b. scan to determine fetal sex
c. minimize exposure time
d. scan for medical indication only
e. minimize exposure intensity

7.43 Which of the following controls affect instrument output intensity?

a. dynamic range and compression
b. transmit and output
c. near gain and far gain
d. overall gain
e. slope and time gain compensation

7.44 Which of the following are correct for a duplex pulsed-Doppler instrument? (More than one correct answer.)

a. tissue anywhere in the Doppler beam is exposed to ultrasound
b. tissue anywhere in the imaging plane is exposed to ultrasound
c. imaging intensities are higher than for conventional real-time instruments
d. Doppler intensities are higher than for continuous-wave fetal monitoring
e. tissue is exposed to the Doppler beam only at the location of the gate

7.45 The tissue of greatest concern with regard to bioeffects in an abdominal scan is

a. spleen
b. pancreas
c. liver
d. kidney
e. fetus

7.46 Which of the following is (are) likely to be exposed to ultrasound during a diagnostic study?

a. patient
b. sonographer

c. sonologist
d. observers in the room
e. more than one of the above

7.47 No bioeffects have been observed in nonhuman mammalian tissues at thermal index values less than

    a. 5
    b. 4
    c. 3
    d. 2
    e. 1

7.48 No bioeffects have been observed in nonhuman mammalian tissues at mechanical index values less than

    a. 0.5
    b. 0.4
    c. 0.3
    d. 0.2
    e. 0.1

7.49 No bioeffects have been observed in nonhuman mammalian tissues at peak rarefactional pressure values (MPa) less than

    a. 0.5
    b. 0.4
    c. 0.3
    d. 0.2
    e. 0.1

7.50 For a given peak pressure, the mechanical index _____ as the frequency increases.

8 Summary

By sending short pulses of ultrasound into the body and using echoes received from tissue interfaces and from within tissues to produce images of internal structures, ultrasound is used as a medical diagnostic tool. Ultrasound is a wave of traveling acoustic variables described by frequency, wavelength, propagation speed, amplitude, intensity, and attenuation. Diagnostic ultrasound commonly uses the frequency range of 2 to 10 MHz. Pulsed ultrasound is used in sonography. It is described, in addition, by the pulse repetition frequency and spatial pulse length. For perpendicular incidence at boundaries, echoes are produced if the media impedances are different. For oblique incidence, refraction occurs if the media propagation speeds are different. Scattering occurs at rough boundaries and within heterogeneous media. The distance to reflectors is found from the round-trip travel time.

Transducers convert electric energy to ultrasound energy and vice versa by piezoelectricity. Axial resolution (equal to one half of the pulse length) can be improved by damping and increasing the frequency. Lateral resolution (equal to the beam's diameter) can be improved by focusing. Disk transducers produce sound beams with near and far zones. Focusing can be accomplished only in the near zone of the comparable unfocused transducer. Arrays can scan, steer, and shape beams electronically, permitting dynamic imaging. Dynamic imaging can also be accomplished with mechanically driven single-element transducers or mirrors.

Pulse-echo systems use the amplitude, direction, and arrival time of echoes to produce images. Imaging systems consist of a pulser, beam former, transducer, receiver, memory, and display. The pulser delivers the energizing voltages to the transducer, which responds by producing ultrasound pulses. Receivers amplify voltages that represent returning

279

echoes and compensate for attenuation. Digital memories store gray-scale image information and permit a display on a television monitor. The number of bits per pixel in the digital memory determines the number of gray shades that can be displayed by the system. Dynamic imaging instruments display a rapid sequence of images (frames). Display artifacts include reverberation, refraction, mirror image, shadowing, and enhancement.

Fluids (gases and liquids) are substances that flow. Blood is a liquid that flows through the vascular system under the influence of the pulsatile pressure provided by the beating heart. The volume flow rate is proportional to the pressure difference between the ends of a tube and inversely proportional to the resistance to flow. The flow resistance increases with viscosity and tube length and decreases (strongly) with increasing tube diameter. Seven (two temporal and five spatial) flow classifications include steady, pulsatile, plug, laminar, parabolic, disturbed, and turbulent. In a stenosis, flow speeds up, pressure drops (Bernoulli effect), and flow is disturbed. If the speed of flow exceeds a critical value, as described by the Reynolds number, turbulence occurs. Pulsatile flow is common in the arterial circulation. Diastolic flow and/ or flow reversal occur in some locations within the arterial system. The fluid's inertia and the vessel's compliance are characteristics that are important in determining flow with pulsatile driving pressure.

The Doppler effect is a change in frequency or wavelength that results from motion. In most medical ultrasound applications, the motion is that of blood flow in the circulation. The change in frequency of the returning echoes with respect to the emitted frequency is called the Doppler shift. For flow toward the transducer, it is positive; for flow away, it is negative.

The Doppler shift depends on the speed of the scatterers of sound, the angle between their direction and that of the sound's propagation, and the operating frequency of the Doppler system. A moving scatterer of sound produces a double Doppler shift. Greater flow speeds and smaller Doppler angles produce larger Doppler shifts but not stronger echoes. Higher operating frequencies produce larger Doppler shifts. Typical ranges of flow speeds (10 to 100 cm/s), Doppler angles (30 to 60 degrees), and operating frequencies (2 to 10 MHz) yield Doppler shifts in the range 100 Hz to 11 kHz for vascular studies. In Doppler echocardiography, in which zero angles and speeds of a few meters per second are encountered, Doppler shifts can be as high as 30 kHz.

Doppler instruments make use of the Doppler shift to yield information regarding motion and flow. Continuous-wave systems provide motion and flow information without a depth-selection capability. Pulsed-Doppler systems provide the ability to select the depth from which the Doppler information is received. Spectral analysis provides visual information on the distribution of the received Doppler-shift frequencies that result from the distribution of scatterer velocities (speeds and directions) encountered. In addition to audible output, the imaging of flow spectra is possible in Doppler systems. Combined (duplex) systems that use dynamic sonography and continuous- and pulsed-wave Doppler are available commerically.

The Doppler spectrum is generated by the range of scatterer velocities encountered by the ultrasound beam. It is derived electronically by using the fast Fourier transform and presented on the display as the Doppler shift versus time, with brightness indicating power. Flow conditions at the site of measurement are indicated by the width of the spectrum, with spectral broadening and a loss of window indicating disturbed and turbulent flow. Flow conditions downstream, particularly distal flow resistance, are indicated by the relationship between peak systolic and end-diastolic flow speeds. Various indices for quantitatively presenting this information have been developed.

Color-flow imaging acquires Doppler- or time-shifted echoes from a cross section of tissue scanned by an ultrasound beam. These echoes are then presented in color and superimposed on the gray-scale anatomic image of nonshifted echoes that were received during the scan. The flow echoes are assigned colors, according to the color map chosen. Red, yellow, blue, cyan, and white indicate positive or negative Doppler shifts (approaching or receding flow). Yellow, cyan, or green is used to indicate variance (disturbed or turbulent flow). Several pulses (the number is called the ensemble length) are needed to generate a color scan line. Linear, convex, and phased arrays are used to acquire the gray-scale and color-flow information. Color controls include gain; depth gain compensation; map selection; variance on/off; persistence; ensemble length; color/gray priority; scale (pulse repetition frequency); baseline shift; wall filter; and the color window's angle, location, and size. Doppler color-flow instruments are pulsed-Doppler instruments and are subject to the same limitations (Doppler angle dependence and aliasing) as are other Doppler instruments. Time-shift instruments have the same angle dependence.

Artifacts with Doppler ultrasound include aliasing, range ambiguity, image and Doppler signal mirroring, spectral trace mirroring, and electrical interference. Aliasing is the most common artifact. It occurs when the Doppler-shift frequency exceeds one half of the pulse repetition frequency. It can be reduced or eliminated by increasing the pulse repetition frequency or Doppler angle, using the baseline shift, reducing the operating frequency, or using a continuous-wave instrument.

Doppler-performance evaluation devices of two types are available: those that use a blood-mimicking fluid and those that use a moving string. They are useful for evaluating the performance (e.g., spectral scale accuracy) of Doppler instruments.

Extensive mechanistic, in vitro, in vivo, and epidemiologic studies have revealed no known risk with the current ultrasound instrumentation used in medical diagnosis. A prudent and conservative approach, however, to ultrasound safety is to assume that there may be an unidentified risk which should be minimized in medically indicated ultrasound studies by minimizing exposure. The output display indices facilitate this conservative approach to patient safety.

Exercises

8.1 Doppler systems convert ＿＿＿＿＿ ＿＿＿＿＿ information to audible sound or visual display.

8.2 A pulser similar to that used in imaging systems is used in Doppler systems. True or false?

8.3 Doppler system transducers (not arrays) may have ＿＿＿＿＿ or ＿＿＿＿＿ elements.

8.4 The receiver in a Doppler system compares the ＿＿＿＿＿ of the voltage generator and the voltage from the receiving transducer.

8.5 The Doppler shift usually is not in the audible frequency range and must be converted by the receiver to a frequency that can be heard. True or false?

8.6 The Doppler shift is determined by the reflector ＿＿＿＿＿ and by the cosine of an angle.

8.7 A component that pulsed-Doppler systems have but continuous-wave Doppler systems do not have is the ＿＿＿＿＿.

8.8 A Doppler system may have as an output a visual ＿＿＿＿＿.

8.9 In a pulsed-Doppler system, the pulse repetition frequency is determined by the generator _____, and the source ultrasound frequency is determined by the _____.

8.10 Pulsed-Doppler systems can give motion information from a particular _____.

8.11 A typical spatial peak temporal average output intensity for a Doppler instrument is 50 mW/cm^2. True or false?

8.12 The sound received by the transducer in a Doppler instrument is in the audible frequency range. True or false?

8.13 Frequencies used in Doppler ultrasound are in approximately the same range as those for pulse-echo imaging. True or false?

8.14 If the incident frequency is 4 MHz, the reflector speed is 100 cm/s, and the angle between the beam and motion directions is 60 degrees, the Doppler shift is _____ kHz.

8.15 There is no problem in Exercise 8.14 with aliasing with a pulse repetition frequency of 10 kHz. True or false?

8.16 If there were a problem in Exercise 8.15, _____ _____ Doppler ultrasound could be used to avoid it.

8.17 Color-flow instruments use

    a. continuous-wave Doppler
    b. pulsed Doppler
    c. compressed Doppler
    d. all of the above
    e. none of the above

8.18 Increasing the frequency

    a. improves the resolution
    b. increases the penetration
    c. increases refraction
    d. both a and b
    e. both a and c

8.19 Increasing the pulse repetition frequency

a. improves resolution
b. increases maximum unambiguous depth
c. decreases maximum unambiguous depth
d. both a and b
e. both a and c

8.20 Increasing the intensity produced by the transducer

a. is accomplished by increasing the pulser voltage
b. increases the sensitivity of the system
c. increases the possibility of bioeffects
d. all of the above
e. none of the above

8.21 Increasing the spatial pulse length

a. is accomplished by transducer damping
b. is accompanied by decreased pulse duration
c. improves the axial resolution
d. all of the above
e. none of the above

8.22 Dynamic imaging is made possible by

a. scan converters
b. mechanically driven transducers
c. gray-scale display
d. arrays
e. both b and d

8.23 If the Doppler shift is 6.5 kHz with a flow speed of 100 cm/s, what pulse repetition frequency is required to detect flow at 200 cm/s?

a. 3.2 kHz
b. 6.5 kHz
c. 13 kHz
d. 26 kHz
e. 52 kHz

8.24 Multiple focus is not used with color-flow imaging because of

a. ensemble length
b. wall filter

c. priority
d. low frame rate
e. a and d

8.25 Ultrasound bioeffects

a. do not occur
b. do not occur with diagnostic instruments
c. are not confirmed below 100 mW/cm^2 spatial peak temporal average
d. both b and c
e. none of the above

8.26 The diagnostic ultrasound frequency range is

a. 2 to 10 MHz
b. 2 to 10 kHz
c. 2 to 10 MHz
d. 3 to 15 kHz
e. none of the above

8.27 Small transducers always produce smaller beam diameters. True or false?

8.28 No reflection occurs if media impedances are equal. True or false?

8.29 No refraction occurs if media impedances are equal. True or false?

8.30 Gray-scale display is made possible by

a. array transducers
b. cathode ray storage tubes
c. scan converters
d. both b and c
e. all of the above

8.31 Attenuation is corrected by

a. demodulation
b. desegregation
c. decompression
d. compensation

8.32 The Doppler effect for a scatterer moving toward the transducer causes scattered sound (compared with the incident sound) received by the transducer to have _____.

   a. increased intensity
   b. decreased intensity
   c. increased impedance
   d. increased frequency
   e. decreased impedance

8.33 An ultrasound instrument that could represent 64 shades of gray would require an eight-bit memory. True or false?

8.34 Continuous-wave sound is used in _____.

   a. all imaging instruments
   b. some imaging instruments
   c. all Doppler instruments
   d. some Doppler instruments
   e. none of the above

8.35 An advantage of continuous-wave Doppler instruments is that they have _____.

   a. no aliasing
   b. depth information and selectivity
   c. bidirectional information
   d. amplitude information
   e. all of the above

8.36 An advantage of pulsed Doppler instruments is that they have _____.

   a. no aliasing
   b. depth selectivity
   c. bidirectional information
   d. amplitude information
   e. all of the above

8.37 A digital memory with one bit per pixel would have a _____ display.

   a. bidirectional
   b. biscattering
   c. bistable

8.38 If a transducer element 19 mm in diameter is focused to produce a minimum beam diameter of 2 mm, the intensity at the focus is approximately _____ times the intensity at the transducer.

    a. 2
    b. 3
    c. 19
    d. 100
    e. 500

8.39 The largest number that can be stored in a pixel of a seven-bit digital memory is _____.

    a. 16
    b. 32
    c. 127
    d. 255
    e. 256

8.40 Digital calipers provide a measurement of distance between _____.

    a. potentiometers
    b. bits
    c. optical encoders
    d. pixels
    e. all of the above

8.41 Which of the following produce(s) a sector scan format?

    a. rotating, mechanical, real-time transducer
    b. oscillating, mechanical, real-time transducer
    c. phased array
    d. oscillating mirror
    e. all of the above

8.42 A digital imaging instrument divides the cross-sectional image into _____.

    a. frequencies
    b. bits
    c. pixels
    d. binaries
    e. wavelengths

8.43 If the thickness of a transducer element is decreased, the frequency is _____.

   a. increased
   b. unchanged
   c. decreased
   d. intensified
   e. none of the above

8.44 In Exercise 8.43, the near-zone length is _____.

   a. increased
   b. unchanged
   c. decreased
   d. intensified
   e. none of the above

8.45 With increased damping, which of the following is increased?

   a. bandwidth
   b. pulse duration
   c. spatial pulse length
   d. Q factor
   e. all of the above

8.46 As frequency is increased, which of the following is (are) decreased?

   a. propagation speed
   b. penetration
   c. imaging depth
   d. more than one of the above
   e. none of the above

8.47 A five-bit memory can store which of the following numbers?

   a. 64
   b. 32
   c. 31
   d. 55
   e. more than one of the above

8.48 Television monitors produce _____ frames per second.

    a. 10
    b. 24
    c. 30
    d. 60
    e. none of the above

8.49 Duplex Doppler instruments include _____.

    a. pulsed Doppler
    b. continuous-wave Doppler
    c. static imaging
    d. dynamic imaging
    e. more than one of the above

8.50 If the Doppler shifts from normal and from stenotic carotid arteries are 4 kHz and 10 kHz, respectively, for which will there be a problem with a pulse repetition frequency of 7 kHz?

    a. normal
    b. stenotic
    c. both
    d. neither

8.51 The problem in Exercise 8.50 is _____.

8.52 Which of the following affects contrast resolution?

    a. number of pixels
    b. number of bits per pixel
    c. pulse duration
    d. frequency
    e. focusing

8.53 Which of the following requires a phased array as a receiving transducer?

    a. dynamic range
    b. dynamic imaging
    c. dynamic focusing
    d. none of the above

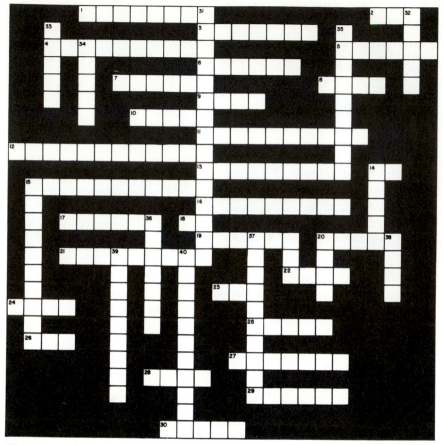

(From Kremkau FW: Diagnostic Ultrasound: Principles, Instruments, and Exercises, 4th edition. Philadelphia, WB Saunders, 1993. Reprinted with permission.)

8.54 Across

1. Referring to sound.

2. Abbreviation for cosine.

3. Not perpendicular to a boundary.

4. Occurs at boundaries with perpendicular incidence.

5. Material through which sound is passing.

6. Pulsed Doppler requires _____ the receiver.

7. The duty _____ is the sound-on fraction.

8. The beam diameter decreases in the _____ zone.

9. The intensity is power divided by _____.

10. Reflector motion produces a Doppler _____.

11. Sound of frequency 20 kHz and higher.

12. Parallel to sound direction.

13. Maximum variation of an acoustic variable.

14. Abbreviation for continuous wave.

15. Attenuation _____ is given in decibels per centimeter.

16. Power divided by area.

17. Reciprocal of frequency.

18. The range equation gives the distance _____ a reflector.

19. Perpendicular to a boundary.

20. Displacement divided by time.

21. The propagation speed depends on density and _____.

22. _____ scale displays several values of spot brightness.

23. The beam's diameter increases in the _____ zone.

24. Force times displacement.

25. The axial resolution depends on spatial _____ length.

26. Abbreviation for sine.

27. The reflected frequency minus the incident frequency equals _____ shift.

28. A traveling variation.

29. Ability to do work.

30. Complete variation of a wave variable.

Down

14. One hertz is one _____ per second.

15. The abbreviation CW stands for _____ wave.

20. A line produced on a display is called a _____ line.

31. (A message for you).

32. Traveling wave of acoustic variables.

33. Transducer assembly containing more than one element.

34. _____ length is the distance from a focused transducer to the minimum beam diameter.

35. Density times propagation speed.

36. Mass divided by volume.

37. Another name for a hydrophone.

38. The pulse duration divided by the pulse repetition period is _____ factor.

39. Reciprocal of period.

40. The ability of an imaging system to detect weak reflections.

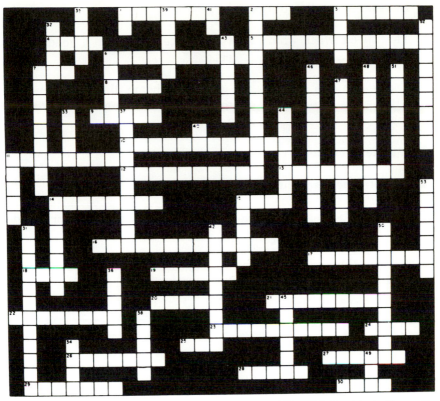

(From Kremkau FW: Crossword puzzle. Med Ultrasound *4*:38, 1980. Reprinted with permission of John Wiley & Sons, Inc.)

8.55 Across

1. The ratio of largest to smallest power that a system can handle is called _____ range.

2. At a distance of one near-zone length from a disk transducer, the beam diameter is approximately equal to disk diameter divided by _____.

3. Passing only reflections that arrive at a certain time after the transducer has produced a pulse is called _____.

4. Continuously displaying moving structures is called _____ time imaging.

5. Increasing small voltages to large ones.

6. The speed with which a wave moves through a medium is called _____ speed.

7. The region of a sound beam where the beam diameter increases with the distance from the transducer is called the _____ zone.

8. Another word for a reflection.

9. Acoustic means having to do with _____.

10. If propagation speeds in two media are equal, the incidence angle equals the _____ angle.

11. A device that stores a gray-scale image and allows it to be displayed on a television monitor is called a scan _____.

12. Conversion of sound to heat.

13. Power divided by area.

14. An echo-free region on a display is called _____.

15. The fraction of time that pulsed ultrasound is actually on is called _____ factor.

16. The American Institute of Ultrasound in Medicine statement on bioeffects says that there have been no _____ confirmed significant bioeffects below 100 mW/cm^2.

17. Density multiplied by sound propagation speed.

18. Displaying several values of spot brightness is called a _____ scale.

19. If no reflection occurs at a boundary, this always means that media impedances are equal in the case of _____ incidence.

20. A few cycles of ultrasound may be called an ultrasound _____.

21. Maximum variation of an acoustic variable or voltage.

22. Reverberations are also called _____ reflections.

23. A device that converts energy from one form to another.

24. Prefix meaning 1000.

25. Abbreviation for megahertz.

26. _____ incidence is when the sound direction is not perpendicular to the boundary of the medium.

27. Ability to do work.

28. Number of complete scans displayed per unit time in a real-time system is called the _____ rate.

29. Perpendicular to the direction of sound travel.

30. A unit for impedance.

Down

1. Abbreviation for decibel.

2. Sound _____ through a medium improves as attenuation decreases.

3. Ratio of output to input electrical power for an amplifier.

6. A Greek prefix meaning pressure.

7. Number of cycles per unit time.

11. One hertz is one _____ per second.

14. An _____ array is made up of ring-shaped elements.

15. Half-intensity _____ decreases with increasing frequency.

31. Along the direction of sound travel (axial).

32. Focusing produces decreased beam _____.

33. A sound _____ is a traveling variation of acoustic variables.

34. Most two-dimensional imaging is done with B _____ displays.

35. To sweep a sound beam to produce an image.

36. Rate at which work is done; rate at which energy is transferred.

37. Sound of frequency greater than 20 kHz.

38. Concentrate the sound beam into a smaller area.

39. A transducer _____ is an assembly containing more than one transducer element.

40. Abbreviation for millimeter.

41. Abbreviation for continuous wave.

42. Frequency unit.

43. A _____ array is made up of rectangular elements in a line.

44. Propagation speed increases with decreasing _____.

45. Material through which a wave travels.

46. Decrease of amplitude and intensity as a wave travels through a medium.

47. Length of space over which a cycle occurs.

48. Change of sound direction on passing from one medium to another.

49. A cathode _____ tube is a common display device.

50. Diffusion or redirection of sound in several directions.

51. Speed, with direction of motion specified.

52. Perpendicular _____ occurs when sound direction is perpendicular to the boundary of the medium.

53. The _____ effect is a frequency change of reflected sound wave caused by reflector motion.

8.56 Identify the physical terms, the common measurement units for which are given.

Across:

1. joule
2. microsecond
3. rayl
4. joule

Down:

5. radian
11. meter/second
12. newton/meter^2
13. watt

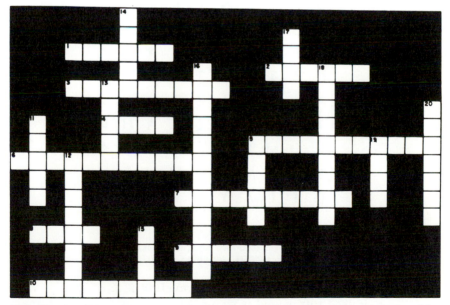

(From Kremkau FW: Ultrapuzzles. Reflections 6:85, 1980. Reprinted with permission of the American Institute of Ultrasound in Medicine.)

5. decibel
6. kelvin
7. millimeter
8. gram
9. milliliter
10. hertz

14. newton
15. decibel
16. meter/second^2
17. centimeter^2
18. watt/centimeter^2
19. second
20. gram/milliliter

8.57 In the following review, blanks need to be filled in. In the figure, begin at the upper left and draw a line to one letter at a time in any direction (horizontal, vertical, or diagonal) to spell out the words for the blanks. All letters are used in a continuous line. Do not cross over your line. Use each letter only once. The words should be found in the same order as they are needed for the blanks.

START

```
W
A  F  R  E  Q  U  S  P  O  P
V  C  I  T  S  E  E  R  A  E
E  A  C  O  U  N  I  G  T  R
E  E  P  S  N  C  A  A  T  I
D  A  T  T  O  T  S  C  N  G
A  U  N  E  I  Z  T  R  E  T
T  I  O  N  M  E  G  A  H  R
R  O  M  E  R  E  D  S  N  A
Y  S  P  M  S  C  U  U  E  N
D  I  L  A  Y  S  E  Q  C  E
                        END
```

(From Kremkau FW: Diagnostic Ultrasound: Principles, Instruments, and Exercises, 4th edition. Philadelphia, WB Saunders, 1993. Reprinted with permission.)

Ultrasound is a _____ of traveling _____ variables. Pulsed ultrasound is commonly used in ultrasound imaging. Pulses contain a range of _____. Soft tissue _____ _____ is 1.54 mm/μs, and the _____ coefficient is 0.5 dB/cm for each _____ of frequency. _____ occurs at rough boundaries and within heterogeneous media. _____ convert electric energy to ultrasound energy and vice versa. Imaging systems consist of pulser, beam former, transducer, receiver, _____, and _____. Dynamic imaging instruments display a rapid _____ of static pictures.

8.58 Find the words, whose definitions follow, that are hidden in the puzzle. They may appear horizontally, vertically, or diagonally.

1. Improper Doppler-shift information from a pulsed-Doppler instrument when the true Doppler shift exceeds one half of the pulse repetition frequency.

2. The presentation of two-dimensional, real-time Doppler- or time-shift information superimposed on a real-time, gray-scale, anatomic, cross-sectional image. Flow directions toward and away from the transducer (i.e., positive and negative Doppler shifts) are presented as different colors on the display.

3. A wave in which cycles repeat indefinitely; not pulsed.

4. The angle between the sound beam and the flow direction.

They may appear horizontally, vertically, or diagonally.

```
J  B  B  E  H  N  B  Y  K  L  Z  R  B  U  F  P  W  F
O  J  M  Y  V  U  P  O  A  I  E  G  L  D  L  M  Q  L
S  J  C  Y  Y  A  B  A  F  P  U  T  O  Z  F  G  E  X
F  C  O  N  P  E  W  F  I  D  R  P  F  M  T  J  C  T
O  Q  L  O  F  H  G  -  L  A  P  T  I  Q  J  A  F  S
E  S  O  C  H  J  S  T  S  L  U  T  F  O  N  I  F  C
I  D  R  O  O  T  V  O  E  U  E  Y  D  L  H  E  O  T
I  N  -  A  E  W  U  R  Q  P  O  V  V  S  D  A  Z  E
O  X  F  H  U  N  -  N  F  A  Y  U  -  T  F  K  V  V
L  F  L  O  D  A  A  D  N  C  O  R  N  O  G  A  D  G
I  N  O  A  N  T  D  N  N  U  E  D  A  I  W  G  S  C
A  T  W  G  L  C  K  E  V  L  J  G  I  -  T  J  C  L
X  I  L  G  A  I  U  F  P  K  L  N  D  W  J  N  U  V
A  E  U  I  E  Q  A  P  G  O  U  E  S  B  C  M  O  W
I  P  M  O  E  E  O  S  K  F  S  B  B  Z  Z  P  D  C
T  A  V  R  T  D  K  S  I  L  X  I  N  Z  I  L  G  C
U  C  F  F  K  H  L  A  U  N  V  N  J  Q  D  N  U  C
Q  Q  Y  Q  G  L  X  P  X  O  G  L  I  M  K  M  U  Q
```

5. Reflected frequency minus incident frequency. Change in frequency caused by motion.

6. Number of cycles per unit time.

7. A wave of pulsed ultrasound.

8. Sound of a frequency greater than 20 kHz.

8.59 Reflections are produced by changes in

    a. stiffness
    b. density
    c. absorption
    d. attenuation
    e. both a and b

8.60 If no reflection occurs at a boundary, this always means that media impedances are equal in the case of

    a. perpendicular incidence
    b. oblique incidence
    c. refraction
    d. both a and b
    e. both b and c

8.61 If the propagation speeds in two media are equal, the incidence angle equals the

    a. reflection angle
    b. transmission angle
    c. Doppler angle
    d. both a and b
    e. both b and c

8.62 Velocity is _____.

    a. speed
    b. direction
    c. acceleration
    d. a and b
    e. all of the above

8.63 If a green tag indicates that flow speed is 20 cm/s but the Doppler angle is 30 degrees and no angle correction is used, the flow speed is actually _____ cm/s.

 a. 23
 b. 17
 c. 40
 d. cos 30
 e. one half of the pulse repetition frequency

8.64 Which of the following can be real time (more than one correct answer)?

 a. A mode
 b. B mode
 c. B scan
 d. M mode
 e. Doppler

8.65 As the operating frequency increases, _____ increases.

 a. Doppler shift
 b. penetration
 c. angle-corrected flow speed
 d. angle correction
 e. all of the above

8.66 The colors used in color-flow displays include

 a. red and blue
 b. yellow and cyan
 c. white and magenta
 d. black and violet
 e. a and b

8.67 If the flow speed doubles and the Doppler angle changes from 0 to 60, the Doppler shift _____.

 a. quarters
 b. halves
 c. does not change
 d. doubles
 e. quadruples

302 Summary

8.68 Which of the following produce(s) a sector scan format?

    a. rotating, mechanical, real-time transducer
    b. oscillating, mechanical, real-time transducer
    c. phased array
    d. linear-sequenced array
    e. more than one of the above

8.69 Which of the following produce(s) a rectangular scan format?

    a. rotating, mechanical, real-time transducer
    b. oscillating, mechanical, real-time transducer
    c. phased array
    d. linear-sequenced array
    e. more than one of the above

8.70 Gray-scale displays present brightness corresponding to echo

    a. frequency
    b. amplitude
    c. bandwidth
    d. impedance
    e. more than one of the above

8.71 A digital scan converter stores _____ corresponding to echo amplitudes.

    a. numbers
    b. electrical charges
    c. lines
    d. frames
    e. none of the above

8.72 The intensity of returning echoes changes with the angle in Doppler-flow measurements. True or false?

8.73 The intensity of returning echoes changes with the flow speed in Doppler ultrasound. True or false?

8.74 As the frequency increases, which of the following (more than one) decrease?

    a. period
    b. wavelength
    c. propagation speed
    d. amplitude

e. intensity
f. attenuation coefficient
g. penetration
h. reflection coefficient
i. transmission coefficient
j. refraction
k. pulse duration
l. spatial pulse length
m. pulse repetition frequency
n. pulse repetition period
o. duty factor
p. near-zone length
q. imaging depth
r. axial resolution
s. impedance

8.75 Fill in the missing values in the table.

Incident Frequency (MHz)	Flow Speed (cm/s)	Angle (°)	Reflected Frequency (MHz)	Doppler Shift (kHz)
2	30	0	(a)	(b)
4	30	0	(c)	(d)
8	30	0	(e)	(f)
2	50	(g)	2.0000	(h)
4	50	(i)	(j)	1.3
8	50	30	(k)	(l)

a. _____   **g.** _____
b. _____   **h.** _____
c. _____   **i.** _____
d. _____   **j.** _____
e. _____   **k.** _____
f. _____   **l.** _____

8.76 Compensation makes up for the fact that echoes from deeper reflectors arrive weaker. True or false?

8.77 In which direction is the blood flow in the red vessel in Figure 1.5 (Color Plate II)?

8.78 If the angle correction is set at 60 degrees but it should be 0 degrees, the display indicates a flow speed of 100 cm/s. The correct flow speed is _____ cm/s.

a. 25
b. 50

c. 100
d. 200
e. 400

8.79 If the angle correction is set at 0 degrees but it should be 60 degrees, the display indicates a flow speed of 100 cm/s. The correct flow speed is _____ cm/s.

a. 25
b. 50
c. 100
d. 200
e. 400

8.80 A color map that progresses from dark red to white uses _____ to indicate the mean Doppler shifts.

a. luminance
b. hue
c. saturation
d. a and c
e. all of the above

Glossary

Absorption.   Conversion of sound to heat.

Aliasing.   Improper Doppler-shift information from a pulsed-Doppler instrument when the true Doppler shift exceeds one half of the pulse repetition frequency.

Amplification.   Increasing small voltages to larger ones.

Amplifier.   A device that accomplishes amplification.

Amplitude.   Maximum variation of an acoustic variable or voltage.

Annular array.   Array made of ring-shaped elements arranged concentrically.

Array.   Transducer array.

Attenuation.   Decrease in amplitude and intensity as a wave travels through a medium.

Attenuation coefficient.   Attenuation per unit length of a wave's traveling distance.

Autocorrelation.   A rapid technique for obtaining the mean Doppler-shift frequency. This technique is used in color-flow instruments.

Axial.   In the direction of the transducer axis (sound-travel direction).

Axial resolution.   Minimum reflector separation along the sound path required for separate echoes to be produced.

B mode.   Mode of operation in which the display records a spot brightening for each echo pulse delivered from the receiver.

B scan.   A brightness image that represents a cross section of the object through the scanning plane.

Backscatter.   Sound scattered back in the direction from which it originally came.

Bandwidth. Range of frequencies contained in an ultrasound pulse or echo.

Baseline shift. Movement of the zero Doppler-shift frequency or zero-flow speed line up or down on a spectral display.

Beam area. Cross-sectional area of a sound beam.

Beam former. The part of an instrument that accomplishes electronic beam scanning, apodization, steering, focusing, and dynamic aperture with arrays.

Bernoulli effect. Pressure reduction in a region of high-flow speed.

Bidirectional. Indicating Doppler instruments capable of distinguishing between positive and negative Doppler shifts (forward and reverse flow).

Bruit. Audible sounds (using a stethoscope) originating in vessels with turbulent flow.

Cathode ray tube (CRT). A display device that produces an image by scanning an electron beam over a phosphor-coated screen.

Cavitation. Production and behavior of bubbles in sound.

Clutter. Noise in the Doppler signal generally caused by high-amplitude, Doppler-shifted echoes from moving heart or vessel walls.

Color flow (CF). The presentation of two-dimensional, real-time Doppler shift or time-shift information superimposed on a real-time, gray-scale anatomic cross-sectional image. Flow directions toward and away from the transducer (i.e., positive and negative Doppler or time shifts) are presented as different colors on the display.

Compensation. Equalizing received echo amplitude differences caused by attenuation and differences in reflector depth.

Compliance. Distensibility. Nonrigid stretchability of vessels.

Composite. Combination of a piezoelectric ceramic with a nonpiezoelectric polymer.

Continuous mode. Continuous-wave mode.

Continuous wave (CW). A wave in which cycles repeat indefinitely. Not pulsed.

Continuous wave Doppler. A Doppler device or procedure that uses continuous-wave ultrasound.

Continuous-wave mode. Mode of operation in which continuous-wave sound is used.

Contrast resolution. Ability of a gray-scale display to distinguish between echoes of slightly different amplitude or intensity.

Convex array. Linear array with a curved (bowed out) shape.

cos. Abbreviation for cosine.

Cosine. The cosine of an angle in a right triangle is the length of the adjacent side divided by the length of the hypotenuse (longest side).

Coupling medium. Gel used to provide a good sound path between the transducer and the skin.

Critical Reynolds number. Reynolds number above which turbulence occurs.

Cross correlation. A rapid technique for determining time shifts in an echo's arrival. This technique is used to determine flow speeds without using the Doppler effect.

Cross talk. Leakage of strong signals in one direction channel of a Doppler receiver into the other channel. Can produce the Doppler spectrum mirror-image artifact.

Crystal. Element.

Cycle. Complete variation of an acoustic variable.

Damping. Material placed behind the rear face of a transducer element to reduce a pulse's duration; also, the process of pulse-duration reduction.

dB. Abbreviation for decibel.

Decibel. Unit of power or intensity ratio; the number of decibels is 10 times the logarithm (to the base 10) of the power or intensity ratio.

Demodulation. Converting voltage pulses from radio-frequency (RF) form to video form.

Density. Mass divided by volume.

Depth gain compensation (DGC). Compensation.

Detail resolution. Ability to image fine detail and to distinguish closely spaced reflectors.

Disturbed flow. Flow that cannot be described by straight, parallel streamlines.

Doppler angle. The angle between the sound beam and the direction of flow.

Doppler effect. Frequency change of reflected sound wave as a result of a reflector's motion relative to a transducer.

Doppler equation. The mathematic description of the relationship between Doppler shift, frequency, Doppler angle, propagation speed, and reflector speed.

Doppler-sample volume. See sample volume.

Doppler shift. Reflected frequency minus incident frequency. Change in frequency caused by motion.

Doppler-shift frequency. Doppler shift.

Doppler spectrum.   The range of frequencies present in Doppler-shifted echoes.

Duplex instrument.   An ultrasound instrument that combines gray-scale sonography with pulsed-Doppler and, possibly, continuous-wave Doppler.

Duty factor.   Fraction of time that pulsed ultrasound is on. Sometimes called duty cycle.

Dynamic focusing.   Continuously variable reception focus that follows the changing position of the transmitted pulse.

Dynamic imaging.   Rapid frame-sequence imaging.

Dynamic range.   Ratio (in decibels) of largest power to smallest power that a system can handle or of the largest to the smallest intensity of a group of echoes.

Echo.   Reflection.

Eddies.   See vortices.

Element.   A small piece of piezoelectric material in a transducer assembly.

Energy.   Ability to do work.

Energy, kinetic.   Energy of motion.

Energy, potential.   Energy of position or state.

Enhancement.   Increase in an echo's amplitude from reflectors that lie behind a weakly attenuating structure.

Ensemble length.   Number of pulses used to generate one color-flow-image scan line; also called packet size, dwell time, or color sensitivity.

Fast Fourier transform (FFT).   Digital computer implementation of the Fourier transform.

Filter.   An electric circuit that passes frequencies within a certain range.

Flow.   To move in a stream. Volume flow rate.

Flow speed.   Rate of motion of a portion of a flowing fluid.

Fluid.   A material that flows and conforms to the shape of its container. A liquid or a gas.

Focal length.   Distance from a focused transducer to the center of a focal region or to the location of the spatial peak intensity.

Focal region.   Region of minimum beam diameter and area.

Focus.   To concentrate the sound beam into a smaller beam area than would exist otherwise.

Focusing, dynamic.   See dynamic focusing.

Force.   That which changes the state of rest or motion of an object.

Fourier analysis.   The application of the Fourier transform to determine the frequency components present.

Fourier transform.   A mathematic technique for obtaining a Doppler spectrum.

Frame.   Single display image produced by one complete scan of the sound beam.

Frame rate.   Number of frames displayed per second.

Freeze frame.   Constant image of the last frame entered into memory.

Frequency.   Number of cycles per second.

Frequency, Doppler-shift.   See Doppler shift.

Frequency spectrum.   The range of frequencies present. In a Doppler instrument, the range of Doppler-shift frequencies present in the returning echoes.

Gain.   Ratio of output to input electric power.

Generator gate.   The electronic portion of a pulsed-Doppler system that converts the continuous voltage of the voltage generator (oscillator) to a pulsed voltage.

Gray scale.   Continuous range of brightnesses between white and black.

Gray-scale display.   Display in which several values of spot brightness may be displayed.

Heat.   Energy resulting from thermal molecular motion.

Hertz.   Unit of frequency, one cycle per second. Unit of pulse repetition frequency, one pulse per second.

Hue.   The color perceived as a result of the frequency of the light.

Hyperechoic.   Having relatively strong echoes.

Hypoechoic.   Having relatively weak echoes.

Impedance (acoustic).   Density multiplied by the sound propagation speed.

Incidence angle.   Angle between the incident sound direction and the line perpendicular to the boundary of the medium.

Inertia.   Resistance to acceleration.

Intensity.   Power divided by area.

kHz.   Abbreviation for kilohertz.

Kilohertz (kHz).   One thousand hertz.

Laminar flow.   Flow in which fluid layers slide over each other in a smooth, orderly manner, with no mixing between layers.
Lateral.   Perpendicular to the direction of sound travel.
Lateral resolution.   Minimum reflector separation perpendicular to the sound path required for separate reflections to be produced.
Linear array.   Array made of rectangular elements in a line.
Linear-phased array.   Linear array operated by applying voltage pulses to all elements but with small time differences.
Linear-sequenced array.   Linear array operated by applying voltage pulses to groups of elements sequentially.
Luminance.   Brightness of a presented hue and saturation.

Mass.   Measure of an object's resistance to acceleration.
Matching layer.   Material placed in front of the front face of a transducer element to reduce the reflection at the transducer's surface.
Mechanical index.   An indicator of nonthermal-mechanism activity. Equal to the peak rarefactional pressure divided by the square root of the center frequency of the pulse bandwidth.
Megahertz (MHz).   One million hertz.
Mirror image.   In sonography, duplication of an object on the opposite side of a strong reflector. In Doppler, duplication of the spectrum on the other side of the baseline.

Noise.   Unwanted acoustic or electric signals.
Nyquist limit.   The Doppler shift above which aliasing occurs (one half of the pulse repetition frequency). One-half PRF.

Operating frequency.   Preferred frequency of operation of a transducer.

Parabolic flow.   Laminar flow with a profile in the shape of a parabola.
Penetration.   Imaging depth.
Phantom.   Tissue-equivalent materials that have some characteristics representative of tissues (e.g., scattering or attenuation properties).
Phase.   A description of progress through a cycle. One full cycle is divided into 360 degrees of phase.

Phase quadrature. Two signals differing by one fourth of a cycle.

Phased array. An array that steers and focuses the beam electronically (with short time delays).

Piezoelectricity. Conversion of pressure to electric voltage.

Pixel. Picture element. The unit into which imaging and Doppler information is divided for storage and display in a digital instrument.

Plug flow. Flow with all fluid portions traveling with nearly the same flow speed and direction.

Poise. Unit of viscosity.

Poiseuille's law. The mathematic description of the dependence of flow rate on pressure, vessel length and radius, and fluid viscosity.

Postprocessing. Signal processing done after memory.

Power. Rate at which work is done. Rate at which energy is transferred.

Preprocessing. Signal processing (e.g., gain, time gain compensation) done before memory.

Pressure. Force divided by area.

PRF. Abbreviation for pulse repetition frequency.

Priority. The gray-scale echo strength below which color-flow information is preferentially shown on a display.

Probe. Transducer assembly.

Propagation speed. Speed with which a wave moves through a medium.

Pulsatility index. A description of the relationship between peak systolic and end-diastolic flow speeds or Doppler shifts.

Pulse. A brief excursion of a quantity from its normal value. A few cycles.

Pulse duration. Time from the beginning to the end of a pulse.

Pulse-echo diagnostic ultrasound. Ultrasound imaging and flow measurement in which ultrasound pulses are reflected and the echoes used to produce a display.

Pulse repetition frequency (PRF). Number of pulses per second. Sometimes called pulse repetition rate.

Pulsed Doppler. A Doppler device or procedure that uses pulsed-wave ultrasound.

Pulsed mode. Mode of operation in which pulsed ultrasound is used.

Pulsed ultrasound. Ultrasound produced in pulse form by applying electric pulses or voltages of a few cycles to the transducer.

Pulsed wave. A wave consisting of a series of pulses each containing a few cycles of ultrasound. Not continuous.

Radiofrequency (RF).   Voltages representing echoes in cyclic form.
Range ambiguity.   Improper placement of late echoes (from a previous pulse) received after the next pulse is emitted.
Range gating.   Selecting the depth from which echoes are accepted based on the echo arrival time.
Real time.   Imaging with a rapid frame-sequence display.
Real-time display.   A display that continuously images moving structures or changing scan planes.
Receiver gate.   A device that allows only echoes from a selected depth (arrival time) to pass.
Reflection.   Portion of sound returned from a boundary of a medium (echo).
Reflector.   Medium boundary that produces a reflection. Reflecting surface.
Refraction.   Change of a sound's direction on passing from one medium to another.
Rejection.   Elimination of voltages below a set level (called the threshold or rejection level).
Resistance (flow).   Pressure difference divided by the volume flow rate for steady flow.
Resonance frequency.   Operating frequency.
Reverberation.   Multiple reflections.
Reynolds number.   A number that depends on the speed of flow and viscosity and predicts the onset of turbulence.

Sample volume.   The region from which Doppler shifts are acquired.
Saturation.   The amount of hue present in a mix with white.
Scan line.   A line produced on a display by moving a spot (produced by an electron beam) across the display face at a constant speed. An echo line written into memory.
Scanning.   Sweeping a sound beam to produce an image.
Scatterer.   An object that scatters sound because of its small size or its surface roughness.
Scattering.   Diffusion or redirection of sound in several directions on encountering a particle suspension or a rough surface.
Sensitivity.   Ability of an imaging system to detect weak echoes. Ability of a Doppler system to detect weak or small Doppler shifts.
Shadowing.   Reduction in an echo's amplitude from reflectors that lie behind a strongly reflecting or attenuating structure.
Signal.   Information-bearing voltages in an electric circuit. An acoustic, visual, electric, or other conveyance of information.

Sound.   Traveling wave of acoustic variables.

Source.   An emitter of ultrasound (transducer).

Spatial pulse length.   Length of space over which a pulse occurs.

Spectral analysis.   Separating frequencies in a Doppler signal for display as a Doppler spectrum.

Spectral broadening.   The widening of the Doppler-shift spectrum, i.e., the increase of the range of Doppler-shift frequencies present because of a broader range of flow speeds encountered by the sound beam. This occurs for normal flow in smaller vessels and for turbulent flow in any vessel.

Spectral display.   Visual display of a Doppler spectrum.

Spectral width.   Range of Doppler shifts or flow velocities present at a given point in time.

Spectrum.   Range of frequencies.

Spectrum analyzer.   A device that derives a frequency spectrum from a complex signal.

Specular reflection.   Reflection from a smooth boundary.

Speed.   Displacement divided by the time over which displacement occurs.

Stenosis.   Narrowing of a vessel.

Stoke.   Unit of kinematic viscosity.

Streamline.   A line representing the path of motion of a particle of fluid.

Strength.   Nonspecific term referring to amplitude or intensity.

Temperature.   Condition of a body that determines transfer of heat to or from other bodies.

Temporal resolution.   Ability to distinguish closely spaced events in time. Improves with an increased frame rate.

Test object.   A device designed to measure some characteristic of an ultrasound system without having tissuelike properties.

Time gain compensation (TGC).   Compensation.

Thermal index.   An indicator of thermal mechanism activity (estimated temperature rise). Equal to a transducer's acoustic output power divided by the estimated power required to raise tissue temperature by 1°C.

Threshold.   See rejection.

Transducer.   Device that converts energy from one form to another.

Transducer array.   Transducer assembly containing more than one transducer element.

Transducer assembly.   Transducer element with damping and matching materials assembled in a case.

Transducer element. Piece of piezoelectric material in a transducer assembly; crystal.
Turbulence. Random, chaotic, multidirectional flow of a fluid with mixing between layers. Not laminar.
Turbulent flow. See turbulence.

Ultrasound. Sound of frequency greater than 20 kHz.
Ultrasound transducer. Device that converts electric energy to ultrasound energy and vice versa.

Variable focusing. Transmit focus with various focal lengths.
Variance. Square of standard deviation. One of the outputs of the autocorrelation process. A measure of spectral broadening.
Vector. A quantity with magnitude and direction.
Velocity. Speed, with direction of motion specified.
Video. Demodulated amplitude voltages representing echoes.
Viscosity. Resistance of a fluid to flow.
Viscosity, kinematic. Viscosity divided by density.
Volume flow rate. Volume of fluid passing a point per unit time (second or minute).
Vortices. Regions of circular flow patterns present in turbulence.

Wall filter. An electric filter that passes frequencies above a set level and eliminates strong low-frequency Doppler shifts (clutter) from the pulsating heart or vessel walls.
Wave. Traveling variation of wave variables.
Wavelength. Length of space over which a cycle occurs.
Window. An anechoic region underneath a region of echo frequencies presented on a Doppler spectral display.
Wrap around. The shift of Doppler information on a spectral display to the wrong side of the baseline (caused by aliasing).

Zero-crossing detector. A simple analog detector that yields the mean Doppler shift as a function of time.
Zero shift. See baseline shift.

Answers to Exercises in the Text

Chapter 1

1.1   d, e
1.2   motion
1.3   a, b, e
1.4   blood, loudspeakers, display
1.5   strip-chart, spectral, color-flow

Chapter 2

2.1   pulses, ultrasound, echoes, image
2.2   pulse echo, or gray scale
2.3   strength (intensity, amplitude)
2.4   parallel
2.5   origin (starting point)
2.6   rectangular
2.7   pie-slice
2.8   pulse, echo, location, strength, location, brightness
2.9   a
2.10 a. 4; b. 1; c. 3; d. 5; e. 2
2.11 propagation speeds, equal
2.12 d
2.13 e
2.14 impedances

2.15   false
2.16   a. 4; b. 3; c. 2; d. 1
2.17   a, d
2.18   c
2.19   focal
2.20   true
2.21   false
2.22   a
2.23   e
2.24   resolution, penetration
2.25   2, 10
2.26   b
2.27   d
2.28   d
2.29   b
2.30   b
2.31   d
2.32   echoes
2.33   strength, direction, time
2.34   display, voltages
2.35   receiver
2.36   beam former
2.37   receiver
2.38   a
2.39   f
2.40   b
2.41   a
2.42   false
2.43   mechanical, electronic
2.44   frame
2.45   pulsed
2.46   false (latter portion)
2.47   increase
2.48   improved, decreases, increased
2.49   freeze, frame
2.50 $1000 \div 20 = 50$ lines per frame (one scan line for each pulse)
2.51   c, d, e
2.52   a. 1; b. 2; c. 2
2.53   separation
2.54   weaker
2.55   b
2.56   true
2.57   refraction (double image)

Chapter **3**

3.1   a, c, d, e, g, h
3.2   capillaries
3.3   a, b, f
3.4   d
3.5   c
3.6   stream
3.7   plasma, erythrocytes, water
3.8   d
3.9   a
3.10 e
3.11 b
3.12 c
3.13 viscosity
3.14 kinematic viscosity
3.15 density
3.16 1.05 g/mL, 0.035 poise, 0.033 stoke
3.17 force
3.18 c
3.19 difference, gradient
3.20 a
3.21 pump
3.22 difference, distance or separation
3.23 pressure, resistance
3.24 d
3.25 decreases
3.26 d
3.27 c
3.28 vessels
3.29 e
3.30 d
3.31 d
3.32 b
3.33 b
3.34 d
3.35 e
3.36 e
3.37 e
3.38 c
3.39 disturbed
3.40 turbulent
3.41 Reynolds

3.42 stenosis
3.43 d
3.44 a
3.45 decrease
3.46 increase
3.47 e
3.48 a
3.49 a
3.50 e
3.51 33 cm/s
3.52 16 cm/s, 960; 64 cm/s, 1920; 16 cm/s, 960
3.53 d
3.54 e
3.55 b
3.56 d
3.57 e
3.58 b
3.59 d
3.60 e

Chapter 4

4.1 Doppler, flow
4.2 frequency or wavelength
4.3 frequency or wavelength, motion
4.4 greater
4.5 less
4.6 equal to
4.7 motion
4.8 0.02, 1.02
4.9 0.026
4.10 -0.026
4.11 reflected, incident, or received, source
4.12 cosine
4.13 0.01, 1.01 (the Doppler shift is cut in half)
4.14 0, 1.00 (no Doppler shift at 90 degrees)
4.15 110
4.16 a. 1.62; b. 0; c. 50; d. 2.5; e. 6.49; f. 0; g. 150; h. 5; i. 14.6; j. 2.81; k. 60; l. 90; m. 100; n. 3.25; o. 100; p. 30; q. 5; r. 0
4.17 c
4.18 0.26 kHz
4.19 0.44 kHz

4.20   1.95 kHz
4.21   100 cm/s
4.22   50 cm/s
4.23   decrease
4.24   increase
4.25   5 MHz
4.26 -5 MHz
4.27   0 MHz
4.28   infinity (shock wave)
4.29   2.5 MHz
4.30   false
4.31   at the blood vessel wall boundary
4.32   yes. Without them the Doppler shifted sound would not be re-flected back to the transducer.
4.33   b ($\sim$5 m/s)
4.34   c
4.35   Doppler angle
4.36   speed, angle
4.37   a
4.38   doubled
4.39   doubled
4.40   decreased
4.41   a. 325 kHz; b. 347 kHz; c. 694 kHz
4.42   4, 10, and 20 MHz
4.43   45 degrees
4.44   10 MHz, 200 cm/s
4.45   5 MHz, 100 cm/s
4.46   5, 0.1
4.47 θ_1, θ_D, θ_3, θ_1, θ_2, 90 degrees
4.48   b
4.49   d
4.50   low
4.51   100
4.52   100
4.53   2
4.54   decreases as the Doppler angle increases
4.55   2, 1

Chapter 5

5.1   false
5.2   direction, bidirectional
5.3   false

5.4   oscillator, transducer, receiver, loudspeakers, spectrum analyzer, memory, display

5.5   amplitude, frequency

5.6   frequency, time

5.7   gray, color

5.8   flow velocities

5.9   true

5.10 gates

5.11 continuous, pulsed

5.12 depths, arrival time

5.13 false

5.14 true

5.15 true

5.16 e

5.17 fast Fourier transform

5.18 FFT

5.19 pulsed

5.20 pulsed

5.21 50 seconds

5.22 100 seconds

5.23 damped, longer, efficient

5.24 c

5.25 c

5.26 e

5.27 b

5.28 continuous-wave and pulsed-wave

5.29 continuous-wave

5.30 pulsed-wave

5.31 duplex

5.32 pulsed-wave

5.33 receiver

5.34 a

5.35 Doppler angle

5.36 cathode ray

5.37 wall, wall thump

5.38 5, 30, gate, pulse

5.39 Nyquist

5.40 range ambiguity

5.41 continuous wave

5.42 false

5.43 false

5.44 mechanical scanner

5.45 c

5.46   components or frequencies, order
5.47   c
5.48   e (a and b)
5.49   shifts
5.50   speeds, directions
5.51   single
5.52   a
5.53   e (more accurately, it is near-plug flow not true plug flow)
5.54   amplitude, power, time
5.55   second
5.56   color, gray scale
5.57   d
5.58   a
5.59   c
5.60   b
5.61   d
5.62   true
5.63   false
5.64   laminar
5.65   b
5.66   e (a, c, or d) (these would each yield a small Doppler shift)
5.67   false
5.68   e
5.69   a
5.70   a
5.71   c
5.72   false
5.73   false
5.74   e (b, c, d)
5.75   false (remember Doppler angle)
5.76   b
5.77   c
5.78   a
5.79   a. 2; b. 1; c. 3
5.80   narrow
5.81   higher
5.82   false
5.83   false (Fig. 5.30)
5.84   c (high-resistance vascular bed)
5.85   true
5.86   varies, compliant, higher, lower
5.87   small Doppler angle
5.88   large Doppler angle

5.89   false (remember Doppler angle)
5.90   e
5.91   b
5.92   c
5.93   e

Chapter 6

6.1   e (a, b, d; black is not a color; magenta is not used)
6.2   e (d because of c)
6.3   a
6.4   false (small Doppler angle causes large Doppler shift)
6.5   e (aliasing at flow speed exceeding about 64 cm/s; see discussion
      of figure in Section 6.4)
6.6   flow, anatomy
6.7   d
6.8   red, blue, blue, red, red, blue
6.9   autocorrelation, mean
6.10   cross-correlation
6.11   false (cosine for both)
6.12   e (spectrum not needed; autocorrelation yields sign, mean Dopp-
      ler shift, and variance)
6.13   no
6.14   false
6.15   b
6.16   c
6.17   e (a, b, or c)
6.18   false
6.19   false (e.g., Fig. 6.18)
6.20   false
6.21   time
6.22   autocorrelation
6.23   cross-correlation
6.24   d
6.25   a and c
6.26   a, b, c
6.27   d
6.28   c and d
6.29   c
6.30   a
6.31   c
6.32   d

6.33 a
6.34 b
6.35 false
6.36 false
6.37 100
6.38 d
6.39 c
6.40 a, b, c
6.41 c
6.42 e (c and d)
6.43 b
6.44 e
6.45 false
6.46 a. 3; b. 2; c. 1; d. 4; e. 5
6.47 e (wall filter setting)
6.48 from right to left
6.49 b
6.50 false (nonzero Doppler angle)

Chapter 7

7.1 a
7.2 e (a, b, d)
7.3 d
7.4 b
7.5 b
7.6 b
7.7 c
7.8 d
7.9 b
7.10 b
7.11 e
7.12 b
7.13 e
7.14 c
7.15 yes (less attenuation, greater penetration, later echoes)
7.16 yes (Doppler shift increases with increasing frequency)
7.17 d
7.18 a
7.19 e (c and d)
7.20 e
7.21 a. 3; b. 4; c. 3; d. 2; e. 1

7.22 b, c, d
7.23 e (b, c, d)
7.24 liquid, string
7.25 a
7.26 false
7.27 d
7.28 false
7.29 false
7.30 b
7.31 no
7.32 yes
7.33 b and d
7.34 c
7.35 c
7.36 e
7.37 e
7.38 e
7.39 d
7.40 b
7.41 d
7.42 c, d, e
7.43 b
7.44 a, b, d
7.45 e
7.46 a
7.47 d
7.48 c
7.49 c
7.50 decreases

Chapter **8**

8.1 Doppler shift
8.2 false
8.3 one, two
8.4 frequencies
8.5 false
8.6 speed
8.7 gate
8.8 display
8.9 gate, voltage generator (oscillator)
8.10 depth

8.11 true
8.12 false
8.13 true
8.14 2.6
8.15 true
8.16 continuous wave
8.17 b
8.18 a
8.19 c
8.20 d
8.21 e
8.22 e
8.23 d
8.24 e
8.25 c
8.26 c
8.27 false (only true near the transducer)
8.28 false (only true for perpendicular incidence or oblique incidence when densities and propagation speeds of the media are equal)
8.29 false (see comment for 8.28)
8.30 c
8.31 d
8.32 d
8.33 false (six bits)
8.34 d
8.35 a
8.36 b
8.37 c
8.38 d (areas are 284 and 3 mm^2)
8.39 c
8.40 d
8.41 e
8.42 c
8.43 a
8.44 a
8.45 a
8.46 d (b and c)
8.47 c
8.48 c
8.49 e (d and a or b)
8.50 c
8.51 aliasing
8.52 b

8.53   c

8.54

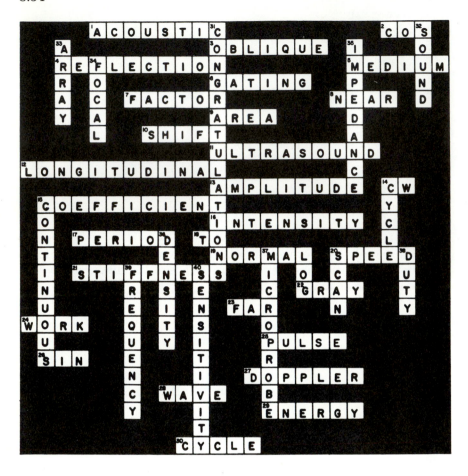

8.55

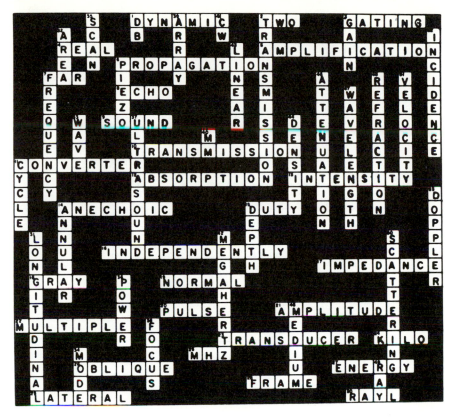

8.56

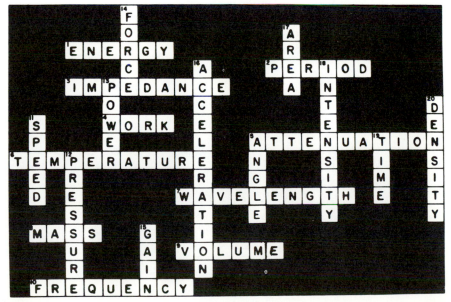

8.57

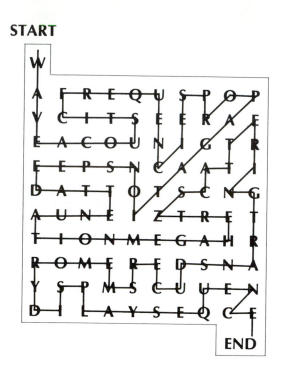

START

END

8.58

```
  .   .   .   E   .   .   .   .   .   .   .   U   .   .   .   .
  .   .   .   .   V   .   .   .   .   .   .   L   D   .   .   .   .
  .   .   C   .   .   A   .   .   .   .   T   O   .   .   .   .
  .   .   O   .   .   .   W   .   .   R   P   .   .   .   .   T
  .   .   L   .   .   .   -   .   A   P   .   .   .   .   F   .
  .   .   O   .   .   .   .   S   L   .   .   .   .   I   .   .
  .   .   R   .   .   .   O   E   U   .   .   .   H   .   .   .
  .   .   -   .   .   .   U   R   .   .   O   .   .   S   .   .   .   E
  .   .   F   .   .   N   .   -   .   .   Y   U   -   .   .   V   .
  .   .   L   .   D   A   .   .   .   C   .   R   N   .   .   A   .
  .   .   O   A   N   .   .   .   N   .   E   .   .   I   W   .   .   .
  .   .   W   G   L   .   .   E   .   L   .   .   .   -   T   .   .
  .   .   L   .   .   I   U   .   P   .   .   D   .   .   N   .   .
  .   E   .   .   .   Q   A   P   .   .   .   E   .   .   .   .   O   .
  .   .   .   E   .   O   S   .   .   S   .   .   .   .   .   .   C
  .   .   R   .   D   .   .   I   L   .   .   .   .   .   .   .
  .   .   F   .   .   .   .   U   N   .   .   .   .   .   .   .
  .   .   .   .   .   .   P   .   G   .   .   .   .   .   .   .
```

8.59 e

8.60 a

8.61 d

8.62 d

8.63 a

8.64 a, b, c, d, e

8.65 a

8.66 e

8.67 c

8.68 e (a, b, c)

8.69 d

8.70 b

8.71 a

8.72 false

8.73 false

8.74 a, b, g, k, l, o, q, r (smaller is better with resolution)

8.75 a. 2.0008; b. 0.8; c. 2.0016; d. 1.6; e. 2.0031; f. 3.1; g. 90; h. 0.0; i. 60; j. 4.0013; k. 8.0046; l. 46

8.76 true

8.77 right to left

8.78 b

8.79 d

8.80 d

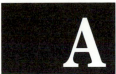

Symbols, Abbreviations, and Equations

The following symbols and abbreviations are used in the equations in this appendix and those in the text.

a	attenuation
A	beam area, cross-sectional area of a tube or vessel
c	sound propagation speed
cos	cosine
d	diameter of a vessel
d_m	maximum unambiguous imaging or Doppler sample depth
DGC	depth gain compensation
f	frequency, source frequency
f_D	Doppler shift
f_e	emitted frequency
f_o	source or operating frequency, emitted frequency
f_r	received frequency
g	gram
Hz	hertz
I	intensity
k	kilo
L	vessel or tube length, sound path length, liter
m	milli, meter
M	mega
n	number of cycles in a pulse
P	power, pressure
PRF	pulse repetition frequency
ΔP	pressure difference
Q	volume flow rate
r	radius of a vessel
R	flow resistance

331

Re	Reynolds number
s	second
SPL	spatial pulse length
TGC	time gain compensation
Δt	echo arrival-time shift
v	speed of a reflector or scatterer, flow speed
v_a	average flow speed
v_m	maximum flow speed
v_r	speed of a receiver
v_s	speed of a source
λ	wavelength
λ_e	emitted wavelength
λ_o	source's wavelength
ρ	density
θ	Doppler angle
θ_D	Doppler angle
θ_i	incidence angle
θ_r	reflection angle
θ_t	transmission angle
ν	viscosity

For convenient reference, the equations (with units of measurement in parentheses) relevant to the material in this book are compiled here. Some (but not all) of them are included in the text.

Chapter 2

$$\text{wavelength (mm)} = \frac{\text{propagation speed (mm/}\mu\text{s)}}{\text{frequency (MHz)}} \quad \lambda = \frac{c}{f}$$

$$\text{spatial pulse length (mm)} =$$

$$\frac{\text{number of cycles in pulse} \times \text{propagation speed (mm/}\mu\text{s)}}{\text{frequency (MHz)}}$$

$$\text{SPL} = \frac{nc}{f}$$

$$\text{intensity (W/cm}^2) = \frac{\text{power (W)}}{\text{area (cm}^2)} \quad I = \frac{P}{A}$$

$$\text{attenuation (dB)} = \tfrac{1}{2} \times \text{frequency (MHz)} \times \text{path length (cm)}$$

$$a = \tfrac{1}{2}fL$$

reflection angle (degrees) = incidence angle (degrees) $\theta_r = \theta_i$

transmission angle (degrees) = incidence angle (degrees) $\times$

$$\left[\frac{\text{medium two propagation speed (mm}/\mu\text{s)}}{\text{medium one propagation speed (mm}/\mu\text{s)}}\right] \quad \theta_t = \theta_i \left[\frac{c_2}{c_1}\right]$$

Chapter **3**

$$\text{volume flow rate (mL/s)} = \frac{\text{pressure difference (dyne/cm}^2)}{\text{flow resistance (g/cm}^4 \cdot \text{s)}} \quad Q = \frac{\Delta P}{R}$$

$$\text{flow resistance} = \frac{8 \times \text{length} \times \text{viscosity}}{\pi \times \text{radius}^4} \quad R = \frac{8L\nu}{\pi r^4}$$

$$\text{volume flow rate} = \frac{\text{pressure difference} \times \pi \times \text{radius}^4}{8 \times \text{length} \times \text{viscosity}} \quad Q = \frac{\Delta P \pi r^4}{8L\nu}$$

volume flow rate =

$$\frac{\text{pressure difference} \times \pi \times \text{diameter}^4}{128 \times \text{length} \times \text{viscosity}} \quad Q = \frac{\Delta P \pi d^4}{128L\nu}$$

$$\text{average flow speed} = \frac{1}{2} \times \text{maximum flow speed} \quad v_a = \frac{1}{2} \times v_m$$

$$\text{Reynolds number} = \frac{\text{average flow speed} \times \text{tube diameter} \times \text{density}}{\text{viscosity}}$$

$$Re = \frac{v_a \times d \times \rho}{\nu}$$

$$\text{volume flow rate} = \text{average flow speed} \times \text{tube area} \quad Q = v_a \times A$$

$$\text{area} = \pi \times \text{radius}^2 \quad A = \pi \times r^2$$

$$\text{average flow speed} = \frac{\text{pressure difference} \times \text{radius}^2}{8 \times \text{length} \times \text{viscosity}} \quad v_a = \frac{\Delta P r^2}{8L\nu}$$

$$\text{pressure} + \frac{1}{2} \times \text{density} \times (\text{flow speed})^2$$
$$= \text{constant energy density (energy per unit volume)}$$

$$\text{pressure drop} = \frac{1}{2} \times \text{density} \times (\text{flow speed})^2$$

$$\Delta P = \frac{1}{2} \times \rho \times v^2$$

$$P_1 - P_2 = 4 v_2^2$$

Chapter **4**

received frequency

$$= \text{emitted frequency} \left[\frac{\text{propagation speed } + \text{ receiver speed}}{\text{propagation speed}} \right]$$

$$f_r = f_o \left[\frac{c + v_r}{c} \right]$$

$$\text{Doppler shift} = \text{source frequency} \left[\frac{\text{receiver speed}}{\text{propagation speed}} \right]$$

$$f_D = f_o \left[\frac{v_r}{c} \right]$$

emitted wavelength

$$= \text{source wavelength} \left[\frac{\text{propagation speed } - \text{ source speed}}{\text{propagation speed}} \right]$$

$$\lambda_e = \lambda_o \left[\frac{c - v_s}{c} \right]$$

emitted frequency

$$= \text{source frequency} \left[\frac{\text{propagation speed}}{\text{propagation speed } - \text{ source speed}} \right]$$

$$f_e = f_o \left[\frac{c}{c - v_s} \right]$$

Doppler shift

$$= \text{source frequency} \left[\frac{\text{source speed}}{\text{propagation speed } - \text{ source speed}} \right]$$

$$f_D = f_o \left[\frac{v_s}{c - v_s} \right]$$

emitted frequency

$$= \text{source frequency} \left[\frac{\text{propagation speed } + \text{ scatterer speed}}{\text{propagation speed } - \text{ scatterer speed}} \right]$$

$$f_e = f_o \left[\frac{c + v}{c - v} \right]$$

Doppler shift

$$= \text{emitted frequency} - \text{source frequency}$$

$$= \text{source frequency} \left[\frac{2 \times \text{scatterer speed}}{\text{propagation speed} - \text{scatterer speed}} \right]$$

$$f_D = f_e - f_o$$

$$= f_o \left[\frac{2v}{c - v} \right]$$

Doppler shift (MHz)

$$= \frac{2 \times \text{operating frequency (MHz)} \times \text{reflector speed (m/s)} \times \cos \theta}{\text{propagation speed (m/s)}}$$

$$f_D = \frac{2 f_o v \cos \theta}{c}$$

$$\text{Doppler shift} = \frac{2 \times \text{scatterer speed}}{\text{wavelength}} \qquad f_D = \frac{2v}{\lambda}$$

$$\text{scatterer speed} = \left[\frac{\text{Doppler shift} \times \text{propagation speed}}{2 \times \text{source frequency} \times \text{cosine Doppler angle}} \right]$$

$$v = \left[\frac{f_D c}{2 f_o \cos \theta_D} \right]$$

scatterer speed (cm/s)

$$= \left[\frac{77 \times \text{Doppler shift (kHz)}}{\text{source frequency (MHz)} \times \text{cosine Doppler angle}} \right]$$

$$v = \left[\frac{77 \times f_D}{f_o \times \cos \theta_D} \right]$$

Chapter **6**

$$v \text{ (cm/s)} = \frac{\Delta t \ (\mu s) \ \text{PRF (Hz)}}{13 \cos \theta}$$

Chapter **7**

maximum flow speed (cm/s)

$$= \frac{3000}{\text{maximum depth (cm)} \times \text{frequency (MHz)} \times \text{cosine Doppler angle}}$$

$$v_m = \frac{3000}{d_m f \cos \theta}$$

APPENDIX

B Comprehensive Examination

This examination should take less than 2 hours to complete (averaging less than 1 minute per question). The answers are found at the end of the examination.

1. Which of the following frequencies is in the ultrasound range?
   a. 15 Hz
   b. 15 kHz
   c. 15 MHz
   d. 17,000 Hz
   e. 17 km

2. The average propagation speed in soft tissues is
   a. 1.54 mm/μs
   b. 0.501 m/s
   c. 1540 dB/cm
   d. 37.0 km/min
   e. 1 to 10 MHz

3. The propagation speed in blood is
   a. 0.330 mm/μs
   b. 1.54 mm/μs
   c. 1.57 mm/μs
   d. 1.75 mm/μs
   e. none of the above

4. Which of the following has a significant dependence on frequency in soft tissues?
   a. propagation speed
   b. density
   c. stiffness
   d. attenuation
   e. impedance

5. The frequencies used in diagnostic ultrasound imaging
   a.   are much lower than those used in Doppler measurements
   b.   determine imaging depth in tissue
   c.   determine imaging resolution
   d.   all of the above
   e.   b and c

6. An echo from a 5-cm deep reflector arrives at the transducer
   _____ μs after pulse emission.
   a.   13
   b.   154
   c.   65
   d.   5
   e.   77

7. A small (relative to the wavelength) reflector is said to
   _____ an incident sound beam.
   a.   focus
   b.   speculate
   c.   scatter
   d.   shatter
   e.   amplify

8. The frequency of an ultrasound transducer is primarily deter-mined by which of the following:
   a.   diameter of the element
   b.   thickness of the element
   c.   speed of sound in tissue
   d.   voltage applied
   e.   all of the above

9. The fundamental operating principle of medical ultrasound transducers is
   a.   Snell's law
   b.   Doppler's law
   c.   magnetostrictive effect
   d.   piezoelectric effect
   e.   impedance effect

10. The axial resolution of a transducer is primarily determined by
   a.   spatial pulse length
   b.   the near-field limit
   c.   the diameter of the transducer
   d.   the acoustic impedance of tissue
   e.   density

11. The lateral resolution of a transducer is primarily determined
    by
    a. spatial pulse length
    b. the near-field limit
    c. the diameter of the transducer
    d. the acoustic impedance of tissue
    e. applied voltage

12. Increasing frequency
    a. improves resolution
    b. increases penetration
    c. increases refraction
    d. a and b
    e. a and c

13. Ultrasound bioeffects
    a. do not occur
    b. do not occur with diagnostic instruments
    c. are not confirmed below $100 \ mW/cm^2$ spatial peak temporal
       average
    d. b and c
    e. none of the above

14. The diagnostic ultrasound frequency range is
    a. 2 to 10 mHz
    b. 2 to 10 kHz
    c. 2 to 10 MHz
    d. 3 to 15 kHz
    e. none of the above

15. What determines the lower and upper limits of the frequency
    range that are useful in diagnostic ultrasound?
    a. resolution and imaging depth
    b. intensity and resolution
    c. intensity and propagation speed
    d. scattering and impedance
    e. impedance and wavelength

16. Reverberation causes us to think that there are reflectors that
    are too great in
    a. impedance
    b. attenuation
    c. range
    d. size
    e. number

17. The standard American television scanning format has
    _____ lines per frame and _____
    frames per second.
    a. 625, 25
    b. 512, 512
    c. 512, 640
    d. 525, 30
    e. 625, 30

18. In an ultrasound imaging instrument, a cathode ray tube is used
    as a
    a. pulser
    b. receiver
    c. memory
    d. display
    e. scan convector

19. The compensation (swept gain, etc.) control
    a. compensates for machine instability during the warm-up
       time
    b. compensates for attenuation
    c. compensates for transducer aging and the ambient light in
       the examining area
    d. decreases the patient's examination time
    e. none of the above

20. A digital scan converter is a
    a. compressor
    b. receiver
    c. display
    d. computer memory
    e. none of the above

21. Enhancement is caused by
    a. strongly reflecting structure
    b. weakly attenuating structure
    c. strongly attenuating structure
    d. frequency error
    e. propagation speed error

22. In a digital instrument, echo intensity is represented in mem-
    ory by
    a. positive charge distribution
    b. a number

c.   electron density of the scan converter writing beam
d.   a and c
e.   all of the above

23.   Which of the following is performed in an imaging receiver?
a.   amplification
b.   compensation
c.   compression
d.   demodulation
e.   all of the above

24.   Increasing the pulse repetition frequency
a.   improves detail resolution
b.   increases maximum unambiguous depth
c.   decreases maximum unambiguous depth
d.   both a and b
e.   both a and c

25.   Attenuation is corrected by
a.   demodulation
b.   desegregation
c.   decompression
d.   compensation
e.   remuneration

26.   What must be known to calculate the distance to a reflector?
a.   attenuation, speed, density
b.   attenuation, impedance
c.   attenuation, absorption
d.   travel time, speed
e.   density, speed

27.   Which of the following improve(s) sound transmission from the transducer element into the tissue?
a.   matching layer
b.   Doppler effect
c.   damping material
d.   coupling medium
e.   a and d

28.   Lateral resolution is improved by
a.   damping
b.   pulsing

c. focusing
d. reflecting
e. absorbing

29. Axial resolution is improved by
a. damping
b. pulsing
c. focusing
d. reflecting
e. absorbing

30. A digital imaging instrument divides the cross-sectional image into _____.
a. frequencies
b. bits
c. pixels
d. binaries
e. wavelengths

31. In general, as a reflector approaches a transducer at constant speed, the positive Doppler-shift frequency
a. increases
b. decreases
c. remains constant
d. b or c
e. none of the above

32. A reduction in diameter produces a(n)
a. increase in flow resistance
b. decrease in area
c. increase in flow speed
d. decrease in flow speed
e. all of the above

33. Which of the following increases vascular flow resistance?
a. decreasing vessel length
b. decreasing viscosity
c. decreasing vessel diameter
d. decreasing pressure
e. decreasing flow speed

34. The Doppler effect occurs as
a. leukocytes move through the plasma
b. erythrocytes move through the plasma
c. erythrocytes move through the serum

    d.   blood moves relative to the vessel wall

    e.   all of the above

35. When a reflector is moving toward the transducer

    a.   propagation speed increases

    b.   propagation speed decreases

    c.   Doppler shift is positive (higher frequency)

    d.   Doppler shift is negative (lower frequency)

    e.   none of the above

36. The Doppler sample volume is determined by

    a.   beam width

    b.   pulse length

    c.   frequency

    d.   receiver gate length

    e.   all of the above

37. Doppler-shift frequencies

    a.   are generally in the audible range

    b.   are usually above 1 MHz

    c.   can be applied to a loudspeaker

    d.   a and b

    e.   a and c

38. The quantitative presentation of frequencies contained in echoes is called

    a.   preamplification

    b.   digitizing

    c.   optical encoding

    d.   spectral analysis

    e.   all of the above

39. The Doppler frequency shift is caused by

    a.   relative motion between the transducer and the reflector

    b.   patient shivering in a cool room

    c.   a high transducer frequency and real-time scanner

    d.   small reflectors in the transducer beam

    e.   changing transducer thickness

40. The Doppler effect is a change in

    a.   intensity

    b.   wavelength

    c.   frequency

    d.   all of the above

    e.   b and c

41. The Doppler shift is zero when the angle between the sound direction and the movement (flow) direction is _____ degrees.
    a. 30
    b. 60
    c. 90
    d. 45
    e. none of the above

42. Duplex Doppler presents
    a. anatomic (structural) data
    b. physiologic (flow) data
    c. impedance data
    d. more than one of the above
    e. all of the above

43. Doppler-shift frequencies are usually in a relatively narrow range above 20 kHz.
    a. true
    b. false

44. Continuous-wave sound is used in
    a. all ultrasound imaging instruments
    b. only bistable instruments
    c. all Doppler instruments
    d. some Doppler instruments
    e. some M-mode instruments

45. An advantage of continuous-wave Doppler over pulsed Doppler is
    a. depth information
    b. bidirectional
    c. no aliasing
    d. b and c
    e. all of the above

46. In Doppler color-flow instruments, hue can represent
    a. sign (+ or −) of Doppler shift
    b. flow direction
    c. magnitude of the Doppler shift
    d. amplitude of the Doppler shift
    e. a, b, and c

47. The Doppler effect for a scatterer moving toward the sound source

causes the scattered sound (compared with the incident sound) received by the transducer to have

a. increased intensity
b. decreased intensity
c. increased impedance
d. increased frequency
e. decreased impedance

48. Duplex Doppler instruments include _____.

a. pulsed Doppler
b. continuous-wave Doppler
c. B-scan imaging
d. dynamic imaging
e. more than one of the above

49. If the Doppler shifts from normal and stenotic arteries are 4 and 10 kHz, respectively, for which will there be a problem (aliasing) with a pulse repetition frequency of 7 kHz?

a. normal
b. stenotic
c. both
d. neither

50. The receiver in a Doppler system compares the _____ of the voltage generator and the echo voltage from the transducer.

a. wavelength
b. intensity
c. impedance
d. frequency
e. all of the above

51. In the Doppler equation

$$f_D = \frac{2\,fv}{c - v}$$

which can normally be ignored?

a. v in the denominator
b. v in the numerator
c. f
d. f_D
e. b and c

52. For which of the following is the reflected frequency less than
     the incident frequency?
     a. advancing flow
     b. receding flow
     c. perpendicular flow
     d. laminar flow
     e. all of the above

53. Doppler ultrasound can measure flow speed in the
     a. heart
     b. veins
     c. arterioles
     d. capillaries
     e. a and b

54. Which of the following are fluids?
     a. gas
     b. liquid
     c. solid
     d. a and b
     e. all of the above

55. The mass per unit volume of a fluid is called its
     a. resistance
     b. viscosity
     c. kinematic viscosity
     d. impedance
     e. density

56. The resistance to flow offered by a fluid is called
     a. resistance
     b. viscosity
     c. kinematic viscosity
     d. impedance
     e. density

57. Viscosity divided by density is called
     a. resistance
     b. viscosity
     c. kinematic viscosity
     d. impedance
     e. density

58. If the following is increased, flow increases.
   a. pressure difference
   b. pressure gradient
   c. resistance
   d. a and b
   e. all of the above

59. Flow resistance depends most strongly on which of the following?
   a. length of the vessel
   b. radius of the vessel
   c. blood viscosity
   d. all of the above
   e. none of the above

60. Proximal to, at, and distal to a stenosis _____ must be constant.
   a. laminar flow
   b. disturbed flow
   c. turbulent flow
   d. volume flow rate
   e. none of the above

61. Added forward flow and flow reversal in diastole are results of _____ flow.
   a. volume
   b. turbulence
   c. laminar
   d. disturbed
   e. pulsatile

62. Turbulence generally occurs when the Reynolds number exceeds
   a. 100
   b. 200
   c. 1000
   d. 2000
   e. a and b

63. As the diameter at a stenosis decreases, the following pass(es) through a maximum
   a. flow speed at the stenosis
   b. flow speed proximal to stenosis
   c. volume flow
   d. Doppler shift at the stenosis
   e. a and d

64. The Doppler shift (kHz) for 4 MHz, 50 cm/s, and 60 degrees is
   a.   0.5
   b.   1.0
   c.   1.3
   d.   2.6
   e.   5.0

65. Physiologic flow speeds can be as much as _____ percent of the propagation speed in soft tissues.
   a.   0.01
   b.   0.3
   c.   5
   d.   10
   e.   50

66. Which Doppler angle gives the greatest Doppler shift?
   a.   −90
   b.   −45
   c.   0
   d.   45
   e.   90

67. Doppler shift frequency is not dependent on
   a.   amplitude
   b.   flow speed
   c.   operating frequency
   d.   Doppler angle
   e.   propagation speed

68. The Fourier-transform technique is not used in color-flow instruments because it is not _____ enough.
   a.   slow
   b.   fast
   c.   bright
   d.   cheap
   e.   none of the above

69. Which of the following on a color-flow display is (are) presented in real time?
   a.   gray-scale anatomy
   b.   flow direction
   c.   Doppler spectrum
   d.   a and b
   e.   all of the above

70. For a 5-MHz instrument and 60-degree Doppler angle, a 100-Hz filter eliminates flow speeds below
   a.   1 cm/s
   b.   2 cm/s
   c.   3 cm/s
   d.   4 cm/s
   e.   5 cm/s

71. For a 7.5-MHz instrument and 0-degree Doppler angle, a 100-Hz filter eliminates flow speeds below
   a.   1 cm/s
   b.   2 cm/s
   c.   3 cm/s
   d.   4 cm/s
   e.   5 cm/s

72. The functions of a Doppler receiver include which of the following?
   a.   amplification
   b.   phase quadrature detection
   c.   demodulation
   d.   rejection
   e.   all of the above

73. A later receiver gate time means a _____ sample volume depth.
   a.   earlier
   b.   shallower
   c.   deeper
   d.   stronger
   e.   none of the above

74. The Doppler shift is typically _____ of the source frequency.
   a.   one thousandth
   b.   one hundredth
   c.   one tenth
   d.   10 times
   e.   100 times

75. Approximately _____ pulses are required to obtain one line of color-flow information.
   a.   1
   b.   10

    c.   100
    d.   1000
    e.   1,000,000

76. There are approximately _____ samples per line on a color-flow display.
    a.   2
    b.   20
    c.   200
    d.   2000
    e.   2,000,000

77. Which of the following instruments can produce aliasing?
    a.   continuous-wave Doppler
    b.   pulsed Doppler
    c.   duplex
    d.   color flow
    e.   more than one of the above

78. For normal flow in a large vessel, a _____ range of Doppler-shift frequencies is received.
    a.   narrow
    b.   broad
    c.   steady
    d.   disturbed
    e.   all of the above

79. Doppler signal power is proportional to
    a.   volume flow rate
    b.   flow speed
    c.   Doppler angle
    d.   cell density
    e.   more than one of the above

80. Stenosis affects
    a.   peak systolic flow speed
    b.   end-diastolic flow speed
    c.   spectral broadening
    d.   window
    e.   all of the above

81. Spectral broadening is a _____ of the spectral trace.
    a.   vertical thickening
    b.   horizontal thickening

    c. brightening
    d. darkening
    e. horizontal shift

82. As stenosis is increased, which of the following increase(s)?
    a. diameter of the vessel
    b. systolic Doppler shift
    c. diastolic Doppler shift
    d. spectral broadening
    e. more than one of the above

83. Flow reversal in diastole (normal flow) indicates
    a. stenosis
    b. aneurysm
    c. high distal flow resistance
    d. low distal flow resistance
    e. more than one of the above

84. About _____ fast Fourier transforms are performed per second on a spectral display.
    a. 3
    b. 10
    c. 100
    d. 700
    e. 1700

85. Each fast Fourier transform appears on a spectral display as a _____.
    a. dot
    b. circle
    c. horizontal line
    d. vertical line
    e. none of the above

86. Hue is _____.
    a. color seen
    b. light frequency
    c. brightness
    d. mix with white
    e. more than one of the above

87. A component *not* included in a continuous-wave Doppler instrument is _____.
    a. loudspeaker
    b. wall filter

    c. oscillator
    d. demodulator
    e. receiver gate

88. On a spectral display, amplitude is indicated by
    a. brightness
    b. horizontal position
    c. vertical position
    d. b and c
    e. none of the above

89. Doppler shift can change because of changes in
    a. velocity
    b. speed
    c. direction
    d. frequency
    e. all of the above

90. A gate-open time of 10 μs corresponds to a sample volume length (mm) of
    a. 10
    b. 7.7
    c. 3.8
    d. 3.3
    e. 2.0

91. The sample volume width is determined by
    a. gate-open time
    b. pulse duration
    c. PRF
    d. PRP
    e. beam width

92. What problem(s) is (are) encountered if the pulse repetition frequency is 10 kHz, the sample volume is located at 10 cm depth, and the Doppler shift is 4 kHz?
    a. aliasing
    b. mirror image
    c. refraction
    d. range ambiguity
    e. more than one of the above

93. What problem(s) is (are) encountered if the pulse repetition frequency is 10 kHz, the sample volume is located at 5 cm depth, and the Doppler shift is 6 kHz?

a. aliasing
b. mirror image
c. refraction
d. range ambiguity
e. more than one of the above

94. What problem(s) is (are) encountered if the pulse repetition frequency is 10 kHz, the sample volume is located at 10 cm depth, and the Doppler shift is 6 kHz?

a. aliasing
b. mirror image
c. refraction
d. range ambiguity
e. more than one of the above

95. The functions of a color Doppler receiver include which of the following?

a. amplification
b. phase quadrature detection
c. demodulation
d. autocorrelation
e. all of the above

96. If all cells in a vessel were moving at the same constant speed, the spectral trace would be a _____ line.

a. thin horizontal
b. thick horizontal
c. thin vertical
d. thick vertical
e. none of the above

97. If the same flow is measured with two transducers (3 and 6 MHz) and the same Doppler shift is observed, what is the Doppler angle with the 6-MHz transducer if it was 70 degrees with the 3-MHz transducer?

a. 60
b. 70
c. 80
d. 90
e. 100

98. For a physiologic flow speed, a 5-MHz beam could produce a Doppler shift of about _____.
    a. 5 kHz
    b. 5 MHz
    c. 5 Hz
    d. depends on continuous-wave or pulsed-wave mode
    e. none of the above

99. Spectral analysis is performed in a Doppler instrument _____.
    a. electronically
    b. mathematically
    c. acoustically
    d. mechanically
    e. more than one of the above

100. The Doppler shift is proportional to
    a. volume flow rate
    b. flow speed
    c. Doppler angle
    d. cell density
    e. more than one of the above

101. Which can be used to evaluate a Doppler instrument's performance?
    a. contrast detail phantom
    b. string test object
    c. flow phantom
    d. b and c
    e. all of the above

102. Place the instruments in the general order of increasing acoustic output: 1. spectral Doppler; 2. sonographic; 3. color flow.
    a. 1, 2, 3
    b. 2, 3, 1
    c. 3, 1, 2
    d. 3, 2, 1
    e. 2, 1, 3

103. If the operating frequency is 5 MHz, the Doppler angle is 60 degrees, the pulse repetition frequency is 9 kHz, and the Doppler shift is 2 kHz, what problem is encountered if the angle is changed to zero?
    a. aliasing
    b. range ambiguity

    c. mirror image

    d. refraction

    e. none

104. When angle correction is applied on a color-flow display, the Nyquist limits (in cm/s) on the color map

    a. increase

    b. decrease

    c. do not change

    d. are irrelevant

    e. are ambiguous

105. When angle correction is applied on a color-flow display, the Nyquist limits (in kHz) on the color map

    a. increase

    b. decrease

    c. do not change

    d. are irrelevant

    e. are ambiguous

106. Flow is _____ if it appears red on a color-flow display.

    a. approaching

    b. receding

    c. turbulent

    d. disturbed

    e. depends on color map

107. Two different colors in the same vessel indicate

    a. flow reversal

    b. sector scan

    c. vessel curvature

    d. aliasing

    e. any of the above

108. The following increase(s) the amount of color appearing in a vessel.

    a. increased color gain

    b. increased wall filter

    c. increased priority

    d. increased pulse repetition frequency

    e. more than one of the above

109. The following decrease(s) the amount of color appearing in a vessel.
   a.   increased wall filter
   b.   increased pulse repetition frequency
   c.   increased ensemble length
   d.   baseline shift
   e.   more than one of the above

110. Which of the following on a color-flow display is (are) presented as a two-dimensional, cross-sectional display?
   a.   gray-scale anatomy
   b.   flow direction
   c.   Doppler spectrum
   d.   a and b
   e.   all of the above

111. Gray compared with white is an example of
   a.   hue
   b.   luminance
   c.   saturation
   d.   b and c
   e.   all of the above

112. Red compared with green is an example of
   a.   hue
   b.   luminance
   c.   saturation
   d.   b and c
   e.   all of the above

113. There are about _____ frames per second produced by a color-flow Doppler instrument.
   a.   10
   b.   20
   c.   40
   d.   80
   e.   more than one of the above

114. The autocorrelation technique yields
   a.   mean Doppler shift
   b.   sign of Doppler shift
   c.   spread around the mean (variance)
   d.   all of the above
   e.   none of the above

115. Increasing ensemble length _____ color sensitivity and accuracy and _____ frame rate.
    a. improves, increases
    b. degrades, increases
    c. degrades, decreases
    d. improves, decreases
    e. none of the above

116. Which control can be used to help with clutter?
    a. wall filter
    b. gain
    c. baseline shift
    d. pulse repetition frequency
    e. smoothing

117. Doubling the width of a color window produces a(n) _____ frame rate.
    a. doubled
    b. quadrupled
    c. unchanged
    d. halved
    e. quartered

118. Steering the color window to the right or left changes
    a. frame rate
    b. pulse repetition frequency
    c. Doppler angle
    d. Doppler shift
    e. more than one of the above

119. Lack of color in a vessel may be caused by
    a. low color gain
    b. low wall filter setting
    c. small Doppler angle
    d. low baseline shift
    e. more than one of the above

120. Which control(s) can help with aliasing?
    a. wall filter
    b. gain
    c. smoothing
    d. pulse repetition frequency
    e. more than one of the above

Comprehensive Examination Answers

Following each answer is the section number in which the subject is discussed. Most answers also have explanatory comments.

1. c. 2.1. Ultrasound is sound of frequency greater than 20 kHz (0.02 MHz). Answer e is not in frequency units.
2. a. 2.1. Propagation speeds in soft tissues are in the range of about 1.4 to 1.6 mm/μs. Answers c and e are not in speed units.
3. c. 4.1. Slightly higher than for soft tissues.
4. d. 2.1. Propagation speed and impedance increase only slightly with frequency.
5. e. 2.1 and 2.2.
6. c. 2.1. The round-trip travel time is 13 μs/cm.
7. c. 2.1. Scattering occurs with rough surfaces and with heterogeneous media (made up of small particles relative to the wavelength). Large, flat surfaces produce specular reflections.
8. b. 2.2. The operating frequency of a transducer is such that its thickness is equal to one half the wavelength in the transducer element material.
9. d. 2.2. Transducer elements expand and contract when a voltage is applied, and conversely, when returning echoes apply pressure to the element, a voltage is generated.
10. a. 2.2. Axial resolution is equal to one half spatial pulse length.
11. c. 2.2. Lateral resolution is equal to beam width. The near-zone length is dependent on the diameter of the transducer and, thus, so is the lateral resolution at any given distance from the transducer.
12. a. 2.1, 2.2. Penetration decreases with increasing frequency, and frequency has no effect on refraction.

13. c. 7.4. This is part of the American Institute of Ultrasound in Medicine's statement on nonhuman in vivo mammalian bioeffects.

14. c. 2.1, 2.2. Frequencies lower than this range do not provide the needed resolution, whereas frequencies greater than this range do not allow for adequate imaging depth for medical purposes.

15. a. 2.1, 2.2. See answer to question 14.

16. e. 2.4. Reverberation adds additional reflectors on the display deeper than the true ones.

17. d. 2.3.

18. d. 2.3.

19. b. 2.3.

20. d. 2.3.

21. b. 2.4.

22. b. 2.3.

23. e. 2.3.

24. c. 7.1. The pulse repetition frequency has no direct effect on detail resolution.

25. d. 2.3.

26. d. 2.1. Distance equals one half the speed times the round-trip time.

27. e. 2.2. The matching layer improves sound transmission by reducing the reflection at the transducer-skin boundary. A coupling medium improves it by removing the air layer between the transducer and the skin.

28. c. 2.2.

29. a. 2.2.

30. c. 2.3.

31. d. 4.1, 4.3. If the transducer is in the path of the reflector, answer c is correct because the Doppler angle is zero. If this is not the case, then b is correct because the Doppler angle will increase (decreasing the Doppler shift) as the reflector approaches.

32. e. 3.2, 3.3. The diameter referred to can be either the entire diameter of the vessel or the diameter of a small portion of it (stenosis). For the former, d is correct. For the latter, c is correct. In either case, a and b are correct.

33. c. 3.2. Poiseuille's equation shows that resistance increases with increasing vessel length, increasing fluid viscosity, or decreasing vessel diameter.

34. d. 4.1. The blood cells move along with the plasma not through it.

35. c. 2.1, 4.1. The propagation speed is determined by the medium not by the motion.

36. e. 5.2.

37. e. 4.1.

38. d. 5.1 and 5.3. Spectral comes from "spectrum," referring to the color spectrum. A prism is an optical spectrum analyzer that breaks down white light into its component colors.

39. a. 4.1.

40. e. 4.1. If the frequency changes, the wavelength changes also.

41. c. 4.3.

42. d. 5.2. Answers a and b are both correct. Anatomic data are provided by the real-time B scan, and physiologic data are provided by the pulsed-Doppler portion of the instrument.

43. b. 4.1. Physiologic Doppler-shift frequencies are usually in the audible frequency range.

44. d. 5.1. All imaging instruments and most Doppler instruments use pulsed ultrasound.

45. c. 5.1, 5.2, and 7.1.

46. e. 6.4.

47. d. 4.1.

48. e. 5.2. They include pulsed-Doppler (and sometimes continuous-Doppler) and dynamic imaging.

49. c. 7.1. Both Doppler shifts exceed one half of the pulse repetition frequency.

50. d. 5.1.

51. a. 4.1 and 4.2. Because physiologic speeds (v) are small compared with the speed of sound (c) in tissues.

52. b. 4.1.

53. e. 3.1. Arterioles and capillaries are too small.

54. d. 3.1.

55. e. 3.1.

56. b. 3.1.

57. c. 3.1.

58. d. 3.2. This is Poiseuille's law. Increasing resistance *decreases* flow.

59. b. 3.2. It depends on the radius to the fourth power.

60. d. 3.3. This is the continuity rule.

61. e. 3.4. Also results of distensible vessels.

62. d. 3.2.

63. e. 3.3. See Figure 3.10.

64. c. 4.1. Assuming a *reflector* moving at 50 cm/s.

65. b. 4.2. That is, about 5 m/s.

66. c. 4.3. Smaller angle, larger cosine, and larger shift.

67. a. 4.1.

68. e. 6.3. Spectrum not needed; it cannot be displayed in a pixel.

69. d. 6.1. The spectrum can be shown *in addition* to the color-flow display.

70. c. 4.1 and 5.1. $$v = \frac{77 \times 0.100}{5 \times 0.5} = 3.08$$

71. a. 4.1 and 5.1. $$v = \frac{77 \times 0.100}{7.5} = 1.03$$

72. e. 5.1.

73. c. 5.2. Thirteen microseconds of delay per centimeter of depth.

74. a. 4.1. Because flow speeds are typically one thousandth of the speed of sound in tissues.

75. b. 6.3. The range is about 4 to 32.

76. c. 6.3. The range is about 40 to 400.

77. e. 7.1. Any pulsed instrument (b, c, or d) can.

78. a. 3.2. This is called plug flow.

79. d. 5.1.

80. e. 3.3 and 5.4. A stenosis generally increases a, b, and c and decreases d.

81. a. 5.4. That is, a widening of the spectrum.

82. e. 3.3 and 5.4. Parameters b, c, and d are increased; a is *decreased*.

83. c. 5.4. The blood flows back out of the high impedance vascular bed during the low-pressure portion of the cardiac cycle.

84. c. 5.3.

85. d. 5.3.

86. e. 6.2. Answer a results from b.

87. e. 5.1.

88. a. 5.4. Gray level or, sometimes, color.

89. e. 4.1. Answer a is b + c.

90. b. 5.2.

91. e. 5.2. Answers a and b determine sample volume length.

92. d. 5.2 and 7.1. Echoes from sample volume arrive after another pulse is emitted.

93. a. 5.2 and 7.1. The shift exceeds the Nyquist limit (5 kHz).

94. e. 5.2 and 7.1. Answers a and d.

95. e. 6.3.

96. a. 5.4.

97. c. 4.3. Cosine of 80 is half the cosine of 70.

98. a. 4.1 and 4.4. Because physiologic flow speeds are about one thousandth of the ultrasound propagation speed (1540 m/s), Doppler shifts are about one thousandth of the operating frequency.

99. e. 5.3. Answers a and b

100. b. 4.1. Also proportional to the *cosine* of the Doppler angle.

101. d. 7.3. Answer a is for gray-scale instruments.

102. b. 7.4.

103. e. 7.1. The shift increases to 4 kHz (still less than the Nyquist limit of 4.5 kHz).
104. a. 6.4 and 7.2. Nonzero Doppler angle increases the calculated equivalent flow speed.
105. c. 6.4 and 7.2. The Nyquist limit is still one half of the pulse repetition frequency.
106. e. 6.4.
107. e. 6.4 and 7.2.
108. e. 6.3. Answers a and c.
109. e. 6.3. Answers a and b (Fig. 7.17D); c increases the amount of color.
110. d. 6.4. Answer c is not strictly part of the color-flow display. Also, it is not a cross-sectional display but rather a frequency versus time presentation.
111. b. 6.2. White is brighter than gray.
112. a. 6.2. Red and green are different hues representing different frequencies of light.
113. e. 6.3. Answers a, b, and c. About 5 to 50 frames per second are displayed.
114. d. 6.3.
115. d. 6.3.
116. a. 6.3. The wall filter removes the lower frequency clutter Doppler shifts.
117. d. 6.4. Twice as many scan lines per frame.
118. e. 6.4. Answers c and d both change because the orientation of the scan line (pulse path) changes.
119. a. 6.3. Answers b and c increase the amount of color.
120. d. 6.3, 6.4, and 7.2. Increasing PRF increases the Nyquist limit, reducing aliasing.

References

1. Kremkau FW: Diagnostic Ultrasound: Principles and Instruments. 4th edition. Philadelphia, WB Saunders, 1993.
2. Nachtigall PE, Moore PWB: Animal Sonar. New York, Plenum Press, 1988.
3. Eden A: The Search for Christian Doppler. New York, Springer-Verlag, 1992.
4. Evans DH, McDicken WN, Skidmore R, et al: Doppler Ultrasound: Physics, Instrumentation, and Clinical Applications. New York, Wiley & Sons, 1989.
5. Smith HJ, Zagzebski J: Basic Doppler Physics. Madison, WI, Medical Physics Publishing, 1991.
6. Powis RL, Schwartz RA: Practical Doppler Ultrasound for the Clinician. Baltimore, Williams & Wilkins, 1991.
7. Kisslo J, Adams DB, Belkin RN: Doppler Color Flow Imaging. New York, Churchill Livingstone, 1988.
8. Merritt CRB (ed): Doppler Color Imaging. New York, Churchill Livingstone, 1992.
9. Guyton AC: Textbook of Medical Physiology. 7th edition. Philadelphia, WB Saunders, 1986, pp. 206–229.
10. Milnor WR: Hemodynamics. 2nd edition. Baltimore, Williams & Wilkins, 1989.
11. Nichols WW, O'Rourke MF: McDonald's Blood Flow in Arteries. Philadelphia, Lea & Febiger, 1990.
12. Beach KW, Lawrence R, Phillips DJ, et al: The systolic velocity criterion for diagnosing significant internal carotid artery stenoses. J Vasc Technol *13*:65–68, 1989.
13. Ku DN, Giddens DP, Phillips DJ, et al: Hemodynamics of the normal human carotid bifurcation: in vitro and in vivo studies. Ultrasound Med Biol *11*:13–26, 1985.
14. Phillips DJ, Beach KW, Primozich J, et al: Should results of ultrasound Doppler studies be reported in units of frequency or velocity? Ultrasound Med Biol *15*:205–212, 1989.
15. Spencer MP, Reid JM: Quantitation of carotid stenosis with continuous wave (CW) Doppler ultrasound. Stroke *10*:326–330, 1979.
16. Bradley EL, Sacerio J: The velocity of ultrasound in human blood under varying physiologic parameters. J Surg Res *12*:290–297, 1972.
17. Goss SA, Johnston RL, Dunn F: Comprehensive compilation of empirical ultrasonic properties of mammalian tissues. J Acoust Soc Am *64*:425–427, 1978.
18. Wells PNT, Luckman NP, Skidmore R, Halliwell M: A second order approximation in the Doppler equation. Ultrasound Med Biol *15*:73–74, 1989 and *16*:423, 1990.
19. Kremkau FW: Source of Doppler shift in blood flow. Ultrasound Med Biol *16*:421–422, 519–521, 1990 and *17*:98, 1991.
20. Thorne GC, Fied-Booth D, Brooks W, et al: Blood flow measurement by Doppler ultrasound: a question of angles. Phys Med Biol *38*:1637–1645, 1993.
21. Fuss EL: The technology of burglar alarm systems. Am Scientist *72*:334–337, 1984.
22. Luckman NP, Evans JM, Skidmore R, et al: Backscattered power in Doppler signals. Ultrasound Med Biol *13*:669–670, 1987.
23. Kremkau FW: Doppler angle error due to refraction. Ultrasound Med Biol *16*:523–524, 1990 and *17*:97, 1991.
24. Kremkau FW: Doppler shift frequency data. J Ultrasound Med *6*:167,1987.
25. Gill RW: Measurement of blood flow by ultrasound: accuracy and sources of error. Ultrasound Med Biol *11*:625–641, 1985.
26. Bracewell RN: The Fourier transform. Sci Am *260*:86–95, 1989.
27. Bracewell RN: Numerical transforms. Science *248*:697–704, 1990.
28. Walker JS: Fast Fourier Transforms. Boca Raton, FL, CRC Press, 1992.
29. Burns PN: The physical principles of Doppler and spectral analysis. J Clin Ultrasound *15*:567–590, 1987.
30. Taylor KJW, Holland S: State-of-the-art Doppler ultrasound I. Basic principles, instrumentation and pitfalls. Radiology *174*:297–307, 1990.
31. Kremkau FW: Doppler principles. Semin Roentgenol *27*:6–16, 1992.
32. Kremkau FW: Principles of color flow imaging. J Vasc Technol *15*:104–111, 1991.
33. Kremkau FW: Color-flow color assignments I. J Vasc Technol *15*:265–266, 1991.

34. Kremkau FW: Color-flow color assignments II. J Vasc Technol *15:*325–326, 1991.
35. Kremkau FW: Color interpretation I. J Vasc Technol *16:*105, 1992.
36. Kremkau FW: Color interpretation II. J Vasc Technol *16:*215–216, 1992.
37. Kremkau FW: Color interpretation III. J Vasc Technol *16:*309–310, 1992.
38. Kremkau FW: Principles and instrumentation. In Merritt CRB (ed): Doppler Color Imaging. New York, Churchill Livingstone, 1992.
39. Kremkau FW: Principles and pitfalls of real-time color-flow imaging. In Bernstein EF (ed): Vascular Diagnosis. 4th edition. St. Louis, Mosby-Year Book, 1993.
40. Kasai C, Namekawa K, Koyano A, et al: Real-time two-dimensional blood flow imaging using an autocorrelation technique. IEEE Trans Son Ultrason *SU-32:*458–464, 1985.
41. Bonnefous O, Pesque P: Time domain formulation of pulse-Doppler ultrasound and blood velocity estimation by cross-correlation. Ultrason Imaging *8:*73–85, 1986.
42. Tegeler CH, Kremkau FW, Hitchings LP: Color velocity imaging: introduction to a new ultrasound technology. J Neuroimaging *1:*85–90, 1991.
43. Pozniak MA, Zagzebski JA, Seanlan KA: Spectral and color Doppler artifacts. Radiographics *12:*25–44, 1992.
44. Gill RW, Kossoff MB, Kossoff G, et al: New class of pulsed Doppler US ambiguity at short ranges. Radiology *173:*272–275, 1989.
45. Mitchell DG, Burns P, Needleman L: Color Doppler artifact in anechoic regions. J Ultrasound Med *9:*255–260, 1990.
46. Boote EJ, Zagzebski JA: Performance tests of Doppler ultrasound equipment with a tissue and blood-mimicking phantom. J Ultrasound Med *7:*137–147, 1988.
47. Walker AR, Phillips DJ, Powers JE: Evaluating Doppler devices using a string target. J Clin Ultrasound *10:*25, 1982.
48. American Institute of Ultrasound in Medicine: Performance Criteria and Measurements for Doppler Ultrasound Devices. Laurel, MD, American Institute of Ultrasound in Medicine, 1993.
49. Kremkau FW: Bioeffects and safety. In Chervenak F, Isaacson G, Campbell S (eds): Textbook of Ultrasound in Obstetrics and Gynecology. Boston, Little, Brown, 1993, pp. 103–110.
50. Kremkau FW: Biologic effects and safety. In Rumack CM, Wilson SR, Charboneau JW (eds): Diagnostic Ultrasound. St. Louis, Mosby Year Book, 1991, pp. 19–29.
51. Bioeffects Committee: Safety Considerations for Diagnostic Ultrasound. Laurel, MD, American Institute of Ultrasound in Medicine, 1991.
52. Bioeffects Conference Subcommittee: Bioeffects and Safety of Diagnostic Ultrasound. Laurel, MD, American Institute of Ultrasound in Medicine, 1993.
53. Frizzell LA: Conclusions regarding biological effects of ultrasound for diagnostically relevant exposures. J Ultrasound Med *13:*69–72, 1994.
54. National Council on Radiation Protection and Measurements: Biological Effects of Ultrasound: Mechanisms and Clinical Applications. Bethesda, MD, National Council on Radiation Protection, 1983.
55. National Council on Radiation Protection and Measurements: Exposure Criteria for Medical Diagnostic Ultrasound: I. Criteria Based on Thermal Mechanisms. Bethesda, MD, National Council on Radiation Protection, 1992.
56. Nyborg WL, Ziskin, MC: Biological Effects of Ultrasound. New York, Churchill Livingstone, 1985.
57. Repacholi MH, Grandolfo M, Rindi A: Ultrasound: Medical Applications, Biological Effects, and Hazard Potential. New York, Plenum Press, 1987.
58. Suslick KS: Ultrasound: Its Chemical, Physical, and Biological Effects. New York, VCH Publishers, 1988.
59. Output Display Standard Joint Task Group: Standard for Real-Time Display of Thermal and Mechanical Acoustic Output Indices on Diagnostic Ultrasound Equipment. Laurel, MD, American Institute of Ultrasound in Medicine, 1992.
60. World Health Organization: Environmental Health Criteria 22: Ultrasound. Geneva, World Health Organization, 1982.

Index

Page numbers in *italics* refer to illustrations; page numbers followed by t refer to tables.

A

Abbreviations, 331–332
Absorption, 15, 52, 253
Acoustic variables, 13
Adder, in phase quadrature detector, *125*, 126
AIUM. See *American Institute of Ultrasound in Medicine.*
Aliasing, 221, 223–225, 226t, *227–228*, 228
  in pulsed-wave instruments, 136
  reduction of, 224–225, *227*, 227t, 233t
American Institute of Ultrasound in Medicine (AIUM), bioeffects statements of, 250–256, 258–259
  safety statement of, 266
Amplification, in sonography, 36
Amplifier, audio frequency (AF), *124*
  radio frequency (RF), *124*
  sample-and-hold. See *Receiver gate.*
Amplitude, 14, *15*, 52
Angle, 102–109
  beam, Doppler shift with, 102, *103–105*, 105–106, 109
  critical, in vascular measurements, 106
  error in, 105–106, 106t, *107, 130–131*, 133
Animal studies, bioeffects studies with, 251–253, 258
Annular array, 28, *30*, 33, 52
Array(s), annular, 28, *30*, 33, 52
  convex, 32, 52
  linear (linear-sequenced), 28, 31–32, *31*
  phased, annular, 33
    linear, 32–33, *32, 33*, 53
Arterioles, resistance in, 68
  sonography in, 77

Artifacts, in color-flow systems, *238–244*, 238–245
  in sonography, 44–50, *45, 46*
  in spectral systems, 221–237
  mirror-image, in Doppler systems, 232–233, *234, 235*
Attenuation, 15, 17, *17*, 52
  artifacts from, 49, *49, 50*
  compensation for, 36, 38, *39*
  frequency with, 15, 17–19
  vs. penetration depth, 18–19, *18*
Attenuation coefficient, 15, 17
Audio frequency (AF) amplifier, *124*
Autocorrelation technique, 182–183, *183*
Axial resolution, 33, *34*, 35, *35*

B

B (brightness) scans, 10
Backscatter, 19
Bandwidth, 110
Beam, steering of, 32–33, *32*
Beam angle, Doppler shift with, 102, *103–105*, 105–106, 109
Beam former, 35–36, *36*, 52
Bernoulli effect, 75, 78
Bidirectional instrument, 122, 162
Biologic effects, American Institute of Ultrasound in Medicine (AIUM) statements on, 250–256, 258–259
  in vivo, 251–253, *259*
  mechanisms of, 253–260
  temperature in, *253*, 253–256, *257*
  ultrasonography in, 248–261, 264
Blood, components of, 64
  function of, 64
  properties of, 64, 65, 65t

367

Blood flow, diastolic, 77
Doppler measurements in, 153, *155,* 156
distal, resistance in, 153, *154,* 156, *157*
disturbed, 69, *70,* 71
Doppler effect in, 96, *97–98,* 99
reversal of, 77, *77, 155*
speed of, Doppler shift with, 99–100, 101–102, 101t, *102,* 105
in stenoses, 72–76, *74, 75*
steady, 65–69, *68–70,* 71–72
turbulent, 71–72, *71*
bruits in, 75, 78
volume flow rate of, 67
windkessel effect in, 76–77
B-mode ultrasonography, 10, 41–42, *42*
Bone, heating of, 254–255
Bone thermal index (TIB), 256
Bruits, in turbulent flow, 75, 78

C
Cathode ray tube, 41–42, *42, 43,* 44, *44*
Cavitation, effects of, 249, 251, 257–259, *258*
mechanical index for, 253, *254,* 258, *259*
Cell studies, bioeffects studies with, 249–251
Chromatids, exchange of, 249–250, *250*
Cine (cine loop) review, *4,* 40, *49*
Clutter, *132–133,* 133–134, 162
Color priority, 186, *192*
Color vision, principles of, 180–181
Color-flow, principle of, 178–180, 210–211
Color-flow artifacts, *238–244,* 238–245
Color-flow imaging, 181–197, 210–211
limiting characteristics of, 189, 191, 193–195, 207–208
Color-flow instruments, 177–218
color-flow imaging in, 181–197, 210–211
components of, 181–183, *182, 183*
displays in, 198–210
Compensation (gain compensation), in sonography, 36, 38, *39,* 52
Compliance, in vessel walls, 76, 78
Composite, 22, 52
Conceptus, sonographic intensities for, 256
Continuity rule, 72–73
Continuous-wave Doppler instrument, components of, 122–125, *123–125,* 128
Continuous-wave transducer, 24

Contrast resolution, 40, 52
Convex array, 32, 52
Coupling medium, transducers with, *23,* 26
Critical angle, in vascular measurements, 106
Critical Reynolds number, 72, 78
Cross correlation, 185–186, 211
Crystal, 23, 52
Cycles, description of, 13, *13,* 52
in acoustic variables, 13, 52
in sampling rate, *142,* 143

D
Damping, *23,* 24, *26,* 52
in axial resolution, 35
Demodulation, 123, *124*
Density, of fluids, 64–65
Depth gain compensation, 36, 38, *39,* 52
Detail (geometric) resolution, 33, *34,* 35, *35,* 52
Digital scan converters, 40
Display. See *Cathode ray tube.*
Doppler angle, 102, *103,* 111
error in, 105–106, 106t, *107, 130–131,* 133
Doppler echocardiography, 76, 106
Doppler effect, 2, 4–5, 89–119
angle in, 102, *103,* 105–106, *107, 108,* 109
applications of, 1
frequency in, 109–111, *110*
in blood flow, 96, *97–98,* 99
information from, 1–2, 2t
speed in, 99–102
Doppler equation(s), 90–91, 93, *96,* 111
Doppler measurement frequencies, 111
Doppler sample volume, 127, *128,* 129
Doppler shift, 112, 124, *124*
beam angle in, 102, *103–105,* 105–106, 109
blood flow speed with, 99–102, 101t, *102,* 105
for moving reflector, 93, *94,* 95
in pulsed-wave instruments, 136
mean of, 181
variance of, 181, 211
with instrument operating frequency, 109, *110*
Doppler shift frequency, 90–91, 93, 95–96, 112
Doppler ultrasound, 63
fetal applications in, 262, 262t
risk assessment in, 265–266

Dual-transducer assembly, 127, *128,* 129
Duplex scanners (instruments), 121, 141
Duty factor, definition of, 14, 52
Dynamic imaging, 42, 44

E

Echo(es), arrival time of, 7–8, 20–21, *21*
  and reflector depths, 137t
  blood flow speed and, 183–185, *184, 185*
Echocardiography, Doppler measurements in, 76, 106
Eddy currents, 71
Electromagnetic interference, 49, *50,* 233–234, *237*
Element, piezoelectric, 23, *23,* 52
  receiving transducer, 123, *123*
  transducer, 23, *23,* 52
Emitted frequency, for moving source, 91, *92,* 93
Enhancement artifact, 48–49, *50,* 52
Ensemble length, 186–187, *193,* 211
Epidemiology, 264
Equations, 332–335
Erythrocytes, function of, 64
  in frequency shift, 110
Extravasation, diagnostic instruments and, 258–259

F

Far zone, of transducer beam, 27, *27*
Fast Fourier transform (FFT), *142,* 143, *144–145,* 162
Fetal Doppler applications, 262, 262t
Fetal tissue, mammalian, bioeffects studies with, 251
Fibroblasts, bioeffects studies with, 249
Filters, high-pass, *132–133,* 133–134, 163
  low-pass, 124–126, *124, 125, 134–135*
Flow. See also *Blood flow.*
  disturbed, 69, *70,* 71, 78
  extended, 76–77
  helical, 69
  impedance of, 76
  laminar, 68–69, *68,* 71, 78
  parabolic, 69, *69,* 78
  plug, 68, *68,* 69, *70,* 78
  pulsatile, 76–77
  resistance to, 67, 78
  steady, 65–72
  tubular, continuity rule in, 72–73

Flow (*Continued*)
  turbulent, 71, *71,* 79
    and flow speed, 71
  volume rate of, 67, 79
Flow impedance, 76
Flow reversal, 77, *77, 155*
Flow speed, 72–75, *74, 75*
  angle estimate in, *130–131,* 133
  phase difference determinations in, 182–183
  vs. fluid pressure, *75*
Fluids, density of, 64–65
  properties of, 64–65
  resistance in, 67, 78
  steady flow in, 65–72
Focal length, of focused transducer, 27, *29*
Focus, in lateral resolution, 35
  long, 33
Focusing sound, 27, *28,* 52
Fourier transform, fast (FFT), *142,* 143, *144–145,* 162
Frame(s), freeze, 38, 40, 53
  memory display, sonographic images as, 42, 44, *44*
Frame rate, in dynamic imaging, 42, 44, 52
  vs. imaging depth, 44
  vs. penetration, 44
Freeze frame, image display by, 38, 40, 53
Frequency, attenuation with, 15, 17–19
  definition of, 13, 53
  emitted, for moving source, 91, *92,* 93
  filtering of, high-pass, *132–133,* 133–134, 163
    low-pass, 124–126, *124, 125, 134–135*
  fundamental, *142*
  mixing, 124–126, *124, 125*
  operating, 24, 53
    with Doppler shift, 109, *110*
  pulse repetition, 14, 24, 53, *135,* 136
  received, for moving receiver, 90–91, *90*
  resonance, 24
  vs. penetration depth, 18–19, *18*
  vs. spatial pulse length, 14
  vs. wavelength, 14
Frequency range, in Doppler measurements, 111
  in sonography, 51
Frequency shift, erythrocytes and, 110
  tissue characteristics in, 110
  transducer electric properties in, 110
Frequency-spectrum processing, 129, *129, 130,* 133
Fundamental frequency, *142*

G

Gain, 36, *37*, 38, *38*
  spectral broadening and, 148, *149*
Gain compensation, 36, 38, *39*, 52
Gated oscillator, 134, *134–135*
Generator gate, 134, *134–135*
Geometric resolution. See *Detail
  (geometric) resolution.*
Glossary, 305–314
Gradient (slope), pressure, 65–66, *66*
Gray-scale imaging, 10, 41–42, *42*

H

Heart valve, stenotic, 76
Hematocrit, 64
Hemodynamics, 63–88
  definition of, 63
  fluids in, 64–65
  pulsatile flow in, 76–77
  steady flow in, 65–69, *68–70*, 71–72
  stenoses in, *71*, 72–76, *74*, *75*
Hertz (Hz), definition of, 13, 53
High-pass wall filter, *132–133*, 133–134,
  163
  range of, 134
Hue, 180–181
Hyperthermia, 256, *257*

I

Imaging depth (penetration), 18–19, *18,
  21, 21*
  vs. frame rate, 44
Imaging instruments, 35–44, *36, 37, 39*
Impedance, acoustic, 19, 53
  in fluid flow, 76
Incidence angle, of wave front, 19
Inertia, 64–65
Instruments, bidirectional, 122, 162
  color-flow, 177–218. See also *Color-
    flow* entries.
    displays in, 198–210
    principle of, 178–180, 210–211
  continuous-wave Doppler, 122–127,
    123–125, 128, 129
  duplex, 121, 141
  governmental regulation of, 261–264
  output intensities of, 260–261, 260t
  pulsed-wave Doppler, *134–135,*
    134–139, 137t, *138, 140*
  sonographic imaging, 35–44, *36, 37, 39*
  spectral, 121–175
    continuous wave in, 122–134
    displays in, 144–159, *150*

Instruments (*Continued*)
  pulsed wave in, 134–141
  spectral analysis in, 141–143
Intensity, instrument output as, 260
  wave, 14–15
Interference artifact, 49, *50*, 233–234,
  237

K

Kilohertz (kHz), 14
Kinematic viscosity, definition of, 65, 79

L

Laminar flow, 68–69, *68*, 71, 78
Lateral resolution, 33, 35
Lesions, focal, 251, *252*
Leukocytes, bioeffects studies with,
  249–250, *250*
  function of, 64
Linear scans, 8, *9*
Linear-phased array (phased array),
  32–33, *32, 33*, 53
Linear-sequenced (linear-switched)
  array, 28, 31–32, *31*
Listening region. See *Sample volume.*
Long focus, phased pulses in, 33
Low-pass filter, 124–126, *124, 125,
  134–135*
Luminance, in color, 181

M

Mass, 64–65
Matching layer, of transducer, *23*, 25, 53
Mechanical index (MI), for cavitation
  effects, 253, *254*, 258, *259*
Megahertz (MHz), 13
Memory, digital, 40–42, *40–43*, 44, *44*
Mirror-image artifact, in Doppler
  systems, 232–233, *234, 235*
  in sonography, 45, *48*, 49, *49*, 53
Motion, Doppler effect in, 2

N

Near zone, of transducer beam,
  26–27, *27*
Nyquist limit, 136, 229, *231*

O

Oblique incidence, sonographic wave
    with, 19
Operating frequency, 24, 53
  with Doppler shift, 109, *110*
Oscillator, 122–123, *123*
Oscillator gate, 134, *134–135*

P

Parabolic flow, 69, *69*
Penetration, 18–19, *18*, 21, *21*
  vs. frame rate, 44
Performance testing, for Doppler
    ultrasound instruments, 245,
    246–247
Phantoms, in performance testing, 245,
    247
Phase quadrature detector, 124–126, *125*
Phased array, annular, 33
Phased array (linear-phased), 32–33, *32,
    33*, 53
Phase-difference determinations,
    182–183
Piezoelectric element, 23, *23*, 52
Piezoelectric principle, 22, *23*, 53
Pixels, 40, 53
Plant tissue studies, 251
Platelets, function of, 64
Plug flow, 68, *68*, 69, *70*, 78
Poise, definition of, 65, 78
Poiseuille's law, 68, 73, 78
Postprocessing, 53
Preprocessing, 53
Pressure, fluid, 65
  gradient of, 65–66, *66*
  volume flow rate and, 67
  vs. flow speed, 75
Pressure difference, 65–66, *66*
Propagation speed, 13, 53
Pulse repetition frequency (PRF), 14, 24,
    35, 53, *135*, 136
Pulse repetition period, 184
Pulsed mode, 24
  transducer assembly in, *25*
Pulsed-Doppler instruments. See *Spectral
    instruments, pulsed wave in.*
Pulsed-Doppler systems. See *Spectral
    instruments, pulsed wave in.*
Pulsed-wave instruments. See *Spectral
    instruments, pulsed wave in.*
Pulse-echo imaging. See *Scanning;
    Sonography (ultrasound imaging).*
Pulse-echo technique, ultrasound
    imaging by, 7–8
Pulser, 35, *36*

Q

Quad (phase quadrature detector),
    124–126, *125*

R

Radio frequency (RF) amplifier, *124*
Range ambiguity, 226t, 228, *231,
    232–233*, 233t
Received frequency, for moving receiver,
    90–91, *90*
Receiver, in continuous-wave Doppler
    systems, 123–124, *123, 124*, 127
  in sonography, 36, *36*, 38
Receiver gate, *134–135*, 136, *140*
  length (depth range) in, 136–137, *140*
Receiving transducer element, 123, *123*
Reflection(s), artifacts from, 45, *45, 48,*
    48–49, *49*
  specular, 19
Reflectors, depth of, echo arrival time
    and, 137t
  Doppler shift with, 93, *94, 95*
Refraction, 19, 53
Refraction artifact, 45, *47, 48*, 53
Resistance, in distal flow, 153, *154*, 156,
    157
  in fluids, 67, 78
Resolution, axial, 33, *34*, 35, *35*
  contrast, 40, 52
  detail (geometric), 33, *34*, 35, *35*
  lateral, 33, 35
  temporal, 44, 54
Resonance frequency, 24
Reverberation artifact, 45, *45, 46*
Reynolds number, 71–72, 78
  critical, 72, 78
  definition of, 71
  vs. viscosity, 71

S

Safety, 248–266
  American Institute of Ultrasound in
    Medicine (AIUM), statement on,
    266
Sample volume, in continuous-wave
    Doppler systems, 127, *128,* 129
  in pulsed-Doppler measurements,
    134–135, 136, 137, *138*
Sample-and-hold amplifier. See *Receiver
    gate.*
Saturation, in color, 181
Scan lines, 8, *8–10*
Scanners, duplex, 121, 141

Scanning. See also *Sonography (ultrasound imaging).*
  automatic, 28, *30,* 31–33, *31–33*
  B (brightness), 10
  B-mode sonography, 10, 41–42, *42*
  electronic, 28, *30,* 31–33, *31–33*
  linear, 8, *9*
  mechanical, 28, *30*
  sector, 8, 10, *10, 11*
Scatterers, Doppler shift in, 93, *94,* 95
Scattering, 19–20, *20,* 53
Sector scans, 8, 10, *10, 11*
Shadowing artifact, 48–49, *49,* 53, 243, *244*
Shock wave(s), 91, 257
Side lobes, of disk transducer, 26
Smoothing (persistence), 186, *193*
Soft-tissue thermal index (TIS), 256
Sonography (ultrasound imaging), 7–61, *9–11, 18.* See also *Scanning.*
  artifacts in, 44–50
  beam former in, 35–36, *36,* 52
  B-mode, 10, 41–42, *42*
  depth range in, 18–19, *18,* 21, *21*
  frequency range in, 51
  instruments of, 35–44, *36*
  pulse-echo imaging in, 7–8
  receiver in, 36, *36,* 38
  transducers in, 22–35, *23, 25*
  ultrasound in, 13–21, *20*
Sound, definition of, 13, 54
  diagnostic, speed of, 65t, 99
  focusing of, 27, *28,* 52
Spatial average exposure intensity, 251
Spatial peak temporal average (SPTA) intensities, *252,* 260, 260t, *261,* 262t
  mechanical index for, 263–264, *263*
  thermal index for, 263–264, *263*
Spatial pulse length, 14, *15*
  vs. frequency, 14
Spectral analysis, 141–143, *142,* 163
Spectral artifacts, 221–237
Spectral broadening, 143, 148, *149,* 163
  receiver gain and, 148, *149*
  vessel diameter in, 150, 153, *153,* 163
Spectral displays, 144–159, *150*
  indices of, 156t
Spectral instruments, 121–175
  continuous wave in, 122–134
  displays in, 144–159, *150*
  pulsed wave in, 134–141
    components of, 134, *134,* 136
  spectral analysis in, 141–143
Spectral traces, 144, 146, *146–147,* 148
  interpretation of, 156–157, 159, *159*
Spectral width, *151,* 163. See also *Bandwidth; Spectral broadening.*

Spectrum analyzer, *134–135,* 163. See also *Spectral analysis.*
Steady flow, in fluids, 65–72
Stenoses, 72–76
  volume flow rate in, 72–74, *74*
Stoke, definition of, 65, 79
Symbols, 331–332

T
Temporal resolution, 44, 54
Thermal indices, for tissue temperature, 255–256
Threshold function (reject), noise elimination with, 127
Time gain compensation, 36, 38, *39,* 52
Time-domain technique, 183–185, *184, 185*
Time-shifted echo technique, 183–185, *184, 185*
Tissue characteristics, frequency shift with, 110
Transducer element, piezoelectric, 23, *23,* 52
  receiving, 123, *123*
Transducers, 22–35, *22–25,* 54
  electric properties of, frequency shifts with, 110
  in continuous-wave Doppler systems, 127, *128,* 129
Tubular flow, continuity rule in, 72–73
Turbulent flow, 71, *71,* 79
  and flow speed, 71
  bruits in, 75, 78

U
Ultrasound, *3,* 4–5, 13–21, 54, 63
  definition of, 13, 54
  Doppler, 63
    fetal applications in, 262, 262t
    risk assessment in, 265–266
  frequency range in, 51
  speed of, 7–8, 20–21, *21,* 99
Ultrasound imaging. See *Sonography (ultrasound imaging).*

V
Velocity, fluid, 106, *108,* 109, 112
Velocity vector, 102, *104–105, 108,* 112
  Doppler shift and, 157, 159, *159*

Viscosity, definition of, 65
  kinematic, 65, 79
Voltage generator, 122–123, *123*
Volume flow rate, flow speed with,
  72–75, *74, 75*
  pressure and, 67
  vs. flow resistance, 67

Wave, 13, 54
Wavelength, definition of, 13, *14,* 54
  vs. frequency, 14
Windkessel effect, 76–77
Window, 148, 163
  spectral broadening and, 148

W
Wall-thump filter, *132–133,* 133–134,
  163

Z
Zero-crossing detector, 126–127, *128*